T0074094

Springer-Verlag Berlin Heidelberg GmbH

Edward H. Phillips • Raul J. Rosenthal (Editors)

Operative Strategies in Laparoscopic Surgery

With 394 Figures

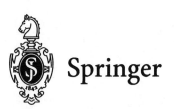

Springer

EDWARD H. PHILLIPS, M.D., F.A.C.S.
Director, Division of Endoscopic Surgery
Cedars Sinai Medical Center
Associate Professor of Surgery
University of Southern California
8700 Beverly Boulevard
Los Angeles, California 90048, USA

RAUL J. ROSENTHAL, M.D.
Division of Endoscopic Surgery
Department of Surgery
Cedars Sinai Medical Center
8700 Beverly Boulevard
Los Angeles, California 90048, USA

ISBN 978-3-642-63358-4

Library of Congress Cataloging-in-Publication Data

Operative strategies in laparoscopic surgery/Edward H.
Phillips, Raul L. Rosenthal (editors). p. cm. Includes biblio-
graphical references and index.
ISBN 978-3-642-63358-4   ISBN 978-3-642-57797-0 (eBook)
DOI 10.1007/978-3-642-57797-0
1. Abdomen –
Endoscopic surgery – Atlases. 2. Digestive organs –
Endoscopic surgery – Atlases. I. Phillips, Edward H., 1947– .
II. Rosenthal, Raul J., 1959– . [DNLM: 1. Surgery,
Laparoscopic – methods – atlases. WO 517 0613 1995]
RD540.066 1995 617.5'5059 – dc20 DNLM/DLC for
Library of Congress 95-24353 CIP

Originally published by Springer-Verlag Berlin Heidelberg
New York in 1995

Drawings: M. Hasler, Arleta, CA, USA
Typesetting: Data conversion by Springer-Verlag

SPIN: 10129864   24/3135 – 5 4 3 2 1 0
Printed on acid-free paper

Dedications

To my wife, Nancy, and my parents, Sophie and Ed,
for their support and many sacrifices.
To my children, Aaron, Rachel, and David, for their
interruptions; soccer, baseball, singing, and schoolwork.
Without which life would not be as wonderful.

Dr. E.H. PHILLIPS

With love! To my parents Inge and Manfred for their
sacrifice in providing me with education.
To my wife Simona and our children Dana and Noam,
for their support, tolerance and long waiting.

Dr. R.J. ROSENTHAL

Preface

The specialty of general surgery has recently undergone a revolution. The application of video-guided surgery to cholecystectomy led to the greatest postgraduate training effort in the history of general surgery. Just several years since the first successful case in 1987, laparoscopic cholecystectomy has become the preferred technique for cholecystectomy throughout the world. Many surgeons felt that this revolution was patient driven, and most were forced reluctantly to learn the technique. Now, virtually every intra-abdominal procedure can be accomplished using laparoscopic guidance. These "advanced" procedures are being performed by ever-increasing numbers of surgeons who have embraced the techniques of laparoscopy not only because of the benefits to their patients, but also because of the finesse and artful skill required in the technique. No longer are laparoscopic operations limited to those requested by patients. They are being developed and perfected by laparoscopic surgeons throughout the world.

Operations such as laparoscopic procedures for cholecystectomy, antireflux surgery, adrenalectomy, splenectomy, gastrostomy, appendectomy in women, liver biopsy, and gynecologic procedures have been accepted as clearly better than their "open" counterparts. Laparoscopic appendectomy in men, hernioplasty, colectomy, gastrectomy, and pancreatectomy are being performed but remain controversial. This surgical atlas is not meant to debate the controversies. Nor is it a textbook in the sense that the physiologic origins and histopathology of the diseases being treated by operation are not (with a few exceptions) discussed.

This is an atlas of laparoscopic strategies. It is meant to provide surgeons and surgeons-in-training who are performing and assisting in these procedures with a proven step-by-step technique employed successfully by the experts in the field. The chapters are brief so that in five minutes or less a resident may review a procedure preoperatively. This atlas contains black and white line drawings to facilitate quick recognition of detail. This atlas should be used in the operating room, the operating room lounge, and in the residents' library.

The views and surgical strategies expressed are those of the authors. In most cases there is more than one way to accomplish the operation detailed. We make no attempt to discuss or even show some of the other approaches, not because they are inferior, but because time and space do not allow. Again, our goal is to show the techniques successfully employed by the authors.

The nature and purpose of this book makes it essential that it be well illustrated. The principal illustrator is Gino Hasler. Without his talents the book could not have been produced, and the editors are grateful to him for his patience and understanding. He had to perform countless revisions of seemingly insignificant detail to satisfy our perfectionism. The editors are also grateful to Mary Semski, who typed the manuscript. We also must thank Springer-Verlag for supporting this project.

Finally, the editors would like to thank all of the authors. Without exception they are incredibly busy. All have ambitious operating schedules, teaching responsibilities, and projects of their own. We appreciate the sacrifices that they and their significant others have made in taking the time to contribute to this book. We know their contributions were made in the name of friendship and their love for the growing field of laparoscopic surgery.

EDWARD H. PHILLIPS
RAUL J. ROSENTHAL

Contents

Contributors

ANNIBALI, RICARDO, M.D.
Consultant Surgeon
Ospedale Valduce
Via Dante 11
22100 Como
Italy

ARREGUI, MAURICE E., M.D., F.A.C.S.
Director of Fellowship in Laparoscopy,
Endoscopy and Ultrasound
St. Vincent Hospital
8402 Harcourt Road, Suite 811
Indianapolis, Indiana 46260
USA

BAFUTTO, M., M.D.
Hospital Samaritano
Praga Walter Santos 1
Setor Coimbra
Goiana, Goias 74530270
Brazil

BEART, ROBERT W., JR., M.D. F.A.C.S., F.A.S.C.R.S.
Professor of Surgery, USC
Head, Division of Colorectal Surgery
University of Southern California
1510 San Pablo Street
Los Angeles, California 90033
USA

BERCI, GEORGE, M.D., F.A.C.S., F.R.C.S., Ed. (Hon.)
Clinical Professor of Surgery
LAC-USC Medical Center
Director, Research and Education
Endocare Center, Midway Hospital
5901 West Olympic Boulevard, Suite 405
Los Angeles, California 90036
USA

BUESS, GERHARD, M.D.
Professor of Surgery
Chirurgische Universitätsklinik
Eberhard-Karls-Universität Tübingen
Hoppe-Seyler-Str. 3
72076 Tübingen
Germany

CAMPS, JOSE, M.D.
Research Fellow
Department of Surgery
Creighton University
601 North 30th Street
Omaha, Nebraska 68131
USA

CARROLL, BRENDAN J., M.D., F.A.C.S.
Attending Surgeon
Cedars Sinai Medical Office Towers
8635 West Third Street, Suite 795 W
Los Angeles, California 90048
USA

CHANDRA, MUDJIANTO, M.D.
Senior Surgical Resident
Department of Surgery, Room 8215
Cedars Sinai Medical Center
8700 Beverly Boulevard
Los Angeles, California 90048
USA

CORNET, DOUGLAS, M.D.
Biomedical Engineer
Department of Surgery
Creighton University
601 North 30th Street
Omaha, Nebraska 68131
USA

CUNNEEN, SCOTT A., M.D.
Department of Surgery
Cedars-Sinai Medical Center
8700 Beverly Boulevard
Los Angeles, California 90048
USA

CURET, MYRIAM J., M.D., F.A.C.S.
Assistant Professor of Surgery
University of New Mexico
School of Medicine
2211 Lomas Boulevard
Albuquerque, New Mexico
USA

CUSCHIERI, ALFRED, M.D., ChM, F.R.C.S.
Professor of Surgery
Head of Department of Surgery
Ninewells Hospital and Medical School
University of Dundee
Dundee, DD1 9SY
UK

DE PAULA, AUREO L., M.D.
Hospital Samaritano
Praga Walter Santos 1
Setor Coimbra
Goiana, Goias 74530270
Brazil

DUBOIS, FRANÇOIS, M.D.
Professor of Surgery
Centre Medico Chirurgical de la Porte Choisy
54 Avenue de Saxe
75015 Paris
France

DUH, QUAN-YANG, M.D., F.A.C.S.
VA Medical Center, Surgical Service 112
4150 Clement Street
San Francisco, California 94121
USA

FALLAS, MOSES J., M.D., F.A.C.S.
Attending Surgeon
Cedars Sinai Medical Office Towers
8635 West 3rd Street, Suite 795 W
Los Angeles, California 90048
USA

FEUSSNER, H., M.D.
Department of Surgery
Klinikum Rechts der Isar
Ismanninger Str. 22
81675 Munich
Germany

FITZGIBBONS, ROBERT J., JR., M.D.
Professor of Surgery
Chief, Division of General Surgery
Department of Surgery
Creighton University
601 North 30th Street
Omaha, Nebraska 68131
USA

FRANKLIN, MORRIS E., JR., M.D., F.A.C.S.
Clinical Professor of Surgery
University of Texas Health Science
Director, Texas Endosurgery Institute
Center San Antonio, Texas
4242 E. Southcross
San Antonio, Texas
USA

GASTINGER, I., M.D.
Department of Surgery
University of Erlangen
Postfach 3560
91023 Erlangen
Germany

GOH, PETER, M.D.
Associate Professor and Chairman
Minimally Invasive Surgical Centre
National University Hospital
5 Lower Kent Ridge Road
Singapore 0511
Republic of Singapore

GORDON, LEO A., M.D., F.A.C.S.
Attending Surgeon
Cedars Sinai Medical Center
8635 West Third Street, Suite 875 West
Los Angeles, California 90048
USA

HASHIBA, K., M.D.
Hospital Samaritano
Praga Walter Santos 1
Setor Coimbra
Goiana, Goias 74530270
Brazil

HIATT, JONATHAN R., M.D., F.A.C.S.
Professor of Surgery, UCLA
Director of Trauma Service
School of Medicine
Department of Surgery
Cedars-Sinai Medical Center
8700 Beverly Boulevard
Los Angeles, California 90048
USA

HUNTER, JOHN G., M.D., F.A.C.S.
Associate Professor of Surgery
Emory University School of Medicine
1364 Clifton Road
Atlanta, Georgia 30322
USA

CONTRIBUTORS

JACOBS, MOISES, M.D., F.A.C.S.
7800 S.W. 87th Avenue
Miami, Florida 33173
USA

KATKHOUDA, NAMIR, M.D.
Associate Professor of Surgery
Department of Surgery
University of Southern California
1510 San Pablo Street, #514
Los Angeles, California 90033-4612
USA

KAVOUSSI, LOUIS R., M.D.
Associate Professor and Chief
Department of Urology
Johns Hopkins Bayview Medical Center
4940 Eastern Avenue
Baltimore, Maryland 21224
USA

KITAJIMA, MASAKI, M.D., F.A.C.S.
Professor of Surgery
Head, Department of Surgery
Keio University School of Medicine, Tokyo,
Japan

KÖCKERLING, F., M.D. Ph.D.
Department of Surgery
University of Erlangen
Postfach 3560
91023 Erlangen
Germany

KOLACHALAM, R.B., M.D.
Providence Hospital
16001 West Nine Mile Road
Southfield, Michigan 48037
USA

KRAEMER, S.J.M., M.D.
Department of Surgery
Klinikum Rechts der Isar
Ismanninger Str. 22
81675 Munich
Germany

KUM, C.K., F.R.C.S. (Edinburgh)
Senior Registrar
Department of Surgery
National University Hospital
5 Lower Kent Ridge Road
Singapore 0511
Republic of Singapore

LIBERMAN, MARK A., M.D.
Clinical Assistant Professor of Surgery
Uniformed Services
University of the Health Sciences
Department of Surgery
Naval Hospital San Diego
San Diego, California
USA

MACHADO, C.A., M.D.
Hospital Samaritano
Praga Walter Santos 1
Setor Coimbra
Goiana, Goias 74530270
Brazil

MARGULIES, DANIEL R., M.D.
Assistant Professor of Surgery
University of Hawaii
School of Medicine
1356 Lusitana Street, 6th Floor
Honolulu, Hawaii 96813
USA

MENTGES, BURKHARDT, M.D.
Chirurgische Universitätsklinik
Eberhard-Karls-Universität Tübingen
Hoppe-Seyler-Str. 3
72076 Tübingen
Germany

MOORE, ROBERT G., M.D.
Instructor, Department of Urology
Johns Hopkins Bayview Medical Center
4940 Eastern Avenue
Baltimore, Maryland 21224
USA

MOUIEL, JEAN
Professor of Surgery
Hopital Saint Roche
5, rue Pierre Devoluy
06000 Nice
France

NGUYEN, N., M.D.
Research Fellow
Department of Surgery
Creighton University
601 North 30th Street
Omaha, Nebraska 68131
USA

NIES, CHRISTOPH, M.D.
Klinik für Allgemeinchirurgie
Philipps-Universität Marburg
Baldinger Str.
35033 Marburg
Germany

OHGAMI, MASAHIRO, M.D., F.A.C.S.
Associate Professor of Surgery
Department of Surgery
Keio University School of Medicine, Tokyo
Japan

OLSEN, DOUGLAS O., M.D., F.A.C.S.
Assistant Clinical Professor of Surgery
Vandenbilt University
2021 Church Street, Suite 502
Nashville, Tennessee 37023
USA

PAZ-PARTLOW, MARGARET, M.A., M.F.A.
Endocare Center
Midway Hospital
5901 West Olympic Boulevard #405
Los Angeles, California 90036
USA

PELLEGRINI, CARLOS A., M.D., F.A.C.S.
Professor and Chairman
Department of Surgery
University of Washington
RF-25 UWMC
1959 Pacific Avenue, N.E., Box 356410
Seattle, Washington 98195-6410
USA

PETERS, JEFFREY H., M.D., F.A.C.S.
Department of Surgery
University of Southern California
1510 San Pablo Street
Los Angeles, California 90033-4612
USA

PHILLIPS, EDWARD H., M.D., F.A.C.S.
Director, Division of Endoscopic Surgery
Cedars Sinai Medical Center
8700 Beverly Boulevard
Los Angeles, California 90048
USA

POLASCIK, THOMAS. J., M.D.
Fellow, Department of Urology
Johns Hopkins Medical Institutions
4940 Eastern Avenue
Baltimore, Maryland 21224
USA

RAMOS, RAOUL, M.D. F.A.C.S.
Clinical Professor of Surgery
UTHSCSA
Colon and Rectal Surgical Associates of San Antonio
8711 Village Drive, Suite 320
San Antonio, Texas 78217-5919
USA

RECK, T., M.D.
Department of Surgery
University of Erlangen
Postfach 3560
91023 Erlangen
Germany

REISSMAN, PETACHIA, M.D.
Cleveland Clinic Florida
3000 West Cypress Creek Road
Fort Lauderdale, Florida 33309
USA

ROSENTHAL, DANIEL, M.D., F.A.C.S.
Clinical Professor of Surgery, UTHSCSA
Colon and Rectal Surgical Associates of San Antonio
8711 Village Drive, Suite 320
San Antonio, Texas 78217-5919
USA

ROSENTHAL, RAUL J., M.D.
Division of Endoscopic Surgery
Department of Surgery
Cedars Sinai Medical Center
8700 Beverly Boulevard
Los Angeles, California 90048
USA

ROTHMUND, MATHIAS, M.D.
Professor and Chairman
Klinik für Allgemeinchirurgie
Philipps-Universität Marburg
Baldingerstr.
35033 Marburg
Germany

CONTRIBUTORS

SALKY, BARRY A., M.D., F.A.C.S.
Professor of Surgery
Chief, Division of Laparoscopic Surgery
Mount Sinai Medical Center
1 Gustav L. Levy Place
New York, New York 10029
USA

SHAPIRO, STEPHEN J., M.D., F.A.C.S.
Attending Surgeon
Cedars Sinai Medical Center
8635 West Third Street, Suite 865 West
Los Angeles, California 90048
USA

SIEWERT, J. R., M.D.
Professor of Surgery
Head, Department of Surgery
Klinikum Rechts der Isar
Ismanninger Str. 22
81675 Munich
Germany

SIMONS, A., M.D.
Department of Surgery
University of Southern California
1510 San Pablo Street
Los Angeles, California 90033
USA

SINANAN, M., M.D., PhD
Assistant Professor
Department of Surgery
University of Washington
RF-25 UWMC
1959 Pacific Avenue N.E., Box 356410
Seattle, Washington 98195-6410
USA

SOPER, NATHANIEL J., M.D., F.A.C.S.
Associate Professor of Surgery
Division of Hepatobiliary Surgery
Washington University School of Medicine
One Barnes Hospital Plaza, Suite 6108
St. Louis, Missouri 63110
USA

STRASBERG, STEVEN M., M.D.
Washington University School of Medicine
University Medical Center
One Barnes Hospital Plaza, Suite 6108
St. Louis, Missouri 63110
USA

UNGEHEUER, ANDREAS, M.D.
Department of Surgery
Klinikum Rechts der Isar
Ismanninger Str. 22
81675 Munich
Germany

WAY, LAWRENCE W., M.D., F.A.C.S.
Professor and Vice Chairman
Department of Surgery
University of California
San Francisco
VA Medical Center
4150 Clement Street
San Francisco, California 94143
USA

WEGENER, MICHAEL E., M.D.
Department of Surgery
Saint Vincent's Hospital and Health Care Center
8402 Harcourt Road, Suite 811
Indianapolis, Indiana
USA

WEXNER, STEVEN D., M.D., F.A.C.S, F.A.S.C.R.S
Chairman Department of Colorectal Surgery
Cleveland Clinic Florida
3000 West Cypress Creek Road
Fort Lauderdale, Florida 33309
USA

ZUCKER, KARL A., M.D., F.A.C.S.
Professor of Surgery
University of New Mexico
School of Medicine
2211 Lomas Boulevard
Albuquerque, New Mexico
USA

SECTION 1

1 Basic Instrumentation and Troubleshooting

M. Paz-Partlow

Introduction

Since its introduction in 1987 laparoscopic cholecystectomy has irrevocably changed general surgery. New techniques have been introduced into the operating room which all surgeons today are expected to know. It is imperative that surgeons in training thoroughly comprehend laparoscopic procedures, equipment, and instrumentation so that they may resolve incipient intraoperative problems in a timely fashion (see Table 1).

Preliminary Preparation

Perioperative Measures

Preliminary preparation begins with review of the procedure and surgeon's preference card. Availability of all essential equipment and instrumentation is assured, including the basic set as well as any special ancillary or consumable instrumentation required. Spares of critical instrumentation should be readily available, ranging from a backup video camera to spare washers and adapters for trocars. Since the patient is often repositioned after the procedure has begun, he should be secured to the operating table with safety straps, adding shoulder braces and footboards if necessary.

Room Layout

Video monitors are positioned to provide convenient viewing in accordance with the surgeon's sight line. A line from the surgeon's eyes through his hands and the operative site intersects with the ideal monitor position. The monitor position must be adjusted for appendectomy, colon resection, or other procedures. All equipment is arranged around the operating table and checked prior to the patient's entry.

Basics

Regardless of the procedure, certain basic instruments are always employed in laparoscopic surgery. These include the Veress needle, trocars, telescope, graspers, and cautery electrodes that can also irrigate and aspirate and an electronic insufflator.

Veress Needle

Although there are now alternative methods, such as the various "laparo-lifts" with which to create a space in which to work, most surgeons begin by introducing a Veress needle into the abdominal cavity through which CO_2 may be infused. The needle consists of a sharp outer sheath and a blunt spring-loaded obturator designed to guard against organ injury upon penetration. Disposable needles are based on the same design, their advantage being a sharper tip and visible introduction mechanisms.

Insufflation

Creation and maintenance of an adequate pneumoperitoneum is essential for performing safe and successful laparoscopic procedures. The scrub nurse confirms patency of the Veress insufflation needle by attaching a 10-cc Luer-Lok syringe and injecting saline through the needle. On electronic insufflators the main power must be turned on. The CO_2 tank is opened with a valve wrench, and adequate tank pressure is verified by the circulating nurse. The initial pressure setting and flow rate are dialed in. Volume reading is reset to zero prior to patient insufflation. To begin gas flow the insufflation "on" button is pressed. Pressure and flow rates can be indicators of problems and should be monitored throughout the procedure. High pressure accompanied by low flow rate may indicate obstruction or occlusion. During initial insufflation this condition may be caused by Veress needle aperture blocking against tissue, and this requires repositioning. If it persists, the CO_2 tubing should be checked for kinking, and all stopcocks, including the trocar inflow, should be opened. Low or no pres-

Table 1. Troubleshooting guide

Symptom	Cause	Solution
1. Pneumoperitoneum loss/poor insufflation	CO_2 tank empty	Change tank; have spare in room
	Open accessory port stopcock(s)	Check all trocars; close open stopcocks
	Trocar seal leak or stopcock leak	Exchange for new one
	Too much suctioning	Stop suction; wait for reinsufflation of abdomen
	Insufflator tubing; loose connections at unit or port	Tighten connections
	Loose Hasson stay sutures	Refasten Sutures
2. Pressure readings too high	Veress needle not in peritoneal space	Reinsert needle
	Tubing blocked (kinked, cart wheel, too small)	Check all tubing
	Stopcock closed	Open stopcock
	"Light" anesthesia	More muscle relaxant
3. Dim image/poor lighting	Cable not well connected at port and/or scope	Tighten connections
	Unit on lowest setting	Increase to maximum
	Burn-out bulb	Replace
	Light cable broken	Replace
	Scope light fibers broken	Replace
	Camera auto-iris compensating for overbright reflection	Switch to "manual" iris or move scope
	Brightness on monitor misadjust to minimum	Push "reset" button for factory settings. Cover fine tuning buttons
4. Overly bright image	"Gain" on camera control unit is set on high	Set to normal
	Light source's "boost" is on	Turn off "boost"
	Brightness on monitor misadjust to maximum	Pusch "reset" button for factory settings
5. No monitor image(s)	Monitor, camera control, or other electronic accessory in cart not switched on	Check all power cords. Turn on all units
	Coaxial cable connections to monitor from camera control unit or last electronic item in chain not coupled correctly	Run coaxial cable "video out" from camera or last item in sequence (i.e., VCR, printer) to "video in" on monitor
	Coaxial cable between first and second cart monitors not connected	Run cable "video out" from cart 1 monitor to "video in" on cart 2 monitor
	Wrong "input" selection made on monitor	Choose the right "input" button on monitor's front

Table 1. (continued)

Symptom	Cause	Solution
6. Inferior monitor image	Scope fogs when introduced into abdominal cavity	Pre-heat scope in warm saline. Keep antifogging solution on sponge in field
	Lens tip smeared with fluids	Clean tip
Intermittend electrical interference, flashes, flickering	Broken coaxical cable	Replace cable
	Inadequate shielding on camera control unit or light source	Isolate electrosurgical unit on separate circuit
	Wet connecting plug on camera cable	Blow dry with compressed air
Fuzzy image	Camera out of focus	Adjust focus ring
	Internal condensation on scope, damaged cover glass	Check lens and camera; exchange
7. Insufficient irrigation/suction	Tubing blocked (kinked, tissue, clots)	Check complete length; flush
	Suction/irrigation tip blocked, valves stuck	Flush with syringe; replace
	Suction tubing not connected to wall or canister	Double check and tighten all connections
	Pressure not dialed in; CO_2 or nitrogen valves not open	Check gas source for correct settings
8. Inappropriate/no cautery current	Insecure grounding pad	Secure pad to patient, ensuring good contact
	Electrosurgical cable partly disconnected to unit or handswitch	Anchor the contacts

sure with normal flow rates often signifies a leak. Tight connection of gas tubing Luer-Loks at all points along the line should be confirmed. Verify that all trocar seals are of appropriate diameter and are firmly seated.

Irrigation Aspiration

Irrigation and aspiration are critically important during laparoscopic procedures, particularly for maintenance of clear visual fields and hemostasis. Variable speed peristaltic irrigation pumps are available with gas sterilizable cartridges. It is important to assure that these cartridges are securely inserted and rotated to the locked position. Irrigation flow is controlled via a foot pedal. Nitrogen gas pumped irrigation systems are also available. After the tank regulator has been appropriately set, irrigation flow is controlled by means of a trumpet valve or stopcock on the irrigation cannula. Many manufacturers incorporate irrigation and aspiration into a single dual-control instrument. These eliminate switching of tubing or instruments and can reduce the number of trocar sites required in some situations.

Trocars

With trocars we create pathways into the abdominal cavity through which to perform surgery. Cannula sleeve diameters are usually 1 mm larger than the instruments to be introduced through them. Two 11-mm and two 5-mm trocars with pyramidal obturators are usually employed for laparoscopic cholecystectomy. The stylets on reusable trocars should be sharpened regularly. Disposable trocars offer sharp stylets and tip shields that may help avoid organ injury. These, however, are not foolproof and do not supplant proper insertion techniques. The newest single-use trocars incorporate anti-splashback features and universal valves that allow instruments ranging from 5 to 11 mm to be introduced without attaching converters. If the patient has had previous surgery, and difficulties are encountered in achieving the pneumoperitoneum, an open laparoscopy may be attempted, using a Hasson cannula. A direct cutdown is made into the abdominal cavity, followed by stay sutures placed in the fascia. The cannula is placed in the abdomen and secured in place with the stay sutures. CO_2 tubing is then attached, and insufflation commences through the Hasson cannula.

Optics/Light Carriers

A 0° telescope is most commonly used for gynecological procedures, while a 30° fore oblique telescope is most often employed in the upper abdomen. By rotating the 30° slowly around the peritoneal cavity, one can peer into gutters and over organs in a manner not possible with the 0°. The main telescope is 10 mm in diameter, although a 5-mm laparoscope is also kept on hand should it be needed due to adhesions or abdominal trauma.

Introducing the telescope "cold" into the abdomen causes it to fog due to higher internal temperature and humidity. To prevent this the telescope is placed in a stainless steel warmer filled with sterile water at body temperature. A sponge soaked with an alcohol-based antifogging solution is attached to the drapes near the scrub nurse to facilitate tip cleaning during the procedure.

Visual clarity is essential for successful laparoscopic intervention. Deficiencies in either the telescope's optical resolution or illumination can be a deciding factor between proceeding laparoscopically or opening the patient. The scrub nurse should visually inspect the telescope for clarity, taking care not to contaminate the eyepiece. One should reexamine it for fogging. The distal cover glass should be free of any chipping or scratches. The scope should be examined visually for dents and also felt for dents. The scope is held to admit light through the cable input, and the distal tip is inspected for fiber bundle transmission. Fiber damage of 25% or greater is unacceptable; the scope must be replaced. Of equal importance is the light carrier, which may be either a fluid or a glass fiber light cable. The quartz rod tips of fluid cables are particularly susceptible to fracture and must be handled with care. Gas sterilization causes the fluid bundle to yellow, resulting in color distortion and light loss. The fluid cable should be inspected for sharp bends and cracks in the plastic sheath.

Glass fiberoptic cables are comprised of tiny glass fibers which can be broken from mishandling. One end of the cable is held to the light, and the distal end is examined for adequate transmission. Significant light loss through broken fibers decreases the illumination to unacceptable levels, and the cable must be replaced. Fiber cables yellow with age and gas sterilization. When this process reaches a level which alters color and transmission, the cable should be removed from service. Tears or cracks in the protective outer sheathing of glass fiber bundles can accelerate this process and should be repaired when possible or the bundle discarded.

Cleanliness is extremely important to continued light cable efficiency. Any contaminate, including water on either end, can cause uneven heat distribution of the high-intensity light and damage the cable.

Dissectors

There is a bewildering variety of accessories available for sharp and for blunt dissection. Serrated, atraumatic graspers in several different weights should be part of the basic set. A 5-mm locking grasper with 1-in. atraumatic jaws is most useful for suspending the gallbladder over the liver. Many surgeons prefer a curved "Maryland" dissector to define the cystic duct and artery, gently separating them. This is available in both 5- and 10-mm sizes. 5- and 10-mm "Kocher" type graspers can be used to pull out the dissected gallblader from the abdomen.

Scissors

Scissors are often used as dissection tools. Blades must be sharp; therefore reusable scissors must be monitored closely and sharpened regularly. Many disposable models are available and are extremely popular with most surgeons since their single use guarantees sharpness, even when doing repeated monopolar coagulation. Blades can be straight, curved, or hooked. Hooked scissors are especially useful when cutting tubular structures such as the cystic duct, for one can lift the duct in the partly closed jaws to ensure the cut's precision. Microhooked scissors are designed specifically to create an opening in the cystic duct prior to cholangiography.

Electrocautery

While almost all graspers and scissors are insulated and can be connected to a cautery generator via cables, electrodes have been designed with assorted tips for monopolar coagulation and sharp dissection. The most useful are the hook, either J or L shaped, and the spatula. The hook is used to define structures in Calot's triangle and to separate the gallbladder from the liver bed, while the spatula can be used to control bleeding and gentle dissection. Reusable versions incorporate suction and irrigation, but the cautery must be activated by footswitch. Their insulation must be carefully inspected after each use to identify possible breaks. Single-use hand switches/electrodes allow the surgeon to perform suction, irrigation, and coagulation all with one hand.

Staplers and Clip Appliers

Although there are times when, for example, a surgeon ligates the cystic duct with an endoloop for added safety, the vast majority of closures are performed with clip appliers. Reusable clip appliers deliver one clip at a time (size varies approximately from 7 to 9 mm) and must then be taken out and reloaded. When clip appliers are used in pairs, the scrub nurse always has one loaded, ready to exchange for the empty one which the surgeon withdraws. It is cost effective and causes minimal delay. Disposable clip appliers come loaded with 20 clips per unit, which can be applied in rapid succession without removing the instrument from the abdominal cavity. Regardless of their cost, 12-mm disposable staplers with either 30- or 60-mm jaws that apply two triple rows of staples and then divide the structure within their jaws have proved invaluable in advanced laparoscopic procedures, such as colon resections and splenectomies. The alternative in these instances would be hand-suturing, time-consuming, difficult techniques which most surgeons have not mastered. Research into various gluing methods, including laser welding, although promising, has not yet come to fruition.

Video Endoscopy/Documentation

The typical video endoscopy setup consists of two video carts. The primary cart includes a monitor, camera controller, character generator, and video cassette recorder. It may also house a still video printer, automatic high-intensity light source, or other equipment. The secondary cart holds the assistant's monitor, perhaps also incorporating the insufflator and other equipment. All elements of this system must be interconnected with coaxial cables to transmit the video image from the camera to each component of the video chain.

To simplify troubleshooting video system problems it is wise to label all coaxial cables with their respective point of equipment connection. It is also advisable to have a schematic diagram of system connections attached to the video cart door. A brief video procedure outlining operative steps for training and reference is also useful. Coaxial cables fail occasionally. A supply of replacement cables easily accessible from the operating room should be available. There are many coaxial plug configurations, the most common being the BNC and RCA phone plug connectors. Since the type of connector may vary from one video device to the next, it is wise to have an assortment of adapters to interchange the various configurations.

The primary video cart may contain six or more components, each with its own AC power cord. It is useful to consolidate these plugs into a UL 544 approved, appropriately rated isolation transformer with multiple receptacles installed on the cart so that only one main power cord need be plugged into the wall.

Basic Video Setup

After the two video carts have been appropriately positioned for the intended procedure, a setup and system check must be performed:

1. Connect the appropriate coaxial cable from cart one to the monitor line input on cart two.
2. Plug in the main power cord.
3. Turn on main power to all system components.

Even if one device, perhaps a video cassette recorder, is not used during the procedure, failure to turn it on may prevent the video signal from reaching the monitors.

VCR

Video cassette recorders from certain manufacturers do not transmit the image to the monitors unless the red record button is pressed. If a 0.75-in. recorder is being used, check that the tape cassette has a red recording plug inserted on the bottom. Cassettes of 0.5 in. must have an unbroken protection tab on the front left to record. If this has been broken, cover it with cellophane tape to enable recording.

A supply of spare unrecorded video cassettes for the system should be kept on hand. Previously recorded tapes should be reviewed to ensure against erasure of prior procedures. If numbers have been logged on the tape, these may be used to find the appropriate location; however, the counters on most machines are not accurate, and a visual search must be conducted to locate the actual end of the previously recorded case.

Some professional VCRs use real-time counters measured in hours, minutes, seconds, and even frames. Because this method of counting is based on the control code laid down on the tape during recording, the numbers advance only when there is recorded information on the tape. When the numbers stop advancing, the recorded portion is over. A brief visual search can locate the precise end point.

The remote control input connector on many video cassette recorders can be wired to accept a momentary switch foot pedal which activates the pause control remotely on the VCR. This enables the surgeon or assistant to control the videotaping during surgery. Once the circulating nurse has started the recording mode, whichever method is employed, responsibility for the recording should be established to avoid failure to document important findings.

Character Generator

Many video chains incorporate a character generator which enables superimposition on the video image of the patient's name, ID number, date, surgeon's name, and other identification data. The information may be stored and retrieved in a memory page.

Automatic Light Source

Many light sources contain an automatic feature which varies the light intensity by monitoring the strength of the video signal. A coaxial cable labeled "light" from the video stack is connected to the video input of the light source, and the automatic feature is selected. Light intensity is adjusted to a suitable range, using care so that light transmitted through a disconnected cable does not cause a fire or patient burn. The current standard is an automatic xenon high-intensity light source. This light unit with its 300-W lamp is still the brightest, most dependable unit available for use with rigid endoscopes. Xenon short-arc technology linked with special ceramic-to-metal sealing techniques comprises the lamp core. Its prealigned internal reflector effects a large collection angle around the arc, maximizing output efficiency. Moreover, it has excellent transmission from the ultraviolet to the infrared. As has been previously described, this unit dispenses automatic light control for video while functioning as a flash generator adequate for still photography.

Monitor

Most manufacturers provide several video monitors to accommodate a variety of video signals from several sources. These inputs are selectable on the front of the monitor. Additional input might be used for signals from other devices, such as a still video printer.

Be certain that the button for the live camera input is selected, usually "line A." If all other steps in the basic checkout have been correctly performed, a live camera image should appear on the monitor. If no camera is connected to the camera control unit, a character generator image is still produced, confirming the appropriate video connections. Newer cameras generate color bars which also allow you to confirm the connection.

Camera

The silicon charge couple device is the basis of most current endoscopic camera systems. To be most useful, the camera must be sturdy, easy to operate, sterilizable (ETO or soaking), and possess excellent optics and light sensitivity at a reasonable price. For general surgery a camera with a built-in zoom lens is most versatile because one can adjust the image size according to the varying telescope diameters.

Cameras, when connected to telescopes, are the eyes of the entire surgical team, and every effort must be made to ensure their proper function. If a sterile camera is to be used, the scrub nurse should check that there are no signs of moisture or condensation behind the sealed connections. Failure to assure tight connections at either end of the light cable can cause light loss severe enough to degrade the video image.

The scrub nurse then attaches the camera endocoupler to the telescope eyepiece. The light source is turned on, and the scrub nurse aims the telescope at a 4 x 4 X-ray sponge. While the video monitor is watched, the light intensity is adjusted, either with the light source intensity control or by moving the telescope back until "bloom" in the highlights is eliminated. The circulating nurse presses the white balance button on the camera control unit, balancing the camera for the light source color temperature. Still pointing the telescope with camera at the 4 x 4, the scrub nurse adjusts the zoom and focus to optimal size and sharpness.

Still Video Printer

While operative procedures on videotape are invaluable for teaching purposes, videotapes have two practical drawbacks as a record-keeping medium for the practicing physician: real-time review and storage. For the purpose of capturing important findings for patient records and consultation, many are turning to the still video recorder/printer, which produces a hard-copy color print of multiple images in 60 s. The circulating nurse confirms that the still video printer recorder power is on, and that the correct monitor input is selected. Image storage and printing are effected from the remote control unit.

To summarize, the basic video cart components are:

- Primary cart
  - 19-in. high-resolution monitor (700 lines)
  - (Two) CCD video camera systems (re: laparoscopic common bile duct exploration, LCBDE)
  - Image enhancement unit
  - Switcher (runs both cameras)
  - S-VHS recorder; foot switch and microphone optional
  - High-intensity xenon light source: 300-W lamp
  - High-flow insufflator

- Second cart
  - Irrigation system
  - 150-W xenon light source (re: LCBDE)
  - Sterile flexible choledochoscope (re: LCBDE)
  - Peel-packed spare graspers, needle holders, light cables, suction tips, etc.
  - Still video printer

This is but a cursory overview of the many components on which one depends when performing laparoscopic surgery. For surgeons in training and for operating room personnel flexibility, life-long learning, and innovative thinking are essential skills in this increasingly complex technological environment.

References

Berci G (ed) (1993) Laparoscopic cholecystectomy and surgical endoscopy. Gastrointestinal endoscopy. Saunders, Philadelphia (Clinics of North America, vol 3/2)

Berci G, Cuschieri A (eds) (1992) Laparoscopic biliary surgery, 2nd edn. Blackwell, Oxford

Cuschieri A, Bueß G (eds) (1992) Operative manual of endoscopic surgery. Springer, Berlin Heidelberg New York

MacFayden B, Ponsky J (eds) (1992) Laparoscopy for the general surgeon. Surg Clin North Am

2 Preoperative and Postoperative Care in Patients Undergoing Laparoscopic Surgery

S.A. Cunneen and D.R. Margulies

Introduction

The selection criteria for patients who are eligible for laparoscopic procedures is dynamic, and as skills and technologies improve, fewer patients are found to have absolute exclusion criteria. Examples of relative exclusion criteria include: the inability to tolerate general anesthesia, an uncorrected coagulopathy, morbid obesity, previous upper abdominal surgery, portal hypertension, severe obstructive lung disease, and pregnancy. There are even arguments that some high-risk patients may be better served with a laparoscopic procedure. For example, in patients with a severe coagulopathy and ascites, a laparoscopic liver biopsy under direct visualization where bleeding can be controlled directly may be less dangerous than one under computed tomography guidance alone. In patients with severe cardiac disease, laparoscopic cholecystectomy has been shown to be as safe as or safer than open cholecystectomy when hemodynamics are monitored carefully.

Preoperative Care

History and Physical Examination

As in the basic tenets of traditional surgery, a careful history and physical examination is performed to define diseases which require surgical intervention and to identify comorbid conditions which may complicate the intraoperative and postoperative course for the patient. A careful history alone results in an accurate diagnosis in approximately 60% of patients presenting for elective surgery. The review of systems should include inquiries into cardiac, respiratory, renal, endocrine, nutritional status, and social habits. Abnormalities in any of these systems may require further laboratory or radiographic studies to define their status.

The physical examination serves further to define the extent of any pathology in each system as well as to identify any physical condition which may complicate or exclude the laparoscopic approach. Examples of such include: murmurs or shortness of breath indicative of valvular heart disease or pulmonary compromise, di-abetic changes, obesity or cachexia, evidence of prior surgery suggesting adhesion formation, or abdominal wall hernias. In combination with the history, the physical examination is diagnostic in 75%–90% of patients.

Laboratory and Radiologic Assessments

Routine Screening. The routine screening examination is similar for patients undergoing the equivalent operation in the traditional fashion. The usual panel includes a complete blood count and urinalysis in all patients. Serum chemistries may be added if the case is major, or if the history suggests the likelihood of an abnormality. A chest X-ray may be added for patients over 40 years of age (yield approximately 20%), and for those who have known cardiac or pulmonary disease. An ECG may be justified in men aged over 40 years of age and in women over the age of 55 years. A clotting profile is indicated when one has elicited a personal history of bleeding, a family history of bleeding, or a history of previous medications that interfere with clotting. In patients with deficiencies of clotting factors or platelets, the appropriate blood products should be administered preoperatively. Drugs which interfere with clotting, for example, heparin, warfarin, and nonsteroidals, should also be stopped at an appropriate interval. If one anticipates significant blood loss during the procedure, preoperative typing of blood should be carried out.

Selective Screening. For *cardiac assessment*, as with open cases, in patients that give a history of having or are suspected of having valvular heart disease or dysrhythmia, an echocardiogram should be obtained. When a patient is suspected to have coronary artery disease, an exercise tolerance test or a thallium-201 exercise test should be performed. When confirmed, plans should be made for intraoperative hemodynamic monitoring. For *pulmonary assessment*, in patients with a history of chronic obstructive pulmonary disease, spirometry should be performed. Reports have demonstrated that the use of a carbon dioxide pneumoperitoneum necessitates a 30% increase in minute ventilation to eliminate the increased carbon dioxide blood levels. This might lead to converting the case to an open procedure if the need should arise. In cases in which an open procedure would not be tolerated, the patient should also be informed that the laparoscopic approach will be abandoned if the procedure proves technically unsafe or impossible.

Postoperative Care

A significant difference exists between the physical state of the patient following a laparoscopic procedure and that after similar open procedures. There is substantially less pain, improved respiratory function, and decreased postoperative bowel dysfunction. The postoperative management reflects these differences.

Feeding Schedule

After nonintestinal surgery it is generally unnecessary to continue gastric suctioning following the procedure. We therefore generally remove the orogastric tube in the operating room upon the completion of the procedure. In biliary procedures a liquid diet can usually be started upon recovery from anesthesia. Exceptions naturally include those possessing prolonged nausea and those with motility disorders. Decreased incidence of this anesthetic side effect has been noted using droperidol or transdermal scopolamine during the operative and perioperative period. In general, most patients tolerate a diet by the first postoperative day. Early feeding is generally well tolerated in cases involving resection of intestine. A nasogastric rather than an orogastric tube is placed intraoperatively, but generally this can be removed by the end of the case in most distal intestinal surgeries. Postoperative ileus is decreased primarily by the nature of the procedure and secondarily by lessened need for postoperative narcotics. In colorectal resection most patients tolerate a diet on the first or second postoperative day, begun without waiting for flatus. Careful attention should be paid to signs and symptoms of dysmotility, such as gastric distention or eructation, to detect those exceptions in which rapid feeding or the lack of nasogastric decompression could be detrimental.

Analgesic Regimen

Postoperative pain is usually minimal and limited to the trocar insertion sites. Some patients note mild shoulder discomfort for up to 1 week following the procedure. This is believed to result from the diaphragmatic stretching during the period of insufflation and/or irri-

tation from intraperitoneal blood or CO_2. Minimizing the rate and peak of insufflation pressures and removing most intraperitoneal blood during the procedure decreases this problem. In the majority of cases the postoperative pain is easily controlled with oral narcotic analgesics. Trocar site pain can be reduced by the local injection of bupivacaine (0.5%) into the fascia and dermis prior to site closure. This can greatly reduce the need for postoperative analgesics.

Discharge Schedule

In general the length of stay has been found to be significantly shorter than in open procedures. In laparoscopic cholecystectomy rates of discharge greater than 90% at 24 h have been reported. In most cases the additional hospital stay was usually necessitated by prolonged nausea and vomiting. Outpatient laparoscopic cholecystectomy has been reported, but early detection of complications may be missed with this approach. Vague symptoms generally begin on the first postoperative day. A high index of suspicion should be adopted in these cases, and a bowel injury should be suspected in any patient experiencing increasing pain after laparoscopy. Aggressive early investigation lowers morbidity. For instance, early detection of colon injuries may eliminate the need for a colostomy and lessen the physiologic complications of sepsis. Consequently, outpatient procedures scheduled in proximity of the weekend are ill-advised. In more advanced procedures the length of stay is dictated by the return of bowel function.

Activities of Daily Living

In general patients are encouraged to assume moderate activity after the first 48–72 h. Additionally, most patients should be able to resume normal activity, including a return to work, after the first week. Results have been variable, but some have reported that 80% of patients were able to tolerate a liquid diet on the first postoperative day, and 70% were discharged by the fourth day, with a complication rate of 15%.

References

Carroll BJ, Chandra M, Phillips EH, Margulies DR (1993) Laparoscopic cholecystectomy in critically ill cardiac patients. Am Surg 59:783–785

Hasnain JU, Matjasko MJ (1993) Practical anesthesia for laparoscopic procedures in surgery laparoscopy. In: Zucker KA,

Bailey RW, Reddick EJ (eds) Surgical laparoscopy – update. Quality Medical, St. Louis

Jackson SH, Schmidt MN, McGuire J (1982) Transdermal scopolamine as a preanesthetic drug and postoperative antinauseant and antiemetic. Anesthesiology 57:330–334

Putensen-Himmer G, Putensin C et al (1992) Comparison of postoperative respiratory function after laparoscopy or open laparotomy for cholecystectomy. Anesthesiology 77(4):675–680

Tan PL, Lee TL, Tweed WA (1992) Carbon dioxide absorption and gas exchange during pelvic laparoscopy. Can J Anaesth 39(7):677–681

3 Pneumoperitoneum

G. Berci

Introduction

Establishing the optimal pneumoperitoneum is the first and most important step of any laparoscopic procedure. There is a definite need to create a protective cushion to facilitate the safe introduction of the trocar and to provide good visibility for the examination and subsequent procedures. The majority of complications in this first phase are the result of inadequate pneumoperitoneum or poor technique. The complications can largely be avoided by adequate training and attention to details.

Technique

Pneumo Needle

This was invented almost seven decades ago by Veress, a thoracic surgeon, for the creation of a pneumothorax to treat a certain type of tuberculosis. It consisted of an outside needle with a spring-loaded blunt stylet which has a side hole. When the needle is passed through the abdominal wall, the blunt stylet is pushed back into the sleeve due to resistance. As soon as the sharp needle tip enters an area without resistance, for instance, the abdominal cavity (but it can be also the lumen of an intestine), the spring pushes the blunt stylet from the sheath into the outside area creating a safer (blunt) tip for further manipulation.

Veress Needle Insertion

It is advisable that before the needle is inserted (one of the most predilected sites is just below the umbilical fold), a small skin incision is made with a scalpel just penetrating the skin (not the underlying muscular layer). Holding the needle with two fingers (Fig. 1), an assistant and the operator with one hand can elevate the abdominal wall by hand or with a towel clip. The needle should be directed toward the pelvic area in the middle (toward the bifurcation of the aorta) and not to either side. The abdominal wall elevation is maintained during the various tests. The scrub nurse and the operator

should check the patency of the needle before inserting it. It is essential that as soon as this needle is introduced anywhere the following tests are performed:

Aspiration Test. A 10-cc syringe filled with saline is attached, and slight aspirations are adminstered, followed by the injection of a small amount of saline. This maneuver must be repeated twice. The reason for this test is as follows. If blood is aspirated, the needle positioning must be changed. If during the second attempt the test is negative, a pneumoperitoneum can be completed, but as soon as the telescope is introduced, close attention should be paid to this area to ensure that the previous puncture holes are not severe, and that no significant pooling of blood is observed. The reason for its being performed twice is that in case of aspiration omentum can be sucked to the tip of the needle. This can be removed by repeated injection of saline. Many injuries (e.g., emboli) can be avoided if this important step is instituted.

Drop Test. A drop of saline is placed into the tip of the Luer lock. If it disappears during the inspiratory phase, the pressure inside the organ is negative. The needle is probably in the proper position.

Hydrostatic Test. A 10-cc syringe is filled with saline, the plunger is removed, and the syringe is attached. The saline should run in with hydrostatic pressure and vary with respiration.

Insufflating Agent. When this procedure was introduced around the turn of the century, the pneumoperitoneum was performed using room air. Later a filter was added. Although air is abundant, it can support combustion when electrocautery is used.

In the earliest stages of diagnostic laparoscopic procedures CO_2 was introduced because it is inexpensive, nonflammable and does not support combustion. Attention must be paid to a drop in pH and an increase in PCO_2 to avoid significant hypercarbia. The majority of operative procedures are performed under general anesthesia, and the anesthesiologist is well aware of this phenomenon. Nevertheless, significant metabolic changes may occur which are difficult to correct with hyperventilation. In this case the insufflation should be stopped and the abdomen desufflated. Cardiac arrhythmias can occur, especially vasovagal reactions to insufflation. All these disadvantages do not outweigh the advantages. CO_2 also has the advantage that it can be absorbed in small amounts from the blood stream if it is injected inadvertently, thus avoiding major sequelae.

N_2O has been used by a few operators because it is nonflammable, although it allegedly supports combustion. It is less painful, and cardiac arrhythmias are less common than with CO_2. In general practice CO_2 is favored as the type of gas. Recently helium was proposed by some investigators. Still others recommend gasless laparoscopy using mechanical abdominal lifters. These techniques are in an early stage, and further investigations are required to assess the efficiency, safety, and cost/benefit ratio.

Insufflator

The apparatus should be checked before the patient is put to sleep. This is a notorious oversight and can be frustrating especially if the CO_2 cylinder is almost empty (or empty) and in the middle of the procedure no more gas is available. Costly time is wasted until another cylinder is located and attached. There should always be a spare CO_2 cylinder at hand.

The early insufflating units were very simple. They consisted of a number of gauges and dials displaying the intra-abdominal pressure, the insufflated volume, and the cylinder (remaining) pressure. A flow meter indicated continuous flow. These units had a tank inside, of up to 10 l, which was filled before the procedure started to measure the used volume. If this inside tank ran out, it was refilled during the procedure. The maximum flow was 3 l, which was inadequate for operative procedures because if the operating time is prolonged, and several trocars are employed, there is an enormous amount of leakage beside the trocars or during the exchange of instruments. Therefore a refill volume of 3 l/min is not sufficient. The present insufflators employ a flow of 10 l/min or more to satisfy the new requirements of therapeutic laparoscopy.

The more complex operative procedures require a larger volume of CO_2 and consequently a change from a mechanical insufflator to an electronically controlled one. Today's insufflators display the intra-abdominal pressure, preset intra-abdominal pressure, and the actual flow and the preset maximum flow. If the preset maximum flow is obtained, the unit shuts off automatically and reopens the flow if the intra-abdominal pressure drops below the preset one. A large variety of these units

are available, with warning signals or audio alarms as well as electronic display of the intra-abdominal pressures on a TV monitor, which is of great help to the operator.

Closed Technique

The selection of the insertion site of the pneumoperitoneum needle and selection of technique is very important, especially in such cases as the operated abdomen, in obese patients, and in those with an umbilical or incisional hernia. In the normal, nonoperated person, there is a choice of several safe sites (Fig. 2). The most common one is the midline, just below the umbilical fold. The skin of the already prepared and draped abdominal wall is slightly incised. The abdominal wall is lifted by the operator and assistant. The pneumo needle is inserted (Fig. 1) and connected to the insufflator after the previously described tests are performed. If it is a diagnostic procedure which should not last longer than 15–20 min, in certain cases it can be performed with IV sedation and local anesthesia. The area of the pneumo needle or trocar insertion is infiltrated with 1% xylocaine without adrenaline. If the pneumo needle is held by its serrated handle, an audible click is heard as the spring-loaded blunt stylet jumps into position as soon as it penetrates the abdominal wall. In the diagnostic case the flow should not exceed 1.5 l/min because if it is performed under local and IV sedation, it should be introduced slowly to provide some time for (hemodynamic and respiratory) adaptation. The same applies for the operative procedure in general anesthesia. It is strongly advised that during the initial phase of the pneumoperitoneum, the operator should first use a low flow insufflation (e.g., 1–1.5 l/min), and only if several trocars are inserted, should the circulating nurse change it to the higher desired flow.

If arrhythmias occur during insufflation, the insufflation should be stopped immediately and the abdomen desufflated. In the case of a pneumo needle the spring-loaded inlet stylet should be removed. If a trocar is already inserted, a valve is opened, and a certain amount of time should be spent in close communication with the anesthesiologist to reintroduce the pneumoperitoneum with a lower flow. If hypertension occurs, the same procedure should be followed, and close observation of the patient's hemodynamic and general conditions are required, again, with close communication with the anesthesiologist. If sudden severe hypotension occurs during the trocar insertion, the operator should suspect a major vessel injury (e.g., aorta), and time should not be wasted in assessing etiology, but immediate exploration should be considered.

If a patient has had certain previous operations, for example, lower midline scar (not uncommon in females after a history of hysterectomy) or upper midline scars, the umbilicus or an optional site can be used for a safe pneumo needle insertion and pneumoperitoneum introduction, or the left subcostal area beside the lateral edge of the rectus muscle can also be employed (Fig. 3 a, b). In the latter case, make sure that the patient does not have splenomegaly.

When the pneumoperitoneum is obtained, a 5-mm trocar can be penetrated into the abdominal cavity and a 5-mm telescope introduced. The abdominal cavity is then observed to select adhesion-free sites for the larger trocar insertion.

Management of Abnormal Veress Needle Aspiration: Results

Blood. When blood is aspirated from the Veress needle, the needle should be withdrawn immediately and reinserted, and if successful pneumoperitoneum can be obtained, the area underneath the needle insertion should be carefully inspected. If there is a small hematoma in the mesentery of the bowel, this can be observed for increase in size without exploration, but if there is a central or pelvic retroperitoneal hematoma, it should be explored. If no evidence of blood is present at the conclusion of the procedure, the underside of the abdominal wall where the trocar was inserted should be inspected.

Yellow Fluid. Aspiration of yellow fluid could indicate a puncture of the lumen of the intestine or bladder. An alternative site should be chosen for insufflation and then trocar insertion and subsequent inspection. Usually a Veress needle puncture of the intestine does not need suture closure. The same is true for the bladder, but insertion of Foley catheter can prevent leakage and secure the healing of the puncture site.

Subcutaneous Emphysema. Leakage of the gas into the subcutaneous tissues is indicated by subcutaneous emphysema. In male patients, in the case of an existing inguinal indirect hernia, the scrotum can be filled with gas and distended as a balloon. In these cases a temporary truss prior to surgery is recommended. An umbilical hernia in an ascitic patient is not a contraindication. If the subcutaneous emphysema is severe because of the prolonged procedure performed in general anesthesia, again, close collaboration with the anesthesiologist is required. It is not rare that the patient's face is involved. These patients should be observed with controlled airways in the recovery area until the picture recedes and spontaneous respiration is guaranteed.

Open Technique

This is an excellent technique to obtain a safe approach for pneumoperitoneum in the difficult or operated abdomen. However, it can be problematic in an obese patient. An incision of 1.5–2 in. incision is made at the selected site down to the peritoneum, usually at the umbilicus (Fig. 4). The posterior sheath of the rectus muscle is lifted up, as is the peritoneum. A careful, small incision is made into the peritoneum, which is slightly enlarged to the opening of the skin incision (Figs. 5–8). A finger is inserted into the abdominal cavity to ensure that there are no adhered intestinal loops. Two retainer stitches are placed on both sides through the fascia. A Hasson cannula with a blunt stylet and a sliding cone on the sleeve is placed into the hole. The cannula is affixed with these two retainer stitches on both sides (Fig. 9).

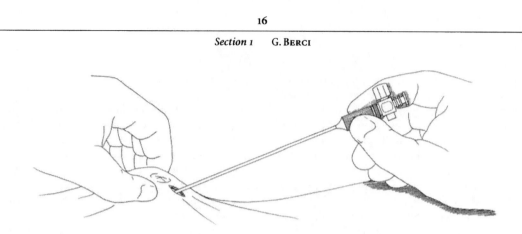

Fig. 1. Technique of Veress needle introduction

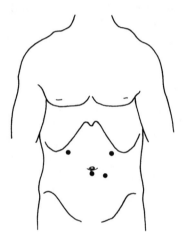

Fig. 2. Trocar sites

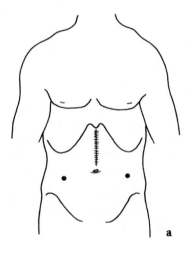

a

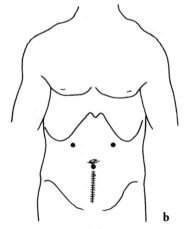

b

Fig. 3 a, b. Alternative trocar sites

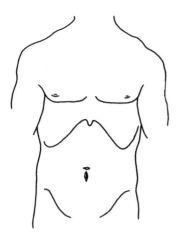

Fig. 4. Hasson technique

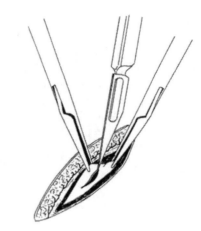

Fig. 7. Hasson technique: peritoneal incision

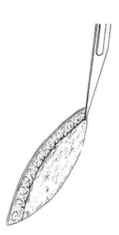

Fig. 5. Hasson technique: skin incision

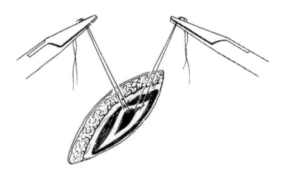

Fig. 8. Hasson technique: stay sutures

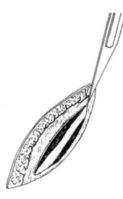

Fig. 6. Hasson technique: incision of the fascia

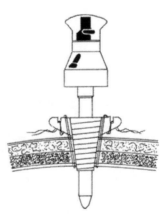

Fig. 9. Hasson technique: trocar fixed to abdominal wall with stay sutures

Comments

The creation of pneumoperitoneum is the first, and one of the most important, steps to create a protective cushion for the insertion of the trocar. Needle injuries can be avoided with appropriate technique. If aspiration is employed routinely, penetration of a blood vessel can be diagnosed immediately and further complications avoided. In the operated abdomen alternate site needle insertion or open laparoscopy as described previously should be the method of choice.

Reference

Berci G, Cuschieri A (1986) Creation of pneumoperitoneum. In: Practical laparoscopy. Baillière Tindall, London

4 Laparoscopy in Trauma and Emergency Surgery

M. Chandra and J.R. Hiatt

Introduction

Determining the presence of organ injury requiring laparotomy is one of the principal tasks in the management of abdominal trauma. For the patient with blunt injury diagnostic peritoneal lavage has been the gold standard because of its sensitivity in identifying intraperitoneal bleeding. However, limitations include the small risk of iatrogenic injury, the possibility of false-negative results with trauma to the retroperitoneum, diaphragm, or intestine, and the failure of the test to identify the specific source of bleeding. Computed tomography has become popular in some centers in recent years because of its ability to demonstrate the site of bleeding and to provide information about the retroperitoneum. Computed tomography has distinct limitations, including the absolute need for hemodynamic stability, removal of the patient from the trauma room, limited sensitivity for hollow visceral injuries, and cost.

In penetrating trauma the approach has been somewhat different. Because of the high frequency of peritoneal penetration and abdominal organ injury, most patients with gunshot wounds have received laparotomy. Knife wounds penetrate peritoneum less often and even then may produce no injuries. Management strategies in patients with knife wounds include routine exploration in those with known peritoneal penetration and various protocols for selective observation, sometimes combined with other tests (usually diagnostic peritoneal lavage for anterior wounds and computed tomography for posterior and flank wounds).

The emergence of laparoscopic cholecystectomy and other laparoscopic procedures has stimulated a new interest in laparoscopic approaches to trauma, particularly in patients with penetrating trauma. In blunt trauma laparoscopy may allow direct visualization of the presence of organ injury, the specific organ injured, and the rate of ongoing hemorrhage. In penetrating trauma diagnostic laparoscopy can identify whether the peritoneum has been violated and can provide information about organ injury and allow for therapeutic hemostasis and repair. When results of laparoscopy are negative, hospitalization which might otherwise be required for expectant observation may be shortened and the cost lowered.

In emergency general surgery laparoscopy has a logical application in the diagnosis of abdominal disease in complex clinical situations. Intensive care patients with abdominal pain and equivocal findings who are poor candidates for laparotomy may benefit from an expeditious procedure, preferably using local anesthesia, to confirm or exclude the presence of peritonitis. All in all, the range of situations in which diagnostic laparoscopy may play a role is expanding as surgeons' facility with the technique increases.

Positioning of the Patient and Team

The patient is positioned supine and draped for all potential procedures at the outset (chest and abdomen in most instances; see Fig. 1).

Technique

The technique for creating pneumoperitoneum is at the discretion of the operator. The Veress needle is inserted in the midline, either infraumbilically or supraumbilically (Fig. 2). The supraumbilical site is used when a pelvic fracture is present to avoid entering a pelvic hematoma. If aspiration returns 10 ml free blood or fluid containing intestinal contents, laparotomy should be performed. The Hasson (open) method may be used in patients with prior abdominal incisions. The telescope is introduced through either a 5- or a 10-mm trocar. A second 5-mm trocar is placed in the right or left subcostal region to allow manipulation of organs with an atraumatic grasper and use of suction and electrocautery (Fig. 3). The upper abdomen is explored in a systematic fashion (Fig. 4). The operating table should be placed in a steep reverse Trendelenburg position to expose the upper abdomen (Fig. 1A). Blind spots are located on the lower aspects of the diaphragm and lateral to the right lobe of the liver. A fan retractor placed through a 5-mm port may be used to retract the liver (Fig. 3). An atraumatic grasper is used to elevate the right and left lobes of the liver, facilitating exposure of undersurfaces, gallbladder, caudate lobe, and porta hepatis. If injury to the biliary tract is suspected, a needle cholangiogram may be performed via the gallbladder. Small liver lacerations may be treated with cautery or hemostatic agents.

The exposure of the spleen is facilitated by turning the operating table to the right lateral position, allowing the splenic flexure of the colon and the omentum to fall away from the spleen. Splenic injury should be considered if blood is observed near the spleen or under the omentum. The pancreas is exposed by opening the gastrocolic omentum in an avascular area. Using atraumatic graspers, the small bowel may be run from the ileocecal valve to the ligament of Treitz. The pelvic organs (Fig. 5), including the bladder, are inspected using Trendelenburg positioning (Fig. 1 B). An additional 5-mm trocar in the suprapubic site may be needed to eval-uate the bowel and pelvic organs. A nonexpanding pelvic hematoma following blunt trauma is usually left undisturbed.

The operative approach to nontrauma patients is similar. Initial aspiration, or subsequent visualization, of fluid which is bloody, turbulent, or frankly purulent may be sufficient to proceed to open exploration or lead one to the offending organ. Immediate Gram's stain of the fluid for white blood cells and bacteria may be performed, and cultures should always be taken.

When laparoscopy has been completed, the surgeon should classify the findings as negative, positive, or equivocal. The two latter categories require the surgeon to determine the need for laparotomy. All 10-mm trocar sites should be closed.

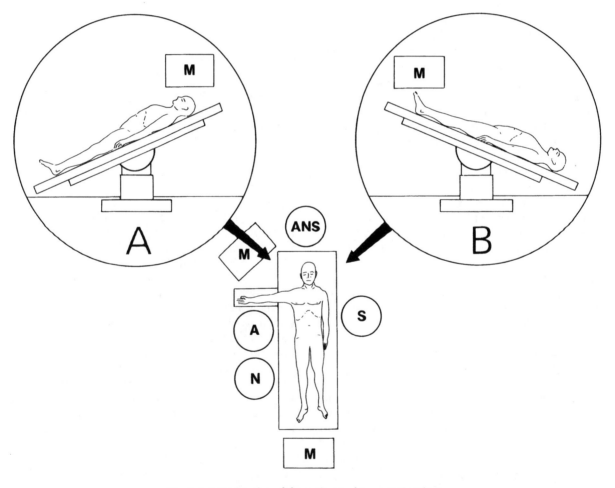

Fig. 1 A, B. Positioning of the patient and team. Patient in supine position. *ANS*, Anesthetist; *S*, surgeon; *A*, assistant; *N*, nurse; *M*, monitor

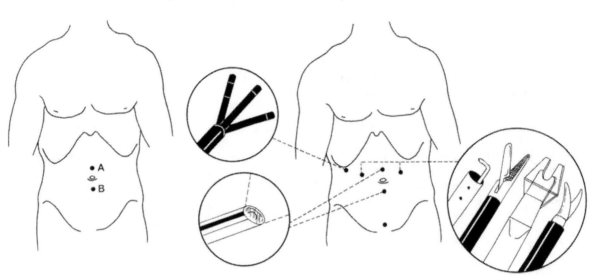

Fig. 2. Trocar sites

Fig. 3. Trocar sites and instrumentation

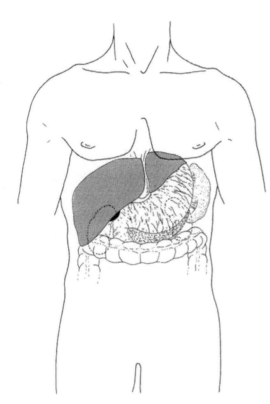

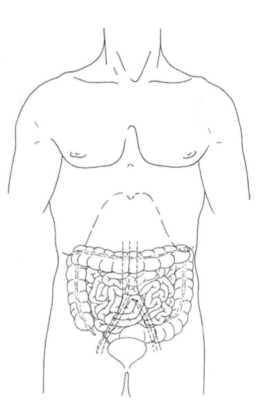

Fig. 4. Exploration sites of the upper abdomen

Fig. 5. Exploration sites of the lower abdomen

Comments

Laparoscopy has an increasing role in trauma and emergency surgery. The primary goal of the procedure is diagnostic, allowing the surgeon to identify or exclude the need for laparotomy. At times specific organ injuries may also be treated through the laparoscope. If nonoperative observation is selected, there should be a clear protocol for monitoring and subsequent evaluation. Growing experience and careful analysis of results should allow even wider application of minimally invasive techniques to these patient populations.

References

Berci G, Dunkelman D, Michel SL (1983) Emergency minilaparoscopy in abdominal trauma. Am J Surg 146:261–265

Carnevale N, Baron N, Delany HM (1977) Peritoneoscopy as an aid in the diagnosis of abdominal trauma: a preliminary report. J Trauma 17:634–641

Gazzaniga AB, Stanton WW, Barlett RH (1976) Laparoscopy in the diagnosis of blunt and penetrating injuries to the abdomen. Am J Surg 131:315–318

Ivatury RI, Simaon RJ, Weksler B, Bayard V, Stahl WM (1992) Laparoscopy in the evaluation of the intrathoracic abdomen after penetrating injury. J Trauma 33:101–109

Sherwood R, Berci G, Austin E, Morgenstern L (1980) Minilaparoscopy for blunt abdominal trauma. Arch Surg 115:672–673

Sosa JL, Sims D, Martin L, Zeppa R (1992) Laparoscopic evaluation of tangential gunshot wounds. Arch Surg 127:109–110

SECTION 2

5 Laparoscopic Intraoperative Cholangiography

D.O. OLSEN

Introduction

Since its introduction by Mirizzi in 1932 intraoperative cholangiography has come to play an integral role in the surgical management of cholelithiasis and choledocholithiasis. The technique not only allows the surgeon a means of evaluating the common duct prior to exploration but also provides an objective means of identifying the ductal anatomy. This should lead to a safer dissection and an accurate placement of clips on the cystic duct. It also allows for immediate identification of ductal injuries when they can best be managed. Although the routine use of intraoperative cholangiography has been advocated, many argue that routine cholangiography is not cost-effective. Every surgeon, however, would agree that cholangiography does play a role in the operative management of gallbladder disease. It is therefore a technique that every biliary tract surgeon needs to be able to perform effectively.

Technique

Cystic Duct Cholangiography

The most versatile of techniques is cystic duct cholangiography. Because the study is performed through the cystic duct, it is useful even with cystic duct obstruction. Since the dissection of the cystic duct has already been completed when the procedure is performed, the cholangiogram serves as an objective study for demonstrating not only the positive identification of the anatomy but also the lack of any ductal injury.

Positioning of the patient and team is shown in Fig. 1 The technique of cystic duct cholangiography begins with isolation of a length of cystic duct high on the neck of the gallbladder. Actual mobilization of the infundibulum and neck of the gallbladder is desired to minimize the problem of inadvertent cannulization of the common bile duct. The serosal attachments of the neck of the gallbladder are first released laterally (Fig. 3). This avoids unnecessary dissection and potential bleeding in the triangle of Calot until the cystic duct is clearly identified. To further mobilize the neck the medial serosal attachments are released, taking care to avoid injury of the cystic artery as it courses along the neck of the gallbladder. Only the thin serosal attachments are divided, avoiding injury to any of the ductal structures if the dissection has been initiated in the wrong location.

With the infundibulum and the neck of the gallbladder completely mobilized, a clip is placed across the neck to prevent any stones from passing down into the cystic duct with further manipulation of the tissues. (If the cystic duct is markedly shortened, the cholangiogram should be shot through the gallbladder itself.) It is important to stress the need to dissect completely the neck and underside of the gallbladder in a continuous circumferential manner to avoid the possibility of missing a right hepatic or common hepatic duct pulled up on the underside of the gallbladder (Fig. 3).

Traction and exposure is maintained on the gallbladder with one grasper on the fundus and one on Hartmann's pouch (see Fig. 4). If an Olsen Cholangiogram Clamp is available (Karl Storz Endoscopy, Culver City, CA; Fig. 4), the approach to the cystic duct is made through one of the lateral ports (Fig. 2). The Olsen Clamp is designed to allow a catheter to be passed down the middle of the clamp, so that once introduced into the duct, the clamp can secure the catheter in place. Exposure is maintained with graspers placed through the epigastric port and the remaining lateral port. A scissor is introduced through the same port that will be used to introduce the cholangiogram clamp, and a small incision is made in the cystic duct as close to the gallbladder as possible.

After making the incision in the cystic duct, the clamp is introduced into the abdomen, with the preloaded cholangiogram catheter. With the clamp introduced into the peritoneal cavity, the catheter is advanced just beyond the end of the clamp and intubated into the small incision that has already been placed in the duct (Fig. 5).

Approaching the duct initially at a perpendicular angle makes the initial introduction of the catheter easier. With the tip of the catheter in the duct, more of the catheter is advanced beyond the clamp, and a slight bend is placed in the catheter, allowing the catheter to come in alignment with the duct. This allows the catheter to be advanced into the duct. The clamp is then advanced over the catheter and the jaws are "clamped" over the cystic duct in a perpendicular fashion. This secures the catheter in the duct and prevents any leakage of contrast.

The cholangiogram is performed in the usual fashion using fluoroscopic technique or a static film technique, if fluoroscopy is not available. The new digital fluoroscopy units yield high-quality films with the advantage of a dynamic study.

Since identification of the ductal anatomy is one of the advantages of cholangiography, it is important to attempt to fill the common hepatic duct along with the intrahepatic ducts. A forceful injection of contrast usually fills the intrahepatic ducts with little difficulty.

When using a static film technique, a two-shot cholangiogram is preferred. The first injection is given using approximately 5 cc full-strength contrast, followed by a second injection of 10 cc 25% (full-strength) contrast. The first injection should give a faint visualization of the distal common duct, allowing visualization of any small stones that may be present. The second injection should fill out the ductal anatomy, allowing identification of not only the ductal anatomy but any filling defects in the upper system. The use of radiolucent disposable trocars in the midclavicular and epigastric positions minimizes the problem of obscuring underlying anatomy with overlying hardware.

Percutaneous Technique

If a cholangiogram clamp is not available, a percutaneous technique can be used. This entails passing the catheter through a needle sheath as a separate puncture, a "fifth" access site (Fig. 2). Since this is made with a 14-gauge needle, the trauma to the patient is minimal. The needle is placed in such a way that the catheter enters the abdominal cavity along the same axis as the cystic duct, facilitating passage of the catheter down the cystic duct (Fig. 6). With the catheter passed through the needle sheath into the abdominal cavity, a scissor is introduced into the abdominal cavity through the epigastric or lateral trocar and used to make a small incision in the cystic duct. Once again, the cystic duct is isolated high on the neck of the gallbladder to eliminate the chance of mistaking the common duct for the cystic duct. One of the advantages of this technique is that a grasper can be used to direct the tip of the catheter into the cystic duct incision and advance the catheter down the duct (Fig. 6). The catheter is secured with a clip, taking care not to overcrimp the clip. This is accomplished by having the assistant inject saline through the catheter as the clip is closed (Fig. 7). The crimp on the clip is halted just as resistance to flow is felt. The injection sequence is the same as described above. The clip is easily removed by grasping the hub of the clip and pulling backwards. Once the clip and catheter have been removed, the laparoscopic cholecystectomy is carried out in the usual fashion.

A number of catheters have become available to facilitate laparoscopic cholangiography. Ureteral catheters work well, but only end-hole catheters should be used so that the catheter does not have to be passed down into the cystic duct far enough to occlude the side holes. The balloon catheter is one which was modified from a vascular irrigation catheter. Because the balloon catheter relies on the cystic duct to secure the catheter when the balloon is distended, the catheter has its limitations when the catheter cannot be fully passed down the duct, or when there is a short cystic duct. The mushroom catheters need only to be wedged into the hole in the cystic duct and held in place with either the clamp or a clip. With their rigid nature, the available metal catheters are easier to manipulate, but they do not conform easily to the slight variations that often occur with trocar placement or differences seen in the anatomy. This, along with their rigidity, can increase the potential risk of trauma to the cystic duct and common duct.

Gallbladder Cholangiography

Intraoperative cholangiography has been described utilizing either of two basic approaches. The direct approach is to perform the cholangiogram directly through the gallbladder (Fig. 8). Drawbacks of this technique include the inability to easily control the amount of contrast infusion and the limitations of obtaining an adequate study if there is cystic duct obstruction. Gallbladder cholangiography is not possible in as many as 20%–30% of cases because of cystic duct occlusion (acute cholecystitis and hydrops of the gallbladder). Without the ability to control the infusion of contrast, poor filling of the intrahepatic bile ducts can be a problem. Furthermore, the cholangiogram is performed before any dissection of the cystic duct has occurred, limiting the ability of this technique to aid in the identification and verification of the ductal anatomy.

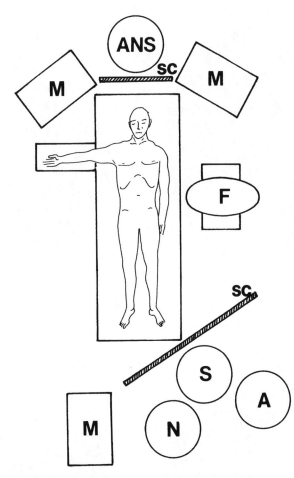

Fig. 1. Positioning of the patient and team. Patient in supine position. *ANS*, Anesthetist; *S*, surgeon; *A*, assistant; *N*, nurse; *M*, monitor; *F*, fluoroscopic equipment; *SC*, lead screen

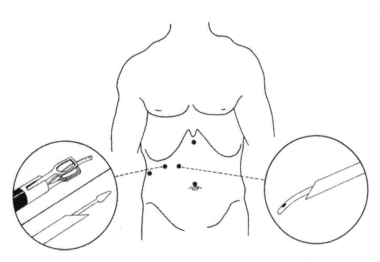

Fig. 2. Trocar sites and instrumentation

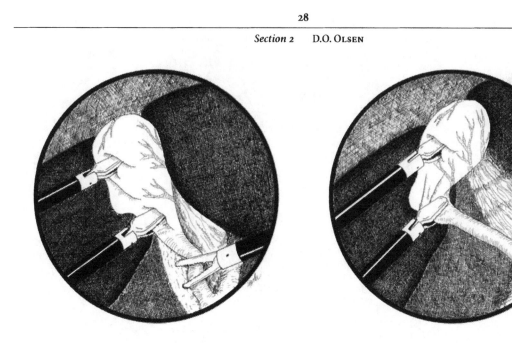

Fig. 3. Dissection of posterior sheath of the hepatoduodenal ligament

Fig. 4. Complete circular dissection of cystic duct

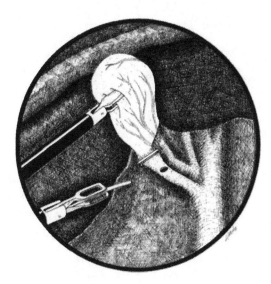

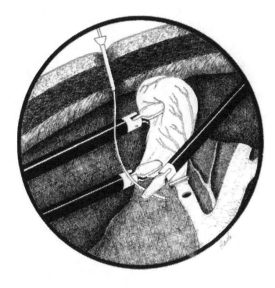

Fig. 5. Cystic duct incision for cholangiography

Fig. 6. Accessory port for insertion of cholangiography catheter

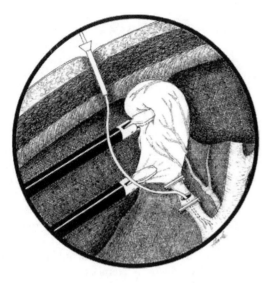

Fig. 7. Cholangiography catheter in place and secured with a clip

Comments

When considering the indications for cholangiography, we are confronted with the issue of a routine vs. selective approach. There are advocates for both views, and the issues have been argued ever since the first description of operative cholangiography. There are both absolute indications and relative indications for the performance of intraoperative cholangiography. These indications are independent of the issue of routine vs. a selective approach.

Cholangiography will always play a role in cholecystectomy, and it is mandatory that the surgeon become proficient in the technique. The selective cholangiographer looks for indications to perform the procedure, while the routine cholangiographer attempts to perform one in all cases. In either respect, the ability to perform cholangiography is a must!

References

Gerber A (1986) A requiem for routine operative cholangiogram. Surg Gynecol Obstet 163:363

Mirizzi PL (1937) Operative cholangiography. Surg Gynecol Obstet 65:702–710

Phillips EH (1993) Routine vs. selective intraoperative cholangiography. Am J Surg 165:505–507

Shively E, Wieman J et al (1990) Operative cholangiography. Am J Surg 159:380–385

Wilson TG, Hall JC, McWatts J (1986) Is operative cholangiography always necessary? Br J Surg 73:637–640

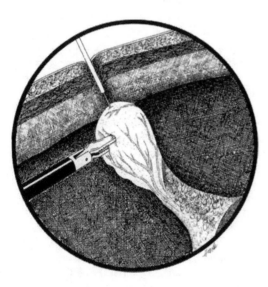

Fig. 8. Puncture of gallbladder fundus for cholecystography

6 Laparoscopic Cholecystectomy: The French Technique

F. Dubois

Introduction

The laparoscopic technique for cholecystectomy, first performed by Phillipe Mouret in Lyon, France, in 1987, was the beginning of a revolution which has spread among general surgeons all over the world. However, it was not until 1989 that several centers in Europe and the United States began clinical work. This simultaneous beginning on both sides of the Atlantic explains why the technique used by the Europeans (French technique) differs in some points from the American one.

Positioning of the Patient and Team

For positioning of the patient and team, see Fig. 1. The so-called French technique, with the patient in the lithotomy position (or double-access position) and the surgeon standing between the legs of the patient, is that most favored one in Europe. The legs of the patient, which are horizontally oriented, are spread out as much as possible to avoid any kind of vein compression. An anti-Trendelenburg position of 15°–20° and a slight rotation on the left facilitate the exposition of Calot's triangle especially in obese patients.

The surgeon is seated between the legs of the patient, allowing him to work in a strictly frontal angle and giving him a better orientation and coordination of his movements (Fig. 1). One assistant standing on the left side of the patient holds the camera and retracting the liver with the lateroxiphoidian port; a second should be positioned on the patient's right side. The surgeon, with the video monitor facing him and above the patient's head, is able to work with both hands as in open surgery. This position is commonly used for all laparoscopic procedures in the upper abdomen.

Technique

Four trocars, two 5 mm and two 10 mm in diameter, are usually used (Fig. 2). The first 10-mm trocar should be inserted in the upper part of the umbilicus in an oblique

direction (45° right to avoid a secondary dehiscence) after the pneumoperitoneum is established. The laparoscope is then inserted, and after thorough exploration of the abdomen the other trocars are inserted under view. The two 5-mm trocars are placed 1 cm under the right costal margin as far as possible from each other. The lateroxiphoidian trocar is used for retraction, aspiration, and irrigation, and the most lateral one for grasping instruments. The fourth trocar (10 mm) is placed under view in the left hypochondrium, taking as an orientation point the features of the round ligament. This trocar site is used for the introduction of scissors, hook, clip appliers, etc. It should be emphasized that the ideal positioning of the trocars is in a lozenge shape, so that an instrument does not disturb the others during its movements. Of course, the positioning of the trocars should be changed regarding previous surgeries, or in obese patients. In the latter all the trocars are placed in the right upper quadrant of the abdomen.

Once the perivesicular adhesions are freed, the neck of the gallbladder is grasped with a forceps and pulled away from the biliary pedicle to unfold and expose the triangle of Calot. This maneuver is essential to separate as much as possible the cystic elements from the hepatic duct and artery. The dissection begins with the posterior aspect of the triangle. The neck of the gallbladder is pulled upward and to the right, and the retractor applied on the biliary pedicle, pushing leftward to expose the posterior aspect of the triangle (Fig. 3).

The peritoneum is opened with scissors or the hook (Fig. 4), and the posterior wall of the gallbladder neck is completely dissected to recognize the junction with the cystic duct. Then the neck of the gallbladder is pushed downward and right, and the probe retracts the liver upward to expose the anterior aspect of the triangle (Fig. 5). The cystic duct and artery are dissected after the anterior sheet of the peritoneum. This dissection should be carried out with smooth instruments very gently from left to right using monopolar electrocautery. Special precautions when using electrocautery in this area are: isolation of the instruments as close as possible to the tip and intermittent use of electrocautery only in tissues elevated by the hook. No monopolar coagulation should be used when working close to the common bile duct.

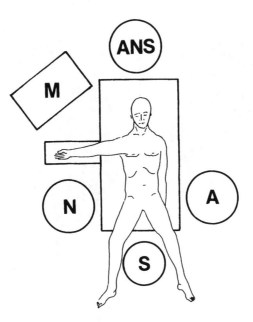

Fig. 1. Positioning of the patient and team. Patient in lithotomy position. *ANS*, Anesthetist; *S*, surgeon; *A*, assistant; *N*, nurse; *M*, monitor

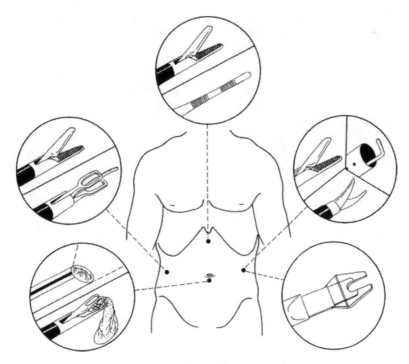

Fig. 2. Trocar sites and instrumentation

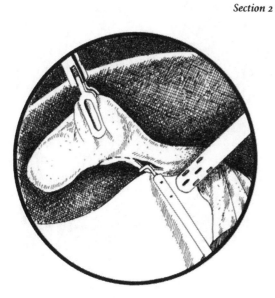

Fig. 3. Incision of hepatoduodenal ligament

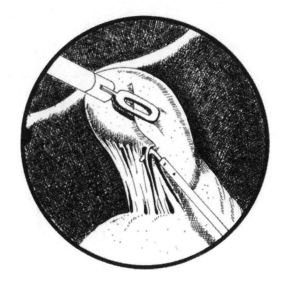

Fig. 4. Dissection of the posterior sheath of the hepatoduodenal ligament

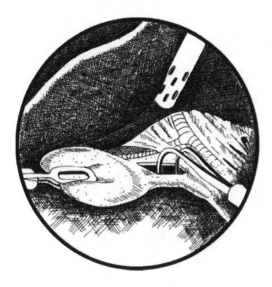

Fig. 5. Dissection of the cystic duct

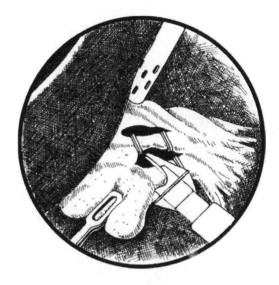

Fig. 6. Closure of cystic duct and artery with clips

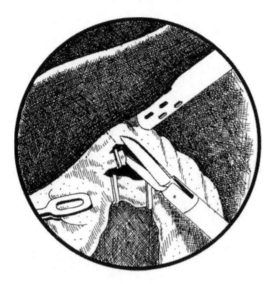

Fig. 7. Transection of tubular structures (cystic duct and artery)

The clamping (Fig. 6) and transection (Fig. 7) of the cystic duct and cystic artery are carried out after the neck of the gallbladder and its junction with the cystic duct are dissected.

The rest of the cholecystectomy is performed as in the American technique (Fig. 8). Cholangiography is performed following selective criteria.

References

Perissat J, Collet D, Beliard R et al (1990) Cholecystectomy par laparoscopic. J Chir (Paris) 127–347

Dubois F, Icard P, Berthelot G (1990) Celioscopic cholecystectomy. Ann Surg 211:60–62

Reddick E, Olsen D (1989) Laparoscopic laser cholecystectomy. Surg Endosc 3:131–133

Phillips EH, Daykhovsky L, Carroll B, Gershman A, Grundfest WS (1990) Laparoscopic cholecystectomy: instrumentation and technique. J Laparoendosc Surg 1:3–15

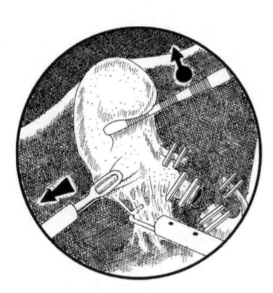

Fig. 8. Excision of the gallbladder from the liver bed

7 Laparoscopic Cholecystectomy: The American Technique

B.J. Carroll

Introduction

Laparoscopic cholecystectomy has become the standard treatment for symptomatic cholelithiasis since its introduction in March 1987 by Mouret in France. Currently there are no absolute contraindications for laparoscopic cholecystectomy, but there are some relative contraindications, the determination of which depends on the operator's experience. These include generalized peritonitis, septic shock from cholangitis, shock from severe acute pancreatitis, cirrhosis with portal hypertension, severe coagulopathies, cancer of the gallbladder, and third-trimester pregnancy.

All patients must be evaluated for history of prior jaundice, pancreatitis, and suspicion of common bile duct stones. Patients should undergo preoperative ultrasound examination of the upper abdomen and blood tests of liver function. In patients with acute cholangitis or septic shock due to suspected common duct stones preoperative endoscopic retrograde cholangiopancreatography should be considered, especially in those over 65 years of age. Intraoperative cholangiography should be performed on all patients to eliminate the need for preoperative diagnostic ERCP and to allow for intraoperative treatment of common duct stones by laparoscopic techniques or by postoperative sphincterotomy. If routine intraoperative cholangiography is not practiced, a very liberal approach to selective cholangiography is indicated: any abnormal liver function test, abnormal amylase, acute cholecystitis, dilated bile duct, or unclear anatomy.

Positioning of the Patient and Team

The patient is positioned in the supine position, with sequential compression devices placed on both legs (see Fig. 1).

Technique

In patients who have had no prior abdominal surgery a Veress needle is placed into the peritoneal cavity in the midline just below the umbilicus. The abdomen is then insufflated with CO_2 to a pressure of approximately 15 mmHg. A 10- to 11-mm trocar is inserted below the umbilicus, and the abdomen is inspected using a 30° angle 10-mm laparoscope (Fig. 2). It is important to inspect immediately below the site of insertion of the Veress needle and the initial trocar since both of these insertions are blind and may cause injury to viscera or blood vessels. All the remaining trocars are placed in the abdomen under direct visualization. A second 10- to 11-mm trocar is inserted immediately below the xiphoid process. The trocar should be guided into the abdomen to the right of the falciform ligament and at the lower edge of the liver. A 5-mm trocar is inserted inferior to the 12th rib as far lateral as possible based on the position of the right colon. A large strong grasper is used to grasp the dome of the gallbladder and elevate it over the liver, exposing the hilum (Fig. 3). This grasper is then affixed to the abdominal wall using a towel clamp so that it remains stable throughout the dissection. A second 5-mm grasper is placed just medial to the first trocar, as lateral as possible and as close to the costal margin as possible. Positioning of this trocar is crucial for parallel insertion of the cholangiogram catheter into the cystic duct.

Dissection of the hilum should start at the gallbladder – cystic duct junction to avoid dissection near the common duct until there is adequate identification of the anatomy (Fig. 4). If the junction is not visible the dissection should start high upon the gallbladder. The overlying fat should be grasped and pulled out and downward until the cystic duct is seen. Meticulous dissection close to the junction of the cystic duct and the gallbladder is safer than early dissection at the junction of the cystic duct and common duct. Once the cystic duct is clearly identified, dissection of the cystic artery can be performed, again close to the cystic duct – gallbladder junction. One clip is placed on the cystic artery (sentinel clip; Fig. 5) and one clip is placed on the cystic duct close to the gallbladder (Fig. 6). A small incision is made in the cystic duct as proximal to the clip as possible (Fig. 7). A no. 4 end hole ureteral catheter is inserted into the cystic duct and is held in place with the cholangioclamp (Fig. 8).

Cholangiography is then performed. The clips on the cystic duct and artery should be identified on the cholangiogram (Fig. 9). Additionally, the length of the cystic duct should be evaluated and the cystic duct – common duct junction confirmed. Visualization of dye flowing into the duodenum is mandatory, as is visualization of the right and left hepatic ducts (see Chap. 5). After the cholangiogram is completed and reviewed, two clips are placed on the "staying" side of the cystic duct, and the cystic duct is divided sharply, not with cautery. Two additional clips are placed on the cystic artery. No specific attempt is made to identify the cystic duct – common duct junction unless a transcystic duct common duct exploration is to be performed.

The gallbladder is grasped at Hartmann's pouch and elevated as it is being withdrawn inferiorly from the liver. Electrocautery is used to separate the gallbladder from the liver bed, and hemostasis is meticulously maintained with electrocautery or small clips (Fig. 10). Once the gallbladder is freed from the liver, the gallbladder is placed into a plastic pouch, and the liver bed and the clips on the duct and artery are reinspected. The abdomen is irrigated with saline solution, and all clots and debris are suctioned from under the right lobe of the liver. All trocar sites are then injected with bupivacaine for postoperative pain relief. The laparoscope is then repositioned in the subxiphoid trocar, and the gallbladder is pulled through the subumbilical trocar site. The open end of the endopouch is exteriorized and the gallbladder is grasped through the open end of the pouch and pulled through the fascia. The gallbladder and gallstones may need to be morcellated and/or the fascial incision extended. After removal of the gallbladder, all trocar sites are inspected for abdominal wall bleeding, and all the 10-mm fascial incisions are closed with Vicryl sutures.

References

Mouret P (1991) From the first laparoscopic cholecystectomy to the frontiers of laparoscopic surgery: their prospective futures. Dig Surg 8:124–126

NIH Consensus Development Panel on Gallstones and Laparoscopic Cholecystectomy (1993) Gallstones and laparoscopic cholecystectomy. JAMA 269 (8):1018–1024

Phillips EH, Berci G, Carroll B et al (1990) The importance of cholangiography during laparoscopic cholecystectomy. Am Surg 56:792–795

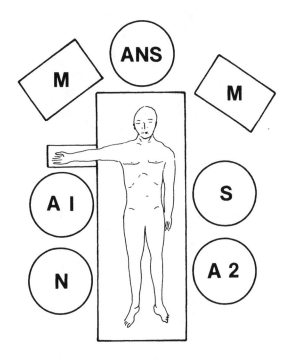

Fig. 1. Positioning of the patient and team. Patient in supine position. *ANS*, Anesthetist; *S*, surgeon; *A1*, *A2*, assistants; *N*, nurse; *M*, monitor

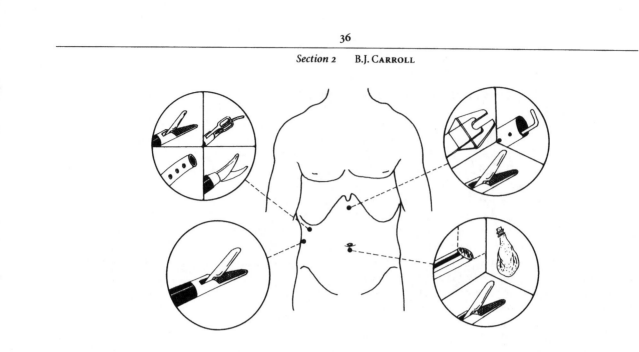

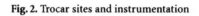

Fig. 2. Trocar sites and instrumentation

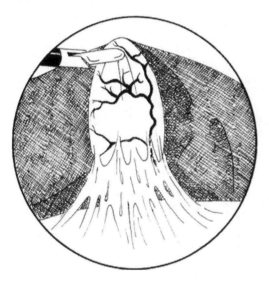

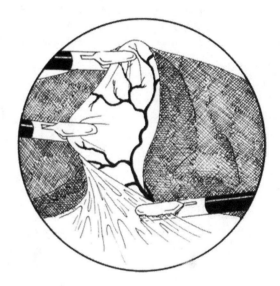

Fig. 3. The gallbaldder is grasped at the fundus and the liver retracted cranially

Fig. 4. Blunt dissection of the hepatoduodenal ligament

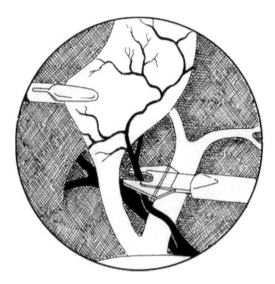

Fig. 5. A sentinel clip is placed on the cystic artery

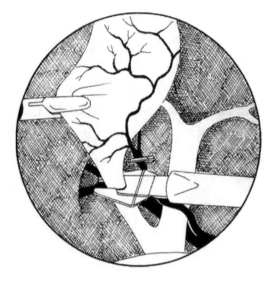

Fig. 6. The cystic duct is closed with a clip

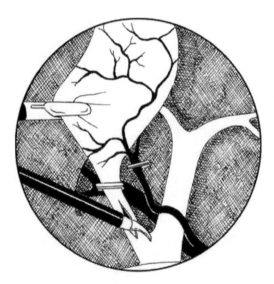

Fig. 7. The cystic duct is incised for the cholangiogram

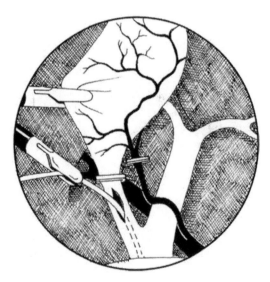

Fig. 8. A cholangiography catheter is introduced in the cystic duct

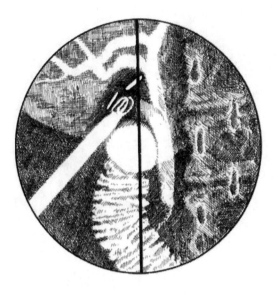

Fig. 9. This figure represents a cholangiogram. Once the sentinel clip has been identified, an imaginary line should be represented along this clip. When dissecting the gallbladder from the liver bed, surgeons should always stay laterally from this line in order to avoid CBD injuries.

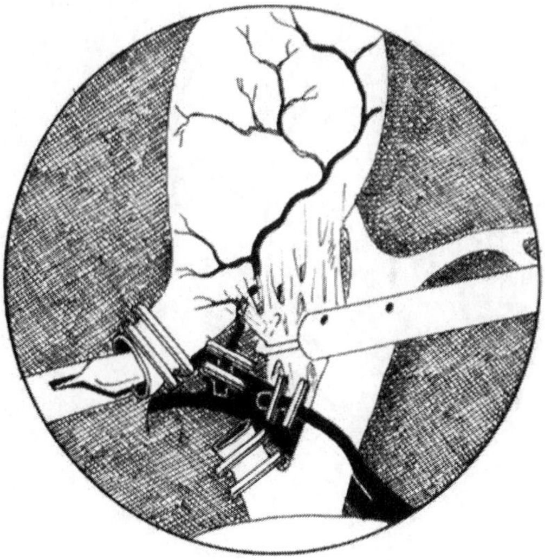

Fig. 10. The tubular structures are transected

8 Laparoscopic Intraoperative Ultrasonography

M.E. Wegener, R.B. Kolachalam, and M.E. Arregui

Introduction

Minimally invasive surgery has progressed to application in complex hepatico-pancreatico-biliary problems as well as to other organ systems. Although indirect palpation can be performed with probes and other instruments during laparoscopy, the sensitive tactile feedback of the surgeon's hands is lost. Common bile duct (CBD) stones, lymph nodes, liver and pancreatic masses cannot be felt or characterized. This greatly limits the diagnostic and therapeutic capabilities of the laparoscopic approach. Laparoscopic ultrasound (LUS) promises to overcome these limitations and may perhaps exceed the sensitivities of manual palpation used with open surgery. Indeed, LUS is not a new technique but an extension of intraoperative ultrasound, which has been demonstrated to be superior to palpation and preoperative imaging techniques in detecting liver masses, finding insulinomas, characterizing tumors, etc. It has also been shown to be as sensitive and accurate as static intraoperative cholangiograms for finding CBD stones.

With the adjunctive use of LUS the surgeon is able to extend his capabilities in advanced laparoscopic procedures. In fact, without ultrasound accurate staging of tumors and optimal management of many disease processes cannot be accomplished. As obstetricians, gynecologists, urologists, vascular surgeons, gastroenterologists, and European and Japanese surgeons have adopted the use of ultrasound, so should general surgeons in the United States take example from this precedent. Ultrasound has been appropriately described as the "surgeon's stethoscope." It is the surgeon performing his own ultrasound who can best use the information obtained, and who can obtain immediate clinical correlation of the findings.

This chapter presents the basic information necessary to understand the principles of ultrasound, anatomy of the liver, biliary tree, and pancreas, and pathology of these systems.

Ultrasound Basics

Ultrasound is based on piezoelectric theory. When subjected to an electrical charge, some crystals change shape. This creates sound waves. Similarly, when sound waves are directed toward these crystals, electrical currents are generated. Lead zirconate is the most commonly used crystal in the formation of sound waves for ultrasound.

Different tissues have inherent densities, which are a function of the number of molecules per cubic unit. These different densities allow sound waves to pass through them at different speeds. This is referred to as the acoustic impedance of the tissue. Solids allow easier transmission of sound waves due to increased density, thereby having a higher acoustic impedance and returning a stronger signal to the crystal. Gases do not echo sound waves well due to the greater dispersion of molecules and therefore do not transmit sound waves well.

There are three basic modes of imaging using ultrasound. A-mode (amplitude modulation) uses a single beam to determine distance. This form of imaging is rarely used. B-mode imaging (brightness modulation), which is the basis of static and real-time imaging, converts multiple A-mode beams into dots of varying intensity depending on the strength of the signal. This allows creation of an image depending on the varying densities of the tissues. M-mode is a variant of the B-mode which plots the B-mode image in a linear fashion with respect to time. This allows a continuum of imaging which allows the motion of an object to be viewed.

Sound waves are measured in cycles per second. A frequency of one cycle per second is the equivalent of one vibration of the crystal in 1 s and is represented as 1 Hz. Sound waves used in ultrasound are generally in the range of 1–30 MHz, whereas audible sound waves are in the range of 20–20 000 Hz. Standard ultrasound probes vary in frequency. The more common probes are 2.3, 3.5, 5, and 7.5 MHz. Increasing frequency improves the visualization by having greater resolution, but has the drawback of having a more shallow depth of penetration.

Transducers are the devices that convert the electrical current to sound waves, and vice versa. There are many different types of transducers, but they can be separated into two fundamental groups, mechanical and electrically steered systems. The more common types of mechanically steered transducers include the rotary wheel and oscillating types. These create arc- or pie-shaped images through the movement of the crystal inside the transducer housing. The electronically steered systems, or arrays, are based on the placement of multiple transducers in sequence and pulse sequencing these to create ultrasound fields. The pattern of arrangement of the transducers determines the shape of the field created.

Biliary Tree

The anatomy of the gallbladder and the extrahepatic biliary system is subject to several anomalies. From the point of view of LUS, the anatomy of the extrahepatic biliary system can be considered at the porta hepatis, suprapancreatic, and intrapancreatic portions. The porta is a fat-filled space separating the anteroinferior margin of the caudate lobe from the medial segment of the left lobe. This space contains the hepatoduodenal ligament, which is composed of loose fibrous tissue, the portal vein, bile duct, hepatic artery, and lymph nodes. The upper border of the porta is formed by the confluence of the right and left hepatic duct to form the common hepatic duct. The lower border of the porta is more variable and is defined by the junction of the cystic duct and the common hepatic duct. Within the porta the common hepatic duct or right hepatic duct arches anteriorly over the hepatic artery and to the right portal vein. Sonographically at this level the artery is seen in transverse cross-section between longitudinal views of the duct anteriorly and portal vein posteriorly (Fig. 1 a, b).

In the hepatoduodenal ligament (suprapancreatic common duct) the portal vein is the most posterior and is the point of orientation. The CBD and the common hepatic duct are ventral and to the right of the portal vein. At the distal end of the ligament the bile duct veers posteriorly as it traverses the pancreas and forms an important landmark for the posterolateral margin of the pancreatic head. The gastroduodenal artery lies anterior to the bile duct and is a landmark for the anterolateral margin of the pancreatic head.

The intraduodenal termination of the bile duct (ampulla of Vater) is approximately 1–2 cm in length and is the most difficult area to visualize sonographically. It is often surrounded by a relatively hypolucent oval area as it courses into the duodenum (Fig. 2).

With current LUS probes the biliary tract may be scanned through a 10-mm port from either the subxiphoid, right subcostal, or the umbilical port. First, a few caveats in the examination are helpful. The bile duct examination is a contact process, requiring good apposition with the transducer. If necessary, irrigation with saline can provide a coupling medium. The portal vein represents an important landmark for identifying the common duct at all levels. Better acoustic contact and a more convenient angle for the examination can sometimes be obtained by partial reduction of the pneumoperitoneum. This serves to decrease the angle of contact from the umbilical port and allows a more parallel contact on the CBD. Lastly, saline irrigation through a cholangiogram catheter in the cystic duct can aid in identifying the intrapancreatic portion of the CBD by creating distention of an otherwise collapsed duct.

The examination begins with the placing of the transducer on the anterior surface of the liver to the right of the falciform ligament. Using the liver as an acoustic window, the portal vein is identified in the porta. The bile duct is then identified anterior to the longitudinal image of the portal vein and the transverse image of the hepatic artery (Fig. 1 a). The best screening maneuvers involve a slow withdrawal of the transducer along its long axis combined with a slight left and right rotation of the transducer along its transverse axis. When the edge of the liver is reached, the transducer is then inserted underneath to the liver to its hilum (porta) as high as possible (Fig. 1 b). Using the same combination of movements (outward, toward the access port and with slight rotation in transverse axis if needed), the common duct is kept continuously in view as it is followed distally, remembering that the bile duct veers laterally and posteriorly as it enters the pancreas. Gentle pressure is applied so as not to collapse the bile duct with the transducer.

Visualization of the intrapancreatic and in particular the intraduodenal segment of the bile duct is the Achilles heel of LUS. This part of the examination is best accomplished looking from a lateral to medial direction by placing and compressing the transducer medially against the lateral wall of the duodenum. One useful tip in this area is finding the confluence of the pancreatic and CBD (Fig. 2). Sonographically the ampulla of Vater is seen as an oval hypolucent area. In our experience, gentle distention of the bile duct with saline injected through the cholangiogram catheter is a useful maneuver in visualizing the distal common duct and the ampulla of Vater.

Gallstones and ductal stones are the predominant pathology identified by routine LUS during laparoscopic cholecystectomy. They are identified by standard ultrasound criteria: echogenic mobile foci, which cast an acoustic shadow (Fig. 3). Unlike laparoscopic intraoperative cholangiography (IOCG), LUS of the biliary tree can be performed in all patients, including during pregnancy. While LUS can always visualize the intrahepatic and the suprapancreatic biliary tree, the intrapancreatic CBD and the ampulla of Vater are very difficult to image in patients with significant intra-abdominal fat or in the presence of pancreatitis. Also, following interventions such as ERCP and sphincterotomy, LUS imaging may be inferior to IOCG for evaluation of the biliary tree because of the acoustic impedance to the transmission of ultrasound waves caused by air in the biliary tree. Sludge in the CBD is better seen with LUS (Fig. 2).

Debris and cholesterolosis in the gallbladder and sludge in the bile duct are seen as echogenic foci 1 mm or less in diameter without acoustic shadows. The exact significance of these two findings is unclear and presently under investigation. Similarly, gallbladder polyps are seen as immobile, echogenic polypoid lesions without acoustic shadowing, identified on the luminal surface of the gallbladder.

The surgeon should always be alert in finding unsuspected gallbladder and bile duct pathology. While LUS diagnosis and staging of gallbladder tumors may prove to be easier, identifying CBD tumors is difficult. This may be suspected when a space-occupying lesion is seen within the lumen of the biliary tree with variable or complex internal echoes making its differentiation from ductal stones relatively straightforward (Fig. 4). Cholangiocarcinoma may show nonspecific ductal wall thickening. In such cases one should then proceed with intraoperative staging by scanning the liver and the draining lymph basin and obtaining biopsies of suspicious lymph nodes. Malignant lymph nodes are typically round and hypoechoic, whereas inflammatory nodes are more oval-shaped with internal echoes. LUS staging, in our experience, is very useful in planning definitive curative operation by providing additional information not obtained by preoperative workup. In tumor staging, remember that negative information by LUS is equally important in the planning of definitive surgery.

Liver

While a detailed description of gross liver anatomy is beyond the scope of this chapter, important anatomical concepts pertaining to ultrasound of the liver need to be addressed. The normal liver parenchyma is uniform, containing fine, homogeneous echoes, and is either minimally hyperechoic or isoechoic compared to the normal renal cortex. The liver is hypoechoic compared with the spleen. In scanning the liver one should be familiar with Couinaud's description of segmental anatomy. Understanding the vascular anatomy of the liver is the key in identifying the hepatic segments. Two fundamental points are worth remembering. First, the major

hepatic veins course between the lobes and segments (interlobar and intersegmental) while portal veins run centrally within the segments (intrasegmental), with the important exception of the ascending portion of the left portal vein. The ascending portion of the left portal vein runs in the left intersegmental fissure, which separates the medial segment of the left lobe from the lateral segment. Second, the portal vein is always surrounded by Glisson's capsule, which gives the portal vein an echogenic wall and allows for its distinction from the hepatic veins, which have an almost imperceptible wall. One other anatomical caveat is that the left portal vein courses anterior to the caudate lobe.

Identification of the portal vein at the porta hepatis is the key to finding the extrahepatic biliary system. The bile duct is anterior to the portal vein, and its size does not fluctuate during respiration. From the porta the bile ducts can be easily followed through the liver parenchyma, remembering that the bile ducts are a part of the portal triad and hence have echogenic walls. Intrahepatic biliary radicals are often poorly seen unless dilated (Fig. 1).

With these important principles in mind, liver scanning can be standardized. A few helpful tips may be useful initially. First, approach the patient from their right side, facing cephalad. Second, all preoperative imaging studies should be available in the operating room for review. Third, dividing the frequency of an ultrasound device into 40 results in a rough guideline to the depth of tissue penetration in centimeters (e.g., 40/10 gives 4 cm tissue penetration for a 10 MHz probe).

LUS can be applied directly to a visible mass to delineate the pathology, or it can be used to scan the liver for occult lesions. To scan the right lobe the transducer is placed as high as possible and close to the diaphragm, and scanning is performed in several parts starting from lateral to medial, and then from medial toward lateral, each time withdrawing the length of the scanning surface mounted upon the probe (usually 3 cm). Depending on the frequency of the probe used and the thickness of the liver examined, it may be necessary to screen from both the anterior and posterior aspects of the liver to ensure complete examination. The left lobe is usually thinner and can often be examined from the anterior aspect alone. The liver should also be scanned craniocaudally, remembering that the major hepatic veins course between the lobes and segments. They are ideal segmental boundaries but are visualized only when scanning the superior aspect of the liver. The middle hepatic vein separates the anterior segment of the right lobe from the medial segment of the left. The right hepatic vein separates the right lobe into anterior and posterior segments. In more caudal sections of the liver, however, the right hepatic vein is not identified. Therefore, in more caudal sections of the right lobe, the boundaries between the anterior and posterior segments become an ill-defined division of the right portal vein into anterior and posterior branches.

In general, sonographic findings of different abnormalities are fairly typical and can be easily recognized with some practice. Liver lesions may be classified as diffuse or discrete based on ultrasound characteristics. Discrete lesions may further be classified broadly as cystic or solid, single or multiple. Benign liver cysts are anechoic or hypoechoic, with a well-demarcated thin wall. Posterior acoustic enhancement is a cyst quality and is due to increased transmission of sound waves through cyst and is seen only when sound waves pass close to the center of the cyst. This sign is seen as bright echoes immediately deep to the cyst wall. Cysts are generally rounded or oval, have sharp walls, have no internal echoes or have fine echoes that are hypoechoic and homogeneous (Fig. 5). The ultrasound features of abscesses are varied. Depending on its stage of evolution, they may appear cystic or solid and echogenic. A few helpful findings include thick walls, fluid interfaces, internal septations, and debris.

The sonographic findings of hepatic adenomas and focal nodular hyperplasia are similar and nonspecific. They may be isoechoic, hypoechoic or hyperechoic (Fig. 6). A central fibrous scar, when seen, is suggestive of focal nodular hyperplasia. A hemangioma is typically well defined, homogeneous, and hyperechoic. Larger lesions may be heterogeneous with central hypoechoic foci. A hemangioma may appear hypoechoic within the background of a fatty infiltrated liver.

Most small (< 5 cm) hepatocellular carcinomas are hypoechoic, corresponding to a solid tumor without necrosis (Fig. 7). Larger lesions are complex or echogenic. Similarly, metastatic lesions may appear echogenic, hypoechoic, target, calcified, cystic, and diffuse. In general, more vascular tumors, such as from renal cell carcinoma, carcinoid, choriocarcinoma, and islet cell carcinoma, tend to be hyperechoic. Similarly, metastases from the gastrointestinal tract tend to be echogenic. Hypoechoic metastases are generally hypovascular. More unusual patterns of metastasis include a bull's eye (target) pattern, cystic pattern, or calcified metastasis. Ultrasound can define the relationship of these lesions to the vascular anatomy of the liver and may delineate satellite nodules, tumor thrombus, and direct vascular invasion (Fig. 7).

Diffuse liver disease is more difficult to identify, since findings are more subtle and often subjective. Increased echogenicity and coarse echo structure are frequent but subjective observations in cirrhosis. Regenerating nodules tend to be hypoechoic and have a thin echogenic border that corresponds to fibrofatty connective tissue.

Fatty infiltration leads to an increase in liver echogenicity and attenuation of the ultrasound beam. It is important that the inexperienced surgeon not adjust the time-gain compensation settings and power to make the fatty liver appear normal. Moderate to severe fatty infiltration is identified by a slight to marked decrease in visualization of the intrahepatic vessels. In severe cases there may be poor penetration of the posterior segment of the right lobe of the liver.

Pancreas

Due to the similar acoustic impedance of pancreatic tissue with the surrounding fat, it is sometimes difficult to obtain good ultrasound images. With LUS the use of higher frequency probes allows one to view the pancreas in much finer detail than could be seen otherwise. The acoustic impedance of the pancreas is slightly lower than that of fat, thereby giving it a slightly darker signal than the surrounding retroperitoneal fat. With age the pancreas may naturally become infiltrated with fat, giving it a slightly higher echogenicity.

Placement of the ultrasound probe in the umbilical port during laparoscopy allows easy access to visualize the entire pancreas. Initially the probe should be placed on the anterior surface of the liver to evaluate the intrahepatic bile ducts, but the best view of the pancreatic head and uncinate process is obtained by placing the probe directly over the gland. The head can easily be viewed in this fashion. The body and tail of the pancreas should be initially evaluated by placing the probe on the anterior wall of the stomach and viewing the structure through the gastric wall. Compression on the stomach should displace the gas (Figure 8). An alternative route is by opening the gastrohepatic or gastrocolic omentum and placing the probe directly on the gland.

The pancreatic duct can be seen throughout the entire gland as a dark echo. The normal size of the major duct is less than 2 mm (Figs. 2, 8). An excellent view of the intrahepatic portion of the CBD and ampulla of Vater can be seen by placing the probe lateral to the duodenum and compressing it medially.

Important peripancreatic structures that should be viewed when ultrasounding the pancreas include the distal CBD, portal vein, superior mesenteric artery, and celiac axis. The portal vein can be seen running obliquely behind the body of the pancreas and can be distinguished from the CBD in that the former passes completely through the gland, whereas the CBD tapers and enters the duodenum. The superior mesenteric artery can be seen running longitudinally behind the midbody of the pancreas. Its origin with the aorta should easily be visualized, as is the celiac axis, which is immediately cephalad to it.

Acute pancreatitis can be seen as a decreased signal secondary to the increased tissue water from edema. Along with this there is an increase in the anteroposterior dimension of the gland (greater than 3 cm). Often the surrounding tissues are also edematous, thereby making the gland more difficult to see. Chronic pancreatitis, in contrast, is demonstrated as a hypoechogenic gland due to the replacement of the normal gland with fibrous tissue. The gland tends to be more irregular. Ductal calculi or tissue calcifications may be seen, as well as a dilated duct (greater than 2 mm).

Cysts of the pancreas are not common but appear similar to cysts in other parts of the body, being well circumscribed and hypoechoic and having good through transmission. The most common cystic lesion of the pancreas are pseudocysts. These may be difficult to differentiate from simple cysts by ultrasound criteria alone but can usually be differentiated from cystadenomas or cystadenocarcinomas in that the latter are usually complex cystic structures (Fig. 9). Some pseudocysts may demonstrate internal echoes signifying early formation with intracystic debris but should alert the physician to the possibility of internal hemorrhage or infection.

Pancreatic tumors present as discrete masses in the substance of the gland. Carcinomas are usually hypoechoic with irregular borders (Fig. 10). The pancreatic and/or bile ducts may also be dilated secondary to compression. In contrast, islet cell tumors are well circumscribed and hypoechoic compared to the surrounding parenchyma (Fig. 11). Biopsies of isoechoic nodules invariably show normal pancreatic tissue.

Peripancreatic adenopathy is not an uncommon finding. Normal lymph nodes, which may be found either surrounding or even in the substance of the gland, are characterized by an isoechoic area surrounded by a rim of hypoechoic tissue. Pathologic lymph nodes may not be as well circumscribed, have lost the rim of hypoechogenicity, may be more hyperechogenic, and tend to be more round than oval.

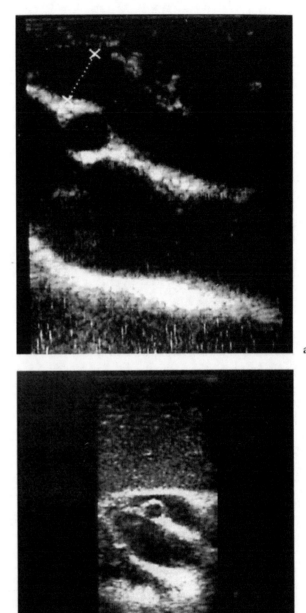

a

b

Fig. 1 a, b. Portal triad. Note transverse view of the hepatic artery between longitudinal views of CBD (*top*) and portal vein (*below*). **a** The probe is directly on portal structures. **b** Transhepatic view with the probe on the liver

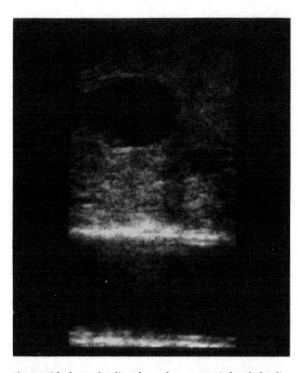

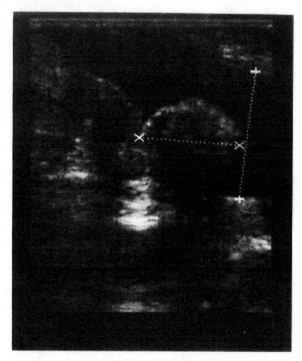

Fig. 2. With the probe directly on the pancreatic head, the distal CBD (*left*) and pancreatic duct (*right*) are seen going through the pancreas. Sludge is seen in the slightly dilated ducts. The vena cava is seen posterior

Fig. 3. CBD duct stone. Note shadowing behind the stone. The dilated CBD is 15 mm

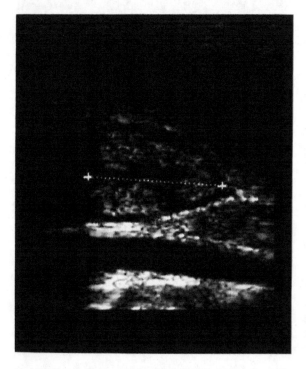

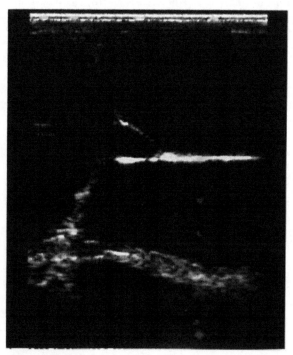

Fig. 4. Villous adenoma of the distal CBD. Note there is no distal shadowing. This tumor recurred after 15 years

Fig. 5. The liver parenchyma replaced by cysts in a patient with polycystic liver disease

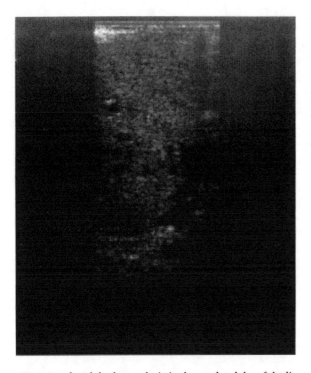

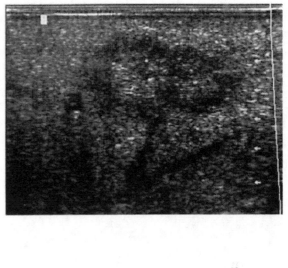

Fig. 6. Focal nodular hyperplasia in the caudate lobe of the liver. A thin rim of hypoechoic tissue delineates the margins. Note the mixed hyper/hypoechogenic nonhomogeneous internal structure

Fig. 7. Hepatic metastasis of a colorectal carcinoma. Note the proximity to the branches of the portal vein. A segment IV resection was performed with ultrasound guidance

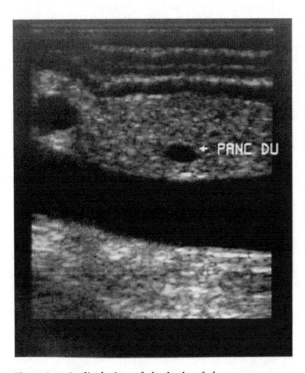

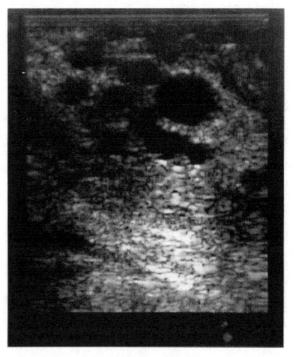

Fig. 8. Longitudinal view of the body of the pancreas seen through the stomach. The portal vein is posterior and the hepatic artery is to the left

Fig. 9. Benign microcystic adenoma of the head of the pancreas

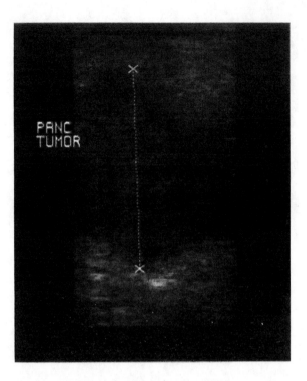

Fig. 10. Adenocarcinoma of the head of the pancreas. Note the complex hypoechoic mass (33 mm) with irregular margins

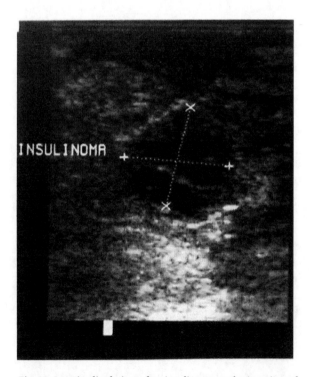

Fig. 11. Longitudinal view of an insulinoma at the junction of the head and body of the pancreas. The mass is hypoechoic with internal septations

Comments

Endoscopic ultrasound is useful as an adjuvant to transabdominal and laparoscopic ultrasound. Endoscopic ultrasound probes are available in linear array and sector scanning. They allow an excellent view of the periluminal anatomy. No controlled studies are available at this time comparing laparoscopic and endoscopic ultrasound. Endoscopic ultrasound is being used in the preoperative staging for resectability of periampullary, pancreatic, gastric, and esophageal tumors.

A new technique has recently been introduced in which extremely high frequency probes are used within the ductal system. Intraductal ultrasound, introduced in Japan, uses a 30-MHz probe to create a real-time image. Excellent wall anatomy can be seen, but there is the severe limitation of a small depth of penetration. The technology exists that also allows for three-dimensional reconstruction of these ultrasound images.

References

Castro D, Arregui M, Brueggemann A (1995) Laparoscopic ultrasound: principles and techniques. In: Arregui M et al (eds) Laparoscopic surgery: principles and techniques. Springer, Berlin Heidelberg New York

Furukawa T, Naitoh Y, Tsukomoto Y et al (1992) New technique using intraductal ultrasonography for the diagnosis of diseases of the pancreatobiliary system. J Ultrasound Med 11 (11):607–612

Sanders R (1991) Clinical sonography: a practical guide, 2nd edn. Little Brown, Boston

Seigel B, Machi J, Beitler J et al (1983) Comparative accuracy of operative ultrasound and cholangiography in detecting common duct calculi. Surgery 94:715–720

9 Laparoscopic Transcystic Duct Common Bile Duct Exploration

E.H. Phillips and R.J. Rosenthal

Introduction

Most transcystic duct techniques of common bile duct (CBD) exploration involve dilation of the cystic duct with balloon dilators or sequential graduated bougies to access the CBD. Biliary flexible endoscopy is our primary approach to the CBD. Nevertheless, balloon trolling of the CBD, fluoroscopically guided wire basket stone retrieval, ampullary balloon dilation with lavage, and transcystic endoscopically assisted sphincterotomy are all techniques that can be employed laparoscopically via the cystic duct without the need for dilation.

Flexible biliary endoscopy with wire basket retrieval of calculi is the preferred technique. It appears to be the safest technique because stone capture and manipulation are performed under direct vision without manipulation of the ampullae. This technique is feasible in 80%–90% of cases. One limitation is that the endoscope can be passed into the proximal bile ducts in approximately only 10% of cases. Multiple stones, small fragile cystic ducts, and stones proximal to the cystic duct – common duct junction usually must be dealt with by choledochotomy, endoscopic sphincteromy, or ampullary balloon dilation. Luckily, these more difficult situations occur infrequently.

Positioning of the Patient and Team

The patient is placed on the operating table in the supine position. The operating team is positioned in the same way as for laparoscopic cholecystectomy (Fig. 1).

Technique

After review of the intraoperative cholangiogram, a strategy for treatment of choledocholithiasis should take into account the number of stones and their location. If the location of the stones and the patient's condition permit, the cystic duct should be dissected bluntly down close to its junction with the common duct. It is often necessary to make an incision in the larger portion of the cystic duct closer to the common duct so that less duct requires dilation. The location of the incision should allow an adequate length of cystic duct stump for closure with an endoloop (Ethicon, Cincinnati, OH) at the end of the procedure. This maneuver increases the success of the procedure. A no. 5 phantom balloon dilating catheter (Insurg, Watertown, MA), which has a balloon that is 4 cm long and 6 mm in outer diameter, is preloaded with a 0.35-in., 150-cm-long hydrophilic guide wire. The assemblage is inserted via a 5-mm trocar in the right anterior axillary line just under the costal margin (Fig. 2). Depending on the laparoscopic cholecystectomy technique employed, it may be necessary to add an additional 5-mm trocar in a better location to intubate the cystic duct.

After X-ray or fluoroscopic confirmation of the guide wire location the balloon dilating catheter or sequential bougies are inserted over the guide wire (Fig. 3). Two-thirds of the balloon should be inserted. The balloon is then inflated slowly with a LeVeen syringe attached to a pressure gauge (Fig. 4). The balloon and cystic duct are observed laparoscopically as the assistant or nurse slowly inflates the balloon as the pressures are read aloud. The balloon should be inflated to the insufflation pressure recommended by the manufacturer (usually 12 atm) and held there for 3 min. If the cystic duct begins to tear, stop the inflation and wait for a minute before attempting further inflation. With patience most cystic ducts can be dilated to 7 mm, but they should never be dilated larger than the inner diameter of the CBD. When exploring a small CBD, care must be taken to choose the proper diameter dilating balloon based on the intraoperative cholangiogram.

The cystic duct must be dilated to the size of the largest CBD stone so that the stone entrapped in the wire basket does not become impacted on removal. Stones larger than 1 cm must usually be fragmented with a dye pulse laser or electrohydraulic lithotripsy or be removed via choledochotomy, which is our usual approach. After the cystic duct is dilated, the balloon catheter is deflated and withdrawn.

The endoscope can be inserted over a guide wire if it is 150 cm long, or the endoscope can be inserted freehand or gently guided with an atraumatic grasping instrument (Fig. 5). The working channel of some endoscopes is eccentric to their cross-section, making insertion over the guide wire difficult.

The endoscope should have bi-directional deflection and a working channel of at least 1.2 mm. An outer diameter of 2.7–3.2 mm is ideal. Smaller scopes compromise the working channel, and larger scopes are more difficult to pass. A camera should be attached to the endoscope, and the image should be projected on a monitor with an A-V mixer (picture in picture), or it should be projected on its own monitor. It is best and most convenient to set up a mobile cart with a monitor, light source, camera box, video recorder, endoscope, wire baskets, balloon dilating catheters, and other instruments needed for a laparoscopic CBD exploration. This cart can function as an emergency laparoscopic cart and/or a backup cart for other laparoscopic procedures. Having all the required instruments in one place decreases the frustration and delays when common duct calculi are encountered.

Once the endoscope is in the cystic duct, irrigation with warm saline should be initiated. Attention must be paid to the temperature of the irrigant, as hypothermia can occur from instillation of cold fluid. The operating surgeon manipulates the scope, inserting and torquing with the left hand while deflecting the end of the scope with the right hand on the deflecting lever.

Once a stone is seen, irrigation is turned off or decreased. Always entrap the stone closest to the scope, and do not bypass any, as they may be irrigated up into the liver. A straight four-wire basket (2.4 F) is preferable. The closed basket should be advanced beyond the stone, opened, and then pulled back to entrap it (Fig. 5). The basket should be closed gently, and the basket and stone should be pulled up lightly against the end of the endoscope so that they can be withdrawn in unison (Fig. 6). This process is repeated until all the stones are removed. A completion cholangiogram is essential. At this point a decision regarding cystic duct tube drainage must be made. Elderly or immunosuppressed patients with cholangitis should have a latex (not silicone) tube placed for postoperative decompression of their biliary system. In patients who are likely to be harboring a retained stone, one should be placed for postoperative cholangiography and, if necessary, percutaneous tube tract stone extraction. If the preexploration intraoperative cholangiogram shows a different number of common duct stones than that found on endoscopy, a tube should be placed. The cystic duct stump must be closed with endoloops as clips may slip off the thinned duct.

Fluoroscopic Wire Basket Stone Retrieval. Fluoroscopic wire basket stone retrieval is feasible if fluoroscopy is available. Special spiral wire baskets with flexible leaders must be used to avoid injuring the CBD.

The basket is placed into the common duct via the cystic duct. It is advanced with fluoroscopic guidance into the distal common duct and opened. Hypaque 25% is injected through the wire basket. It is then pulled back until the stone is captured. The advantage of not having to dilate the cystic duct is offset by the problem of extracting the wire basket with the captured stone through the nondilated cystic duct. In our experience, this technique is not as successful as other transcystic duct techniques, and it can lead to an impacted basket and stone that requires choledochotomy for its removal. Nevertheless, it can be an easy and successful technique in selected patients – those with relatively few common duct calculi whose size is close to the inner diameter of the cystic duct.

Biliary Balloon Catheter Stone Retrieval. Especially in cases with a dilated cystic duct, biliary balloon catheter stone retrieval is occasionally helpful. A biliary balloon catheter can be passed blindly or under fluoroscopic control via the cystic duct into the distal common duct or the duodenum. The balloon is inflated gently, and the catheter is then withdrawn, modulating the pressure on the balloon. This is often successful via choledochotomy but has the potential to pull the stone into the common hepatic duct out of reach of an endoscope when used via the cystic duct.

References

Arregui ME, Davis CJ, Arkush AM, Nagan RF (1992) Laparoscopic cholecystectomy combined with endoscopic sphincterotomy and stone extraction or laparoscopic choledochoscopy and electrohydraulic lithotripsy for management of cholelithiasis with choledocholithiasis. Surg Endosc 6:10–15

Cotton PB, Vennes J, Geenen JE et al (1991) Endoscopic sphincterotomy complications and their management: an attempt at consensus. Gastrointest Endosc 37 (3):383–386

Neoptolemos JP, Carr-Locke DI, Fossard DP (1987) Prospective randomized study of preoperative endoscopic sphincterotomy versus surgery alone for common bile duct stones. BMJ 294:470–474

Phillips EH, Carroll BJ, Pearlstein AR et al (1993) Laparoscopic choledochoscopy and extraction of common bile duct stones. World J Surg 17:22–28

Phillips EH, Rosenthal RJ, Carroll BJ, Fallas MJ (1994) Laparoscopic transcystic duct common bile duct exploration. Surg Endosc 8:1389–1394

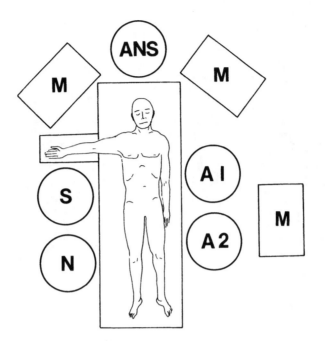

Fig. 1. Positioning of the patient and team. Patient in supine position. *ANS*, Anesthetist; *S*, surgeon; *A1, A2*, assistants; *N*, nurse; *M*, monitor

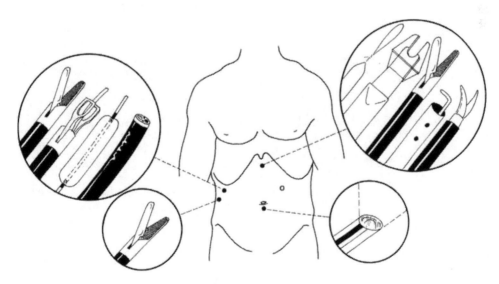

Fig. 2. Trocar sites and instrumentation

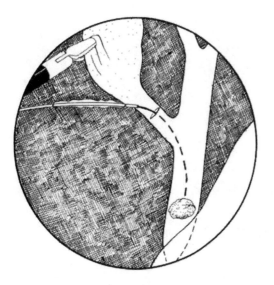

Fig. 3. Positioning of guide wire in preparation of advancing balloon dilating catheter for cystic duct dilation

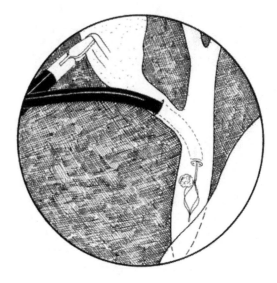

Fig. 5. Advancing wire basket through choledochoscope for stone entrapment

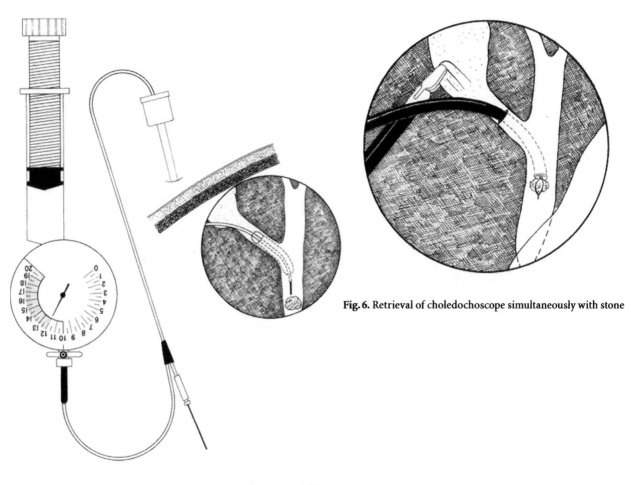

Fig. 6. Retrieval of choledochoscope simultaneously with stone

Fig. 4. Balloon catheter attached to LeVeen syringe during dilation of cystic duct

10 Laparoscopic Transcystic Ampullary Balloon Dilation

E.H. PHILLIPS

Introduction

In an effort to enhance our ability to lavage small stones and debris from the common bile duct (CBD) and to rid the CBD of small stones when an endoscope cannot be inserted into a small fragile cystic duct, we applied the technique of balloon dilation of the sphincter of Oddi (LTBDS) via the cystic duct. Although our series is small, initial results indicate that LTBDS is a useful adjunct to laparoscopic CBD exploration techniques. However, it should be used when the only alternative to LTBDS is endoscopic sphincterotomy.

Positioning of the Patient and Team

The patient is placed on the operating table in supine position. The operating team is positioned in the same way as for a laparoscopic cholecystectomy (Fig. 1).

Technique

When CBD duct stones are discovered at fluorocholangiography during laparoscopic cholecystectomy, our first choice is to approach them with a flexible endoscope via the cystic duct. In those patients with stones and/or debris less than 4 mm in diameter that cannot be extracted by endoscopic wire basket or lavage, LTBDS can be performed. This is especially useful in a patient with a small fragile cystic duct.

A 6-mm-diameter balloon dilating catheter, no. 5 phantom (Microvasive, Watertown, MA) is inserted via the right subcostal trocar (Fig. 2) over a floppy-tipped 0.035-inch hydrophilic guide wire (Guidewire; Microvasive). The wire is advanced through the incision in the cystic duct. The wire is gently passed into the CBD and then the duodenum, under fluoroscopic control. The balloon catheter is advanced over the guide wire through the cystic duct into the CBD and passed through the sphincter of Oddi. Radiopaque markers on the balloon catheter identify its position spanning the sphincter (Fig. 2).

Care is taken to avoid repeated in-and-out manipulations through the sphincter. Using a LeVeen syringe, the balloon is dilated slowly under fluoroscopic view with 50% Hypaque only to the diameter of the largest stone in the CBD, and never larger than the inner diameter of the CBD (Fig. 3). After 3 min (using a pressure not greater than 12 atm) the balloon is deflated. Forceful irrigation through the cystic duct is then performed with warm saline solution (Fig. 4), and completion cholangiography is obtained. The cystic duct is then ligated with an endoloop, and a drain is placed in Morison's pouch. Placement of a cystic duct tube should be considered in cases in which percutaneous access or follow-up cholangiography might be required.

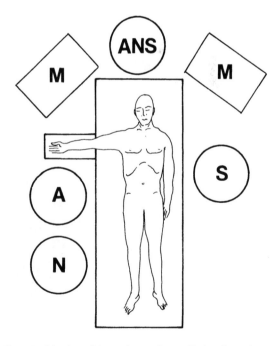

Fig. 1. Positioning of the patient and team. Patient in supine position. *ANS*, Anesthetist; *S*, surgeon; *A*, assistant; *N*, nurse; *M*, monitor

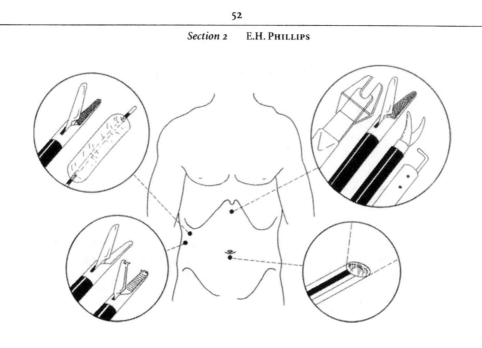

Fig. 2. Trocar sites and instrumentation

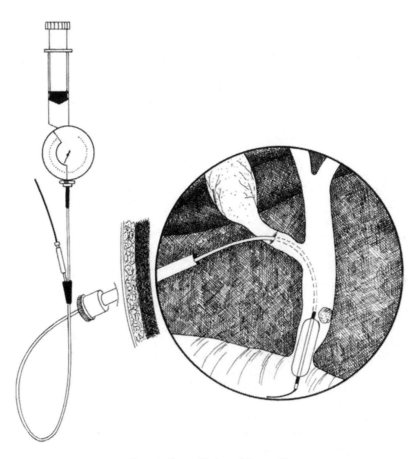

Fig. 3. Balloon dilation of the papilla

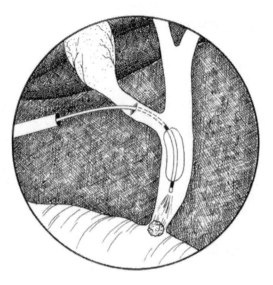

Fig. 4. Flushing of the CBD

Comments

Any manipulations of the papilla of Vater can produce hyperamylasemia and/or clinical pancreatitis. In our experience, 17 of 20 patients (85%) had successful LTBDS with clearance of stones from the CBD. Hyperamylasemia occurred in 15% of cases, and clinical mild pancreatitis occurred in three patients. Though LTBDS appears to have a lower rate of clinical pancreatitis than endoscopic retrograde methods of sphincter dilation, surgeons should take this risk into consideration when employing this technique.

References

Carroll BJ, Phillips EH, Chandra M, Fallas MJ (1993) Laparoscopic transcystic duct balloon dilatation of the sphincter of Oddi. Surg Endosc 7:514–517

Foutch R, Sivik M (1985) Therapeutic endoscopic balloon dilation of the extrahepatic biliary ducts. Am J Gastroenterol 80 (7):575–579

Kozarek R (1988) Balloon dilation of the sphincter Oddi. Endoscopy 8 (3):387–394

Staritz M, Ewe K, Meyer K (1983) Endoscopic papillary dilation for the treatment of common bile duct stones and papillary stenosis. Endoscopy 15:197–198

Vernava A, Andrus C, Herrman V, Kaminski D (1987) Pancreatitis after biliary tract surgery. Arch Surg 122:575–580

11 Laparoscopic Antegrade Transcystic Sphincterotomy

K.A. ZUCKER and M.J. CURET

Introduction

The management of common bile duct (CBD) stones in the era of laparoscopic surgery, especially in individuals with complex choledocholithiasis, often presents a challenge. Currently employed techniques of laparoscopic guided transcystic common bile duct exploration or even direct attempts via a choledochostomy may be unsuccessful in patients with multiple extra- and intrahepatic calculi, or if one or more stones are impacted at the ampulla. In these circumstances surgeons have often felt compelled to convert to an open laparotomy or depend on the success of postoperative endoscopic retrograde cholangiography and sphincterotomy.

In an attempt to extend the benefits of minimally invasive surgery to individuals with complex biliary tract disease, an innovative physician from Brazil, A.L. De Paula, has described a technique which combines the modalities of laparoscopic common bile duct exploration and endoscopic sphincterotomy.

For antegrade sphincterotomy additional equipment includes a side-viewing duodenoscope, a desired selection of endoscopic sphincterotomes, an appropriately sized guide wire, and a cautery cable compatible with the sphincterotome. This equipment is rarely kept in the operating room, and we therefore arrange for a portable endoscopy cart to be kept available in the gastrointestinal suite which contains the above equipment.

Indications for performing laparoscopic antegrade sphincterotomy vary from surgeon to surgeon. De Paula recommends this procedure in any patient with multiple bile duct stones, a greatly enlarged CBD (e.g., >20 mm), ampullary dyskinesia, or any evidence of impaired bile duct emptying. In our institution we perform antegrade sphincterotomy only in those patients with complex choledocholithiasis in whom we have failed to clear the bile ducts using fluoroscopic or choledochoscopic (transcystic or via a separate choledochostomy) means of CBD exploration. In the last 400 patients undergoing laparoscopic biliary tract surgery at the University of New Mexico Medical Center we have performed antegrade sphincterotomy in only 13 (3%).

Positioning of the Patient and Team

The patient is place in supine position (Fig. 1).

Technique

Antegrade sphincterotomy is usually performed after an attempt has been made at laparoscopic CBD exploration. When attempting laparoscopic CBD exploration we usually insert a fifth cannula (5.0 mm) high in the right upper quadrant to facilitate passage of the catheters, choledochoscope, etc. (Fig. 2). The transcystic approach is our preferred means of exploring the ducts, although if necessary we make a separate opening along the anterior aspect of the CBD. Either method of accessing the CBD, however, can also be used for introducing the devices required for performing antegrade sphincterotomy.

The first step attempts to pass the sphincterotome directly into the distal CBD and across the ampulla. Several different types of endoscopic sphincterotomes are commercially available; however, we have found that a 30-mm short-nose sphincterotome (Microvasive, Watertown, MA) works in nearly every case. De Paula prefers a Classen-Demling type sphincterotome designed originally for intubating the ampulla following a Billroth II gastrectomy.

The sphincterotome is introduced through the right upper quadrant (the fifth) port using a suture introducer to minimize CO_2 leakage (Fig. 3). A grasping forceps is inserted through the subxiphoid sheath and then used to guide the sphincterotome into the lumen of the cystic duct or through the anterior choledochostomy. While the sphincterotome is being maneuvered into the biliary tree, a second member of the team passes a side-viewing duodenoscope through the mouth and into the esophagus (a video endoscope is preferred so that the surgeon manipulating the sphincterotome can also see the view afforded by the duodenoscope). Any nasogastric or orogastric tubes, esophageal stethoscopes, or temperature probes must be first removed and care taken to avoid dislodging the endotracheal tube while inserting this large flexible endoscope.

Occasionally it is necessary to elevate the jaw of the patient with one hand while introducing the duodenoscope. This maneuver opens the pharynx allowing the endoscope easier passage into the esophagus. The scope is then guided into the stomach, through the pylorus, and into the duodenum. At this point glucagon should be administered (0.5–1.0 mg IV) to minimize duodenal peristalsis. The duodenoscope is then positioned directly across from the ampulla (Fig. 4). Often it is difficult to distend the duodenum with air (via the insufflation channel of the scope) because the muscle relaxation of the general anesthetic encourages free reflux of air back into the stomach and out the esophagus. To counter this we have found gentle compression of the neck to seal the proximal esophagus around the duodenoscope helpful.

As the sphincterotome passes through the ampulla its movement should be readily visible by the endoscopist. The surgeon then withdraws and manipulates the sphincterotome (usually by twisting it) until the cutting wire is bowed at the 12 o'clock position (Fig. 5). A blend of cutting and coagulation current is applied until the sphincter and overlying mucosa are divided up to the first transverse fold of the duodenum. A gush of bile and/or stones usually signifies a successful sphincterotomy. The sphincterotome is then removed and a red rubber catheter guided into the CBD. The ducts are then flushed copiously with saline to wash out any remaining stones or debris. If desired, the choledochoscope can be reinserted to explore the ducts, and on occasion we have used this device to flush the duct (by irrigating through the working channel) and even push stones out through the widened ampulla.

If one or more stones are impacted in the distal CBD or ampulla, it may prove difficult to pass the sphincterotome antegrade into the duodenum. In these cases we advance the choledochoscope as far distal as possible and then maneuver a much smaller guide wire through the working channel and across the ampulla (Fig. 6). The choledochoscope is then removed and the sphincterotome passed over the guide wire and into the duodenum. The guide wire is pulled back and the sphincterotome bowed to expose the cutting wire which is maneuvered into position as described earlier.

If sphincterotomy is successful, we do not routinely insert a T-tube for postoperative biliary decompression. Bile should flow very easily across the widened ampulla even if there has been extensive instrumentation of the biliary tree. Often a small amount of bleeding is observed from the site of sphincterotomy. In most cases this bleeding stops spontaneously, but on occasion the endoscopist must inject epinephrine or coagulate smaller vessels.

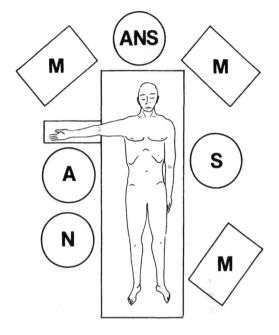

Fig. 1. Positioning of the patient and team. Patient in supine position. *ANS*, Anesthetist; *S*, surgeon; *A*, assistant; *N*, nurse; *M*, monitor

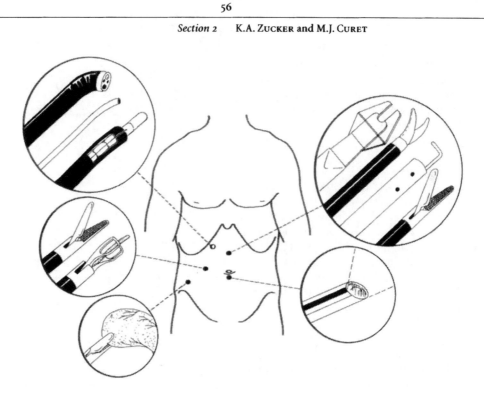

Fig. 2. Trocar sites and instrumentation. A fifth cannula
(5.0 mm) may be placed in the right upper quadrant to facilitate introduction of the choledochoscope, sphincterotome, etc.

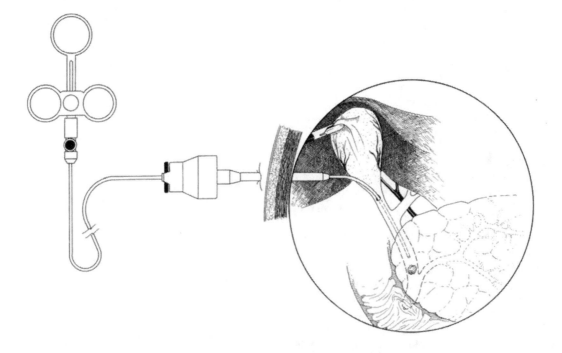

Fig. 3. A standard endoscopic sphincterotome is inserted
through the right upper quadrant 5.0-mm cannula using a suture introducer to minimize gas leakage

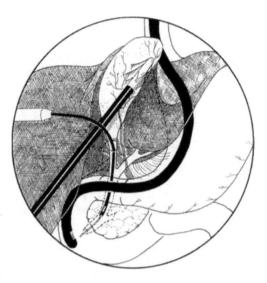

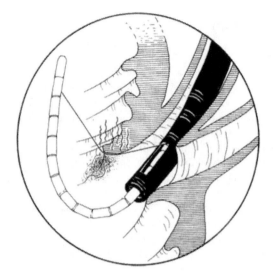

Fig. 4. The side-viewing duodenoscope is positioned directly opposite the ampulla so that the sphincterotome may be guided into proper position under direct vision

Fig. 5. The sphincterotome is bowed, which exposes the cutting wire, and maneuvered until it is at the 12 o'clock position

a
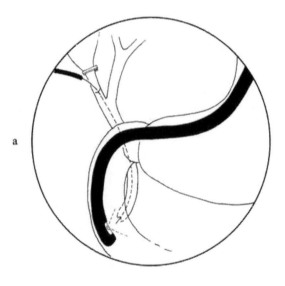

b
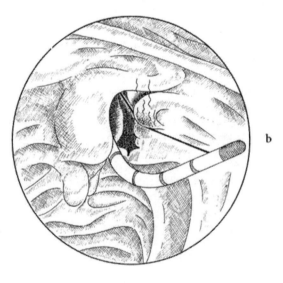

Fig. 6. a A guide wire may be used to facilitate passage of the sphincterotome across the ampulla. **b** A blend of coagulation and cutting current is used to divide the sphincter up to the first transverse fold of the duodenum

Comments

Laparoscopic antegrade sphincterotomy has a number of advantages over conventional methods of endoscopic sphincterotomy. First, the sphincterotome is passed antegrade rather than retrograde so that the device passes quickly through the bile ducts and across the ampulla. De Paula reported a mean time of 17 min to perform this procedure, and in our series we were able to complete antegrade sphincterotomy in just over 25 min (excluding the time spent at attempted CBD exploration). Inadvertent cannulation of the pancreatic duct is also eliminated, and other complications associated with endoscopic retrograde cholangiography such as the creation of false passages, perforation of the bile duct or duodenum and the so-called "trapped basket or sphincterotome" should be dramatically reduced.

Another important aspect is patient expectation. Individuals prefer complete management of all of their biliary tract problems at one setting (preferably with laparoscopic surgery) rather than multiple procedures before or after cholecystectomy. Antegrade sphincterotomy is, however, associated with a number of disadvantages as well. Operative and anesthesia time is prolonged, although with experience this should be less than 25 min, as mentioned above. Surgeons who are already skilled at laparoscopic CBD exploration become adept at this technique very quickly. Antegrade sphincterotomy does require additional equipment, in what is often already a crowded operating room, and an experienced individual is required to operate the endoscope. In our institution many of the surgeons are experienced endoscopists and are qualified to perform endoscopic retrograde cholangiography and sphincterotomy but in most institutions a gastroenterologist is required for this function. Despite some disadvantages we believe that laparoscopic antegrade sphincterotomy will have an increasingly important role in the surgical management of complex choledocholithiasis.

References

Zucker KA (1993) Laparoscopic cholangiography and management of choledocholithiasis. In: Zucker KA, Bailey RW, Reddick EJ (eds) Surgical laparoscopy – update. Quality Medical, St. Louis, pp 145–193

Flowers JL, Zucker KA, Graham SM, Scovill WA, Imbembo AL, Bailey RW (1992) Laparoscopic cholangiography: results and indications. Ann Surg 215 (3):209–216

De Paula AL, Hashiba K, Bafutto M, Zago R, Machado MM (1993) Laparoscopic antegrade sphincterotomy. Surg Laparosc Endosc 3 (3):157–160

Curet MJ, Martin DE, Pitcher DT, Zucker KA (1995) Laparoscopic antegrade sphincterotomy for complex choledocholithiasis. Ann Surg 221(2):149–155

Graham SM, Flowers JL, Bailey RW, Zucker KA, Imbembo AL (1992) Utility of planned perioperative endoscopic retrograde cholangiopancreatography and sphincterotomy in the era of laparoscopic cholecystectomy. Endoscopy 24:788–789

Phillips EH (1994) Laparoscopic approaches to the common bile duct. In: Greene F, Ponsky J (eds) Endoscopic surgery. Saunders, Philadelphia, pp 327–344

12 Laparoscopic Choledochotomy

M.E. FRANKLIN

Introduction

For many years calculus disease of the common duct has been the purview of the general surgeon. Only in recent years, with the advent of laparoscopic surgery and the advances in ERCP, has this disease process been approached by the gastroenterologist as a primary procedure. The reasons for this are multiple: the reluctance of the general surgeon to approach this disease laparoscopically, a lack of equipment, a lack of skills to perform the surgery, a feeling by most general surgeons that this is no longer their territory or is required of them. It is the feeling of the author that choledocholithiasis and indeed many diseases of the common bile duct should be approached by the general surgeon and treated with a single procedure rather than subjecting the patient to multiple procedures. Additionally, cholangiography is an integral part of laparoscopic cholecystectomy – not only to identify unsuspected common bile duct stones but also to identify the anatomy and aid in avoiding or at least identifying common bile duct injuries.

The methods for common bile duct exploration once a diagnosis of common bile duct stones has been made are varied, and the present discussion does not dwell upon the pluses and minuses of the transcystic approach versus the choledochotomy approach but rather describes the technique which has been improved for more than 100 years and is now applied to laparoscopic cholecystectomy, e.g., a choledochotomy approach to the common bile duct.

Contraindications for common bile duct exploration performed via choledochotomy at the time of laparoscopy are primarily those related to the size of the common bile duct and skill of the individual surgeon. We have used 6 mm as the lower limits of the duct size for an approach via choledochotomy. Patients with extremely small stones and extremely small ducts are those in whom a transcystic duct approach or a postoperative endoscopic sphincterotomy is perhaps the best approach.

Positioning of the Patient and Team

Patient positioning is essentially the same as that for laparoscopic cholecystectomy (Fig. 1). The patient should be securely strapped to the operative table to allow for safe positioning in multiple directions (e.g., severe Trendelenburg and reverse Trendelenburg as well as right and left tilt).

An operating table which allows fluoroscopy is extremely advantageous in laparoscopic cholecystectomy, not only for intraoperative cholangiography but also for intraoperative manipulation of the choledochoscope and direct visualization of stones should a choledochoscope not be available. It allows for fluoroscopic wire basket extraction of common duct calculi in selected cases.

A third monitor is helpful unless one has a light and image switching system or an electronic system which allows the picture to be placed on either monitor. It is the opinion of the author that a monitor needs to be available not only for the choledochoscope but also for view of the abdominal cavity in order to direct equipment into the common bile duct after the choledochotomy is made.

Technique

The equipment needed for laparoscopic choledochotomy is essentially the same as that for a laparoscopic cholecystectomy with the exception that special allowance must be made for a choledochoscope. Many common bile duct explorations, particularly for solitary large stones, can be performed without a choledochoscope if milking of the common bile duct stone into the choledochotomy can be performed. However, this technique cannot be relied upon accurately to locate and/or remove all stones on a consistent basis. Therefore we recommend use of a 10.5-F (3.3-mm) choledochoscope which can be flexed in two directions with greater than 30° flexing capability and a 1.2 mm working channel. Special equipment for a choledochotomy is really not necessary. A laparoscopic knife and/or microscissors should be readily available in all biliary laparoscopic sets.

The anesthesiologist should be alerted that the procedure may take somewhat longer, and that the patient's temperature may drop. Attempts must be made to warm all irrigating fluids as well as to carefully monitor not only end expired CO_2 levels but also the patient's temperature to prevent complications of these two problems.

Cannula positioning is virtually the same as that for a standard laparoscopic cholecystectomy, and it is the rare patient who requires an additional cannula (Fig. 2). If so, the additional cannulae should be placed in the left upper quadrant in the midclavicular line, midway between the umbilicus and xiphoid for retraction of a large duodenum or prominent retroperitoneum.

Laparoscopic choledochotomy should not be performed without first performing an intraoperative cholangiogram.

After completion of the cholangiogram and ascertaining the exact location and number of common bile duct stones a choledochotomy can be made at the point most desirable for extraction of the stones. The choledochotomy is placed in the anterior aspect of the common bile duct preferably below the junction of the cystic duct into the common bile duct. This seems to allow the greatest maneuverability and has in our experience not compromised the lumen of the duct when the choledochotomy is closed.

As the dissection is carried out to expose the common bile duct, it is important to look for the inevitable vein or artery that crosses the common bile duct and avoid injury to these structures if at all possible. If there is doubt as to the location of the common bile duct, meticulous dissection following the cystic duct down to the common bile duct is indicated. If the common bile duct still cannot be found, or if the patient has had a previous cholecystectomy, needle aspiration can indeed be performed with an intraperitoneally placed needle. Intraoperative ultrasound is an additional method which can be exceptionally helpful in identifying the duct and locating stones. After location of the common bile duct a vertical choledochotomy should be made. If a bypass is anticipated, the choledochotomy should be as low as possible, preferably near the duodenum. If a choledochojejunostomy is the surgeon's choice of bypass procedure, the choledochotomy can obviously be made almost anywhere along the anterior surface of the common bile duct. It must be emphasized that the gallbladder should be left intact during the common bile duct exploration, as this is the primary method of upward traction upon the common bile duct. If the gallbladder is absent, the edge of the common bile duct and the adventitial layer can act as a traction site as well with placement of stay sutures in the common duct. We do not, however, routinely use stay sutures as we have found them to be unnecessary and time consuming.

The length of the choledochotomy should be just greater than the diameter of the largest stone. However, we prefer initially to make a very small incision (approximately 3.5–4 mm in length) to afford a tight fit around the choledochoscope as this prevents undue loss of irrigation fluid during the procedure and allows better distention of the common bile duct. A larger choledochotomy can always be made at any time to accommodate the removal of a larger stone.

Prior to the introduction of the choledochoscope via the subxyphoid trocar it is advisable to have all accessories available and checked. The irrigation fluid should be attached to the working channel of the scope prior to introduction of the choledochoscope to ensure a more expeditious exploration of the common bile duct. Great care should be taken upon introduction of the choledochoscope through an access cannula. We strongly recommend using a pretied loop passer or other shield to protect the choledochoscope during its ingress and egress through the trocar. Immediately after entering the abdominal cavity the choledochoscope should be visualized. Upon entering the abdominal cavity the choledochoscope should be oriented so that flexion is in a vertical manner, as this expedites the passage through the choledochotomy (Fig. 3). The common bile duct should be entered at a right angle and the scope turned after entering the common bile duct. Explore the proximal common bile duct initially. It must be remembered that many times this segment of the duct is extremely short. After checking the right and left hepatic ducts the scope is slowly withdrawn to the choledochotomy site and flexed in the opposite direction for distal common bile duct visualization. The vast majority of stones are in the distal common bile duct; however, it is an error to assume that stones are only in this location despite their localization here on the cholangiogram. Stones in the distal bile duct may float into the common hepatic duct during manipulation.

Stones which are very near the choledochotomy may result in extreme frustration as an inadequate amount of scope can be introduced to expeditiously place a basket around a given stone. These stones should be milked to the choledochotomy and plucked from the common bile duct with a grasper. After removal of several of the most proximal stones the choledochoscope can be reintroduced and the basket used to capture the remaining stones. The sphincter should be visualized with the choledochoscope after all stones have been removed, and in the case of a prior sphincterotomy and/or a very large sphincter opening the choledochoscope frequently falls into the duodenum. The stones do not need to be removed individually from the abdominal cavity at the time of the common bile duct exploration but perhaps placed in a sterile bag, such as a condom or a commercially available bag, for subsequent removal as a group.

After clearing all stones and debris in the distal common bile duct, the proximal duct should be viewed again, and a second cholangiogram should then be taken through the choledochoscope or a T-tube. This can be facilitated quite easily through the working port of the scope with the use of the C-arm and ascertains the clearance of the common bile duct prior to withdrawal of the choledochoscope. Care must be taken to remove the choledochoscope through the protective shield in order to avoid "instrument" injury from trocar valves.

After removal of the choledochoscope, preparations are made for T-tube placement. We frequently use an 8- or 10-F T-tube which has been tailored with a long and short end. The entire T-tube is brought into the abdominal cavity, and the long tail is allowed to extend over the top of the liver. The long end of the cut T-tube is introduced into the distal aspect of the common bile duct and the short end into the proximal end. After the T-tube is well situated in the common bile duct, the T-tube is pushed cephalad to lessen the chances of inadvertent dislodgement of the tube during the suturing process (Fig. 4). We uniformly use interrupted sutures not only with open but with laparoscopic common bile duct exploration and currently favor use of an absorbable suture such as Vicryl or Polysorb. An RB 1 needle seems to be quite appropriate, and we prefer to straighten this needle to some extent for the placement of the initial suture. A pretied loop is very advantageous (Fig. 5a) for the first suture, which is placed immediately below the neck of the T-tube as the T-tube is being pushed cephalad. This results in trapping the T-tube and lessening the chance of subsequent dislodgement. The sequence for suture placement after T-tube insertion is outlined in Fig. 5 b–d.

Care must be taken to ensure as close to a watertight seal as is possible without causing ischemia to the segment of the duct. It is better to have a small leak than to have an ischemic duct, and thus we have avoided using running sutures except in the instance of an extremely long choledochotomy. We routinely take a cholangiogram after T-tube insertion by exteriorizing the long limb of the T-tube through the subcostal port and obtaining a final cholangiogram (Fig. 4). The T-tube is then brought back into the abdominal cavity again, placed on top of the liver, and the cholecystectomy is completed. After complete hemostasis is achieved, the choledochotomy site is reinspected, the cystic duct is reinspected to assure a lack of leaks, and a 10-mm closed suction drain is placed and brought out through the lateral umbilical port after the gallbladder has been placed in an extraction bag. The T-tube is brought out through the subcostal port and all 10-mm trocar sites are closed with through-and-through 0 Vicryl/Polysorb suture.

References

Arregui ME, Davis CJ, Arkush AM, Nagan RF (1992) Laparoscopic cholecystectomy combined with endoscopic sphincterotomy and stone extraction or laparoscopic choledochoscopy and electrohydraulic lithotripsy for management of cholelithiasis with choledocholithiasis. Surg Endosc 6:10–14

Berci G, Morgenstern L (1994) Laparoscopic management of common bile duct stones. A multi-institutional SAGES study. Surg Endosc 8:1168–1175

Carroll BJ, Fallas MJ, Phillips EH (1994) Laparoscopic transcystic choledochoscopy. Surg Endosc 8:310–314

Franklin ME, Pharond D, Rosenthal D (1994) Laparoscopic common bile duct exploration. Surgical laparoscopy and endoscopy 4(2):119–124

McSherry CK (1994) Laparoscopic management of common bile duct stones. Surg Endosc 8:1161–1162

Phillips EH, Rosenthal RJ, Carroll BJ, Fallas MJ (1994) Laparoscopic transcystic common bile duct exploration. Surg Endosc 8:1389–1394

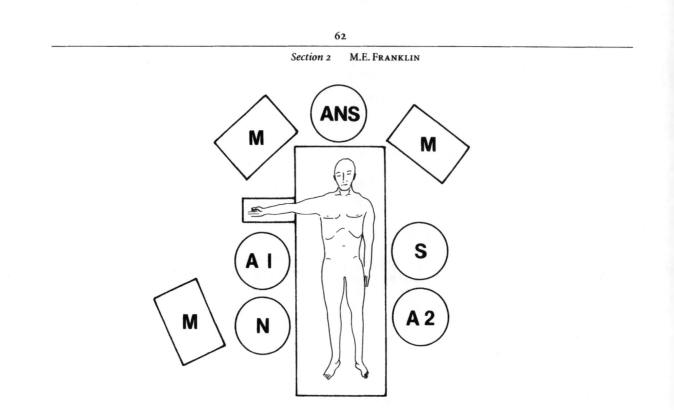

Fig. 1. Positioning of the patient and team. Patient in supine position. *ANS,* Anesthetist; *S,* surgeon; *A1, A2,* assistants; *N,* nurse; *M,* monitor

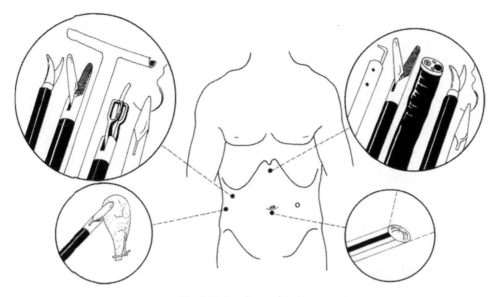

Fig. 2. Trocar sites and instrumentation

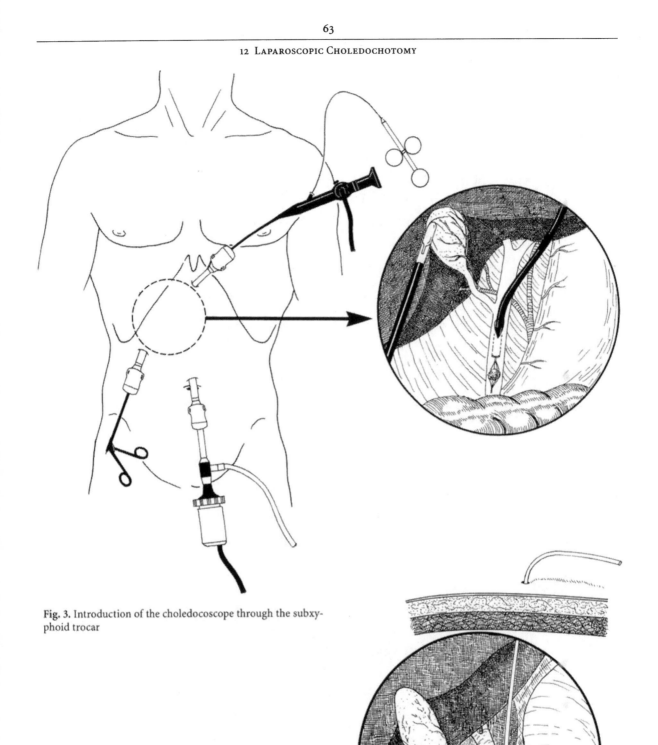

Fig. 3. Introduction of the choledocoscope through the subxyphoid trocar

Fig. 4. A T-drain is placed into the choledochotomy after stone removal and brought out through a subcostal trocar site

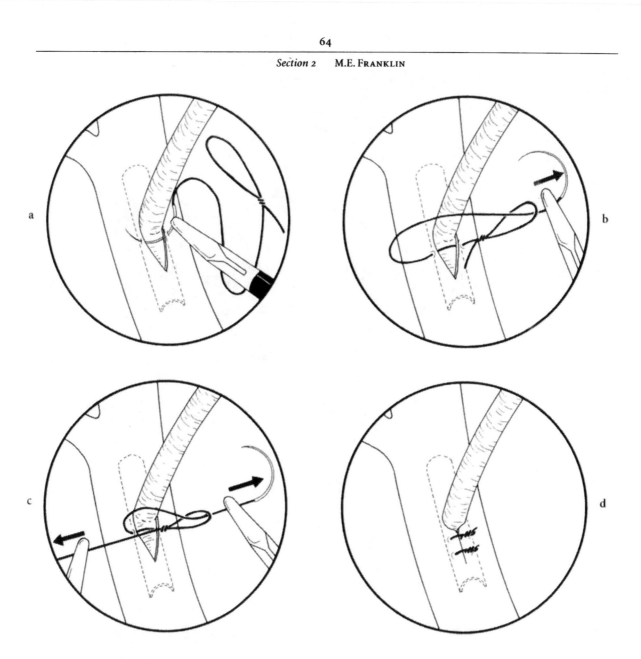

Fig. 5 a–d. The T-tube is sutured in place

13 Avoiding and Classifying Common Bile Duct Injuries During Laparoscopic Cholecystectomy

N.J. Soper and S.M. Strasberg

Introduction

Injuries to the bile duct are a serious problem and are potentially life threatening. They can cause major morbidity, prolong hospitalization, increase cost, and lead to litigation. Compared with open cholecystectomy, the incidence of injuries to the bile duct seems to be increased in laparoscopic cholecystectomy (LC). However, ductal injuries are highest during the learning curve.

During open cholecystectomy the risk of bile duct injury is low, with an incidence of approximately 0.125%. In an exhaustive review of common bile duct injuries occurring during LC we reported the risk of bile duct injury with LC to be some three to four times greater than with open cholecystectomy, although it is difficult to arrive at a precise figure, and the injuries associated with LC occur early in the surgeon's experience. However, as the overall risk is still less than 1%, bile duct injury remains infrequent in each individual surgeon's practice. This demonstrates the vigilance required in every LC over prolonged periods of surgical practice to reduce the injury rate to acceptable levels.

The most widely used system to classify bile duct injuries during open cholecystectomy is the Bismuth classification of major injuries to the bile duct. This classification is based primarily on the length of remaining bile duct and does not include bile leaks from the cystic duct stump or the liver bed; it also neglects lateral injuries to the bile duct and isolated occlusion of the right hepatic duct. These injuries have all been reported following LC, and we have therefore proposed a new classification for bile duct injury during LC.

Classification of Bile Duct Injuries During Laparoscopic Cholecystectomy

Type A Injury: *Bile Leak from a Minor Duct Still in Continuity with the Common Bile Duct.* In most cases the leaks occur from the cystic duct or from the liver bed. The two injuries are combined because their presentation and management are almost identical. They may be thought of as lateral injuries to the biliary tract in which biliary communication between hepatic parenchyma

and the major bile ducts and duodenum remains intact (Fig. 1).

Type B Injury: *Occlusion of Part of Biliary Tree.* This injury is almost always the result of an injury to an aberrant right hepatic duct (Fig. 1). In about 2% of patients the cystic duct enters the right hepatic duct rather than the common bile duct – common hepatic duct junction. The right duct then joins the main ductal system. Such an aberrant duct has a similar appearance to a cystic duct at the point where it joins the main duct and is in danger of being mistaken for the cystic duct or cystic artery and divided.

Type C Injury: *Bile Leak from Duct Not in Communication with the Common Bile Duct.* This injury is almost always the result of transection of an aberrant right hepatic duct with drainage of bile into the peritoneal cavity. Usually it is thought to be an artery. It is clipped near the common hepatic duct and cut off flush with the liver bed. Both type B and type C injuries, as opposed to type A injuries, result in disconnection of a part of the hepatic parenchyma from the main biliary tree. Type C injuries are usually diagnosed in the early postoperative period due to bile accumulation with a biloma (Fig. 1).

Type D Injury: *Lateral Injury to Extrahepatic Bile Ducts.* As with type A injuries, all hepatic parenchyma remains in communication with the distal end of the biliary tree and duodenum (Fig. 1). The separate classification is justified because the consequences of type D injuries are potentially greater than type A injuries. Type D injuries often require repair and may result in stenosis of the bile duct.

Type E Injury: *Circumferential Injury of Major Bile Ducts (Bismuth Classes I–V).* These injuries involve circumferential injury of one or more main bile ducts as described by Bismuth and illustrated in Fig. 1. Subclassification in the first four Bismuth classes relates to the upper level of injury, while class V is a combined injury to the common hepatic duct and an aberrant right duct. Type E injuries cause "separation" of hepatic parenchyma from the lower ducts and duodenum. This separation is usually the result of resection or ablation with cautery. This is the most serious type of bile duct injury and is associated with the greatest morbidity and mortality.

Risk Factors for Biliary Injury

Training and Experience. An early case series of over 1500 LCs suggested that the high rate of ductal injury (0.5%) is mainly a result of the "learning curve" effect. In that study most injuries occurred within the first 13 procedures performed by a surgeon. It is too early to determine whether the biliary injury rate subsides to acceptable levels once the learning period has passed, but it seems wise to take all measures to eradicate the problem.

Local Operative Risk Factors. As laparoscopic operations depend upon the transmitted video image with little tactile feedback to the surgeon, anything interfering with clear visualization may increase the risk of bile duct injuries. These include acute inflammation, chronic inflammation with dense scarring, operative bleeding obscuring the field, and fat in the portal area.

Aberrant Anatomy. Aberrant anatomy is a common and well-recognized danger in biliary operations. The biliary anomaly most likely to be involved in ductal injury is variants of the right hepatic duct, previously referred to in type B and C injuries.

Exposure of the Operative Field. It is also likely that use of the gallbladder itself to give cephalad retraction to the liver and expose the porta hepatis may align the cystic duct with the common bile duct, leading to the illusion that the common bile duct is the cystic duct.

Direct Causes of Laparoscopic Biliary Injuries

The immediate causes of biliary injuries may be classified as either misidentification of an anatomic structure or technical. Misidentification of the bile duct as the cystic duct results in type D or E injuries. Misidentification may also occur when there is an aberrant right duct, leading to type B and C injuries. The exact events that occur after misidentification of the common duct are variable. At least one clip is placed on the common duct, in the belief that it is being placed on the distal end of the cystic duct. The clip that the surgeon believes is being applied to the proximal end of the cystic duct may also be placed on the misidentified common duct or on

the cystic duct. In a common scenario described by Davidoff and coworkers as the "classical" injury, the common duct is mistaken to be the cystic duct, receives all three clips (one proximal and two distal), and is divided (Fig. 2). Then, to excise the gallbladder, the common hepatic duct must be divided. This is often associated with injury to the right hepatic artery. The common hepatic duct may be either clipped or divided, which results in complete obstruction or bile leak. Often the second transection point is above the bifurcation and is described in the operative note as encountering a "second cystic duct" or "accessory duct." Other contributing factors to misidentification are a short cystic duct, "tethering" of the infundibulum of the gallbladder to the common bile duct by inflammatory bands (Fig. 3), and a large stone contained in Hartmann's pouch. The small caliber common bile duct is also in danger of being misidentified; bile ducts may normally be as narrow as 3 mm in the adult.

Technical errors may also cause biliary injury. The most frequent technical causes of ductal injuries in the laparoscopic era seem to be failure to occlude the cystic duct securely, too deep a plane of dissection of the gallbladder off the liver bed, and thermal injuries to the bile duct.

Prevention of Biliary Injuries

Laparoscopic cholecystectomy should be performed only by trained surgeons who have received adequate instruction and are operating with appropriate equipment. Difficult cases should be avoided early in one's experience, and conversion to "open" surgery should be considered good judgment and not a failure.

Avoidance of Misidentification of Ducts

Many guidelines have been suggested to avoid misidentification of ducts, including instructions for directing traction on the gallbladder, use of operative cholangiography, and the need to identify or not to identify the common bile duct–cystic duct junction. The key issue is that misidentification is a result of failure conclusively to identify the tubular structures before clipping or division. Injuries should be avoidable by adhering to certain principles.

Because the cystic duct and artery are the structures to be divided, it is these structures that must be conclusively identified in every LC. Accordingly, the cystic duct and artery should not be clipped or cut until conclusively identified. To achieve conclusive identification the hepatocystic triangle must be dissected at the lower end of the gallbladder (Fig. 4). At the completed dissection only two structures should be seen to be entering the gallbladder, and the bottom of the liver bed should be visible. It is not necessary to see the common duct. It is helpful to view the hepatocystic triangle both from its traditional ventral aspect by applying traction on the gallbladder infundibulum in a lateral direction (to bring the cystic duct out of alignment with the common bile duct) and to view the dorsal aspect of the triangle by applying traction to the infundibulum in a superior and medial direction (Fig. 5 A, B). When the neck of the gallbladder has been freed from the surrounding tissue, and the cystic structures are clearly seen arising from the gallbladder wall itself, the critical view of safety has been achieved, and the cystic structures may be occluded because they have been conclusively identified.

These principles are similar in rationale to those enunciated for years by expert biliary surgeons for open cholecystectomy. The surgeon should be proficient in a variety of dissection techniques, including pulling techniques, gentle spreading with forceps, and blunt dissection with a nonactivated spatula cautery tip or anchored pledgets. The plane of dissection should always be maintained on the gallbladder wall or the cystic duct. Staying on or close to the gallbladder during clearance of the hepatocystic triangle is a key feature of safe dissection.

Routine operative cholangiography has been recommended to avoid ductal injury. However, even when a cholangiogram is obtained, misinterpretation can occur prior to major bile duct injuries. The usual misinterpretation of normal is that only the lower part of the biliary tree is visualized, without filling of the hepatic ducts. This often means that the common bile duct has been cannulated, and that a clip has been placed across it that so contrast cannot flow proximally into the hepatic ducts. When only the lower part of the duct is seen, one may reposition the catheter or administer morphine to increase sphincter of Oddi tone and allow cholangiographic visualization of the intrahepatic bile ducts. Failure to fill the proximal ducts must be interpreted as abnormal until proven otherwise and is a reason to convert to an open procedure. Routine cholangiography prevents conversion of a type D injury (due to catheterization of the common bile duct with a cholangiocatheter) to the far more serious type E injury of resection of a portion of the common bile duct when it is noted that the common bile duct has been cannulated.

Presentation of Bile Duct Injuries Following Laparoscopic Cholecystectomy

There are important differences in the presentation of type A and type E injuries. Type A injuries almost always present in the first postoperative week, although they have been reported as late as 2–3 weeks postoperatively. There are two common modes of presentation for type A injuries. About two-thirds of patients present with a symptom complex of abdominal pain coupled with fever and abdominal tenderness caused by bile collecting locally or generally in the peritoneal cavity. About one-third of patients present with bile leaking externally through an incision. However, a few patients present only with vague symptoms, such as anorexia or failure to thrive. It is important to be aware of this third mode of presentation because such patients may be ignored or misdiagnosed. An important matter differentiating type A from type E injuries is that jaundice occurs quite uncommonly in type A injuries, although mild hyperbilirubinemia is frequent, as is an elevated alkaline phosphatase level.

Type E injuries are more likely to be appreciated during operation, as is carried out in approximately 25% of cases. Intraoperative recognition occurs either because of observation of bile in the operative field, indicating a cut bile duct, or secondary to abnormalities seen on cholangiography. As with type A injuries, most type E injuries are discovered within 30 days of operation. However, unlike type A injuries, about 5% of type E injuries present one or more months postoperatively. About 50% of cases present with a combination of jaundice and pain. About 25% of patients present with painless jaundice, which is the sole manifestation in the very late presentations. Some patients present with pain, fever, and sepsis, while a few present with an external bile leak.

Type B injuries (in which a portion of the biliary tree is occluded) may present long after operation with pain or cholangitis in the occluded segment or remain asymptomatic with liver atrophy involving the occluded segment. Type C and D injuries are less well characterized, but when patients with these injuries are not diagnosed by intraoperative bile leak, they present much as type A injuries.

Investigation of a Biliary Injury in the Postoperative Period (see Table 1). In general when the patient presents with pain, fever, and sepsis, but not jaundice (likely a type A injury with bile in the peritoneal cavity), the presence or absence of a bile collection should be established by ultrasound or computerized axial tomogra-

Table 1. Comparison of diagnostic techniques for investigating laparoscopic biliary injuries

Test	Major functions	Characteristics	Negative outcomes	Cost
Hepatobiliary scintigraphy	Detect bile leak	Can be used with low levels of jaundice. Poor localization of site of leakage. Good screening test	Non-invasive	Low
Ultrasound	Detect biloma, detect dilated bile ducts	Localizes bile collections well. Bowel gas interferes. Some user dependency. Good screening test when injury suspected. Can be combined with percutaneous aspiration	Non-invasive	Low
Fistulagram	Detect site of leak and presence of biloma	Very useful when established external fistula exists	Non-invasive	Low
CT scan	Detect biloma, detect dilated bile dutcts	Can be combined with percutaneous aspiration	Non-invasive	Moderate
ERCP	Detect exact site of leak or obstruction	Can be combined with sphincterotomy and drainage to treat Type A and D injuries. Important planning step for many operative procedures	Invasive	Expensive
Percutaneous transhepatic cholangiography	Detect exact site of leak and obstruction. Demonstrates intrahepatic biliary anatomy	Decompresses ducts, can be used for some Type A and D injuries and E injuries with stricture. Important planning step for surgery and for treatment of cholangitis. Catheders guide operative dissection	Invasive	Expensive

phy with percutaneous aspiration if a collection is present. When this occurs, catheter drainage should be instituted unless the collection is simply serous fluid. If bile is found, hepatobiliary scintigraphy can determine whether the bile leak is active. If an active leak is found, ERCP is used to demonstrate the site and type of problem. If it is a type A injury, sphincterotomy and intubation can be performed at the same time. If it is a more serious injury, the choice is between stenting or operation, depending on the type of injury.

Management of Biliary Injuries

Injuries Recognized at the Initial Operation

Management depends on the type of injury and the time of diagnosis. The usual injury discovered at an operation is to the main bile ducts, type C, D, or E. Early repair of these injuries is desirable, but the repair is often difficult and may require dissection and suturing techniques that are not commonly used by many surgeons who perform cholecystectomies. The keys to successful repair are the ability to dissect hepatic ducts up to and above the bifurcation and into the hepatic parenchyma, if necessary, and the ability to perform a mucosa-to-mucosa anastomosis without tension between a defunctioned loop of jejunum and one or several hepatic ducts, sometimes of small caliber, while maintaining intact blood supply. Direct duct-to-duct repair should be reserved for clean transections with little or no loss of ductal tissue, an uncommon event in laparoscopic injuries, and duct-to-duodenal anastomoses should be avoided. If a laparoscopic biliary injury is created and recognized at the time of operation by a surgeon not expert at the repair required, drainage of the right upper quadrant with referral to a hepatobiliary unit is preferable to attempting a complex biliary repair. When the injury is discovered in the postoperative period, it is increasingly advisable to refer the patient, as it is essential that the first repair be technically perfect.

Biliary Injuries Found in the Postoperative Period

Management depends on the type of injury, the type of initial management and its result, and the time elapsed since the initial operation or repair.

Type A Injuries. The treatment is to drain the intraperitoneal bile collection, and if bile leakage is continuing, intrabiliary pressure is reduced by endoscopic techniques, such as ERCP and placement of a stent. The vast majority of patients may be successfully managed without laparotomy in this fashion.

Type B Injuries. These injuries may remain asymptomatic or present as late as 10 or more years after the initial injury with pain or cholangitis. Patients who are symptomatic require treatment, usually hepaticojejunostomy and, more rarely, segmental hepatic resection when biliary enteric anastomosis is not possible.

Type C Injuries. In the case of type C injuries to major ducts drainage of the bile collection is required and either biliary-enteric anastomosis or ligation of the transected duct. If the duct is very small (< 2 mm), the biliary enteric anastomosis is unlikely to be unsuccessful, and ligation may be preferable.

Type D Injuries. Most injuries have been repaired at the time of the initial operation or shortly thereafter by suture of the duct over a T-tube. Whether the T-tube should be brought out through the injury or via separate incision in the duct depends on the exact nature of the injury. When its location and length are similar to an intended choledochotomy, and the injury is fresh, there is no reason to make a second opening in the duct. However, in most cases, a second stab opening for the T-tube is recommended. Some cases of type D injuries in which the cut in the bile duct is very small might be managed by external drainage and biliary intubation or by suture closure alone.

Type E Injuries. Short strictures, and occasionally clip occlusions, may be treated primarily by nonoperative means, including balloon dilatation and stents placed either by ERCP or percutaneously through the liver. Operation is required for failure of stent therapy and when there is ductal discontinuity.

The optimal timing of reconstruction is variable. Operation can be performed immediately if the patient is stable. If the duct is stented or drained, and bile collections are drained, there is no rush to repair the injury. It is best to wait until the inflammation can be expected to have subsided. Another reason for waiting is that with cauterization or devascularization injuries the process may progress over several months. It is best to wait for definitive reconstruction until stabilization of the injury has occurred.

References

Bismuth H (1982) Postoperative strictures of the bile duct. In: Blumgart LH (ed) Surgery of the liver and biliary tract, vol 5. Churchill-Livingstone, Edinburgh, pp 209–218

Branum G, Schmitt C, Baillie J et al (1993) Management of major biliary complications after laparoscopic cholecystectomy. Ann Surg 217:532–541

Brunt LM, Soper NJ (1993) Laparoscopic cholecystectomy: early results and complications. Comp Surg 12:25–53

Davidoff AM, Pappas TN, Murray EA, Hilleren DJ, Johnson RD, Baker ME, Newman GE, Cotton PB, Meyers WC (1992) Mechanisms of major biliary injury during laparoscopic cholecystectomy. Ann Surg 215(3):196–202

Hunter JG (1991) Avoidance of bile duct injury during laparoscopic cholecystectomy. Am J Surg 162:71–76

McSherry CK (1987) Cholecystostomy and cholecystectomy. In: Way LW, Pellegrini CA (eds) Surgery of the gallbladder and bile ducts. Saunders, Philadelphia, pp 335–349

Smadja C, Blumgart LH (1988) The biliary tract and the anatomy of biliary exposure. In: Blumgart LH (ed) Surgery of the liver and biliary tract, vol I. Churchill-Livingstone, Edinburgh, pp 11–22

Soper NJ (1991) Laparoscopic cholecystectomy. Curr Probl Surg 28:581–655

Soper NJ, Flye MW, Brunt LM et al (1993) Diagnosis and management of biliary complications of laparoscopic cholecystectomy. Am J Surg 165:663–669

Strasberg SM, Hertl M, Soper NJ (1995) An analysis of the problem of biliary injury during laparoscopic cholecystectomy. J Am Coll Surg 180:101–125

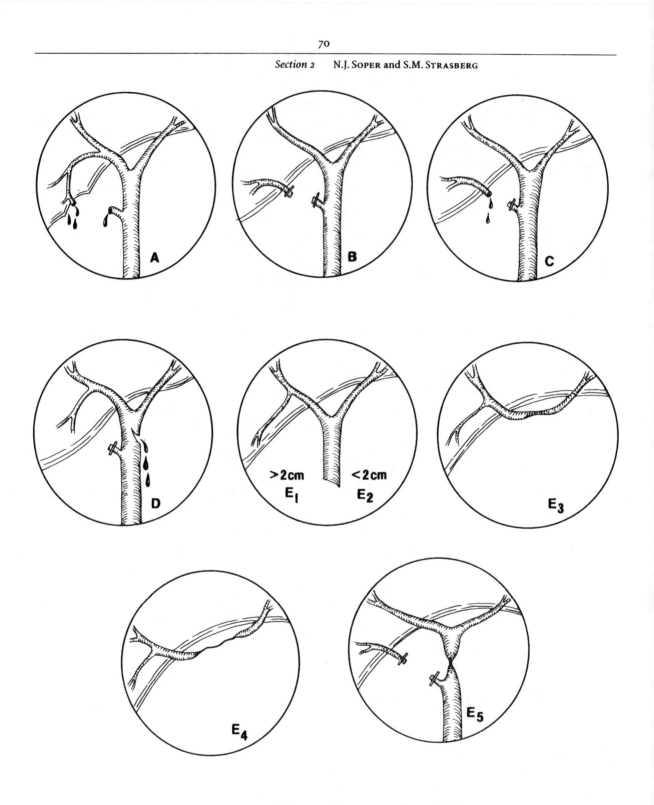

Fig. 1. Proposed classification of laparoscopic injuries to the biliary tract; type E injuries are subdivided according to the Bismuth classification. (From Strasberg et al. 1993)

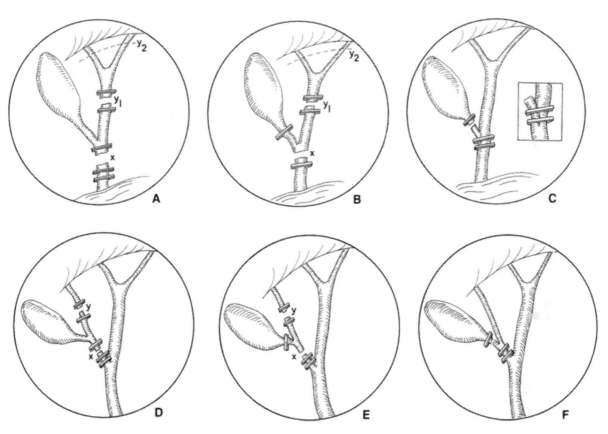

Fig. 2 A–F. Patterns of biliary injury. **A** "Classical" type E injury in which the common duct is divided between clips (X). The ductal system is divided again later to remove the gallbladder (Y1, E1 and E2 injuries; Y2, E3 or E4 injuries). **B, C** Variants of the injury may occur. **D, E, F** Represent variants of injury to aberrant right hepatic duct, producing type B and C injuries. (From Strasberg et al. 1993)

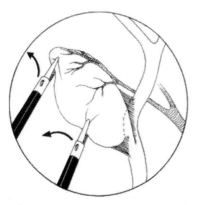

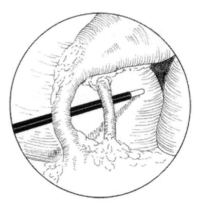

Fig. 3. Area of common duct frequently mistaken for cystic duct when the infundibulum is "tethered" to hepatic duct by adhesions or inflammation. (From Brunt and Soper 1993)

Fig. 4. Critical view of safety during laparoscopic cholecystectomy. The hepatocystic triangle is dissected free of all tissue except for the cystic duct and artery, and the base of the liver bed is exposed. (From Strasberg 1995)

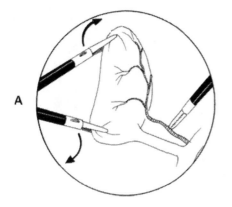

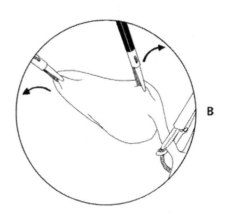

Fig. 5 A, B. Exposure of hepatocystic triangle during laparoscopic cholecystectomy. **A** "Classical" ventral aspect exposed by lateral traction on infundibulum and superior traction on fundus. **B** Dorsal aspect exposed by superomedial traction on infundibulum and lateral traction on fundus. (From Soper 1991)

SECTION 3

14 Laparoscopic Anatomy of the Abdominal Wall

R. ANNIBALI and R.J. FITZGIBBONS, JR.

Introduction

The recent introduction of laparoscopic surgical techniques has challenged the surgeon with a totally new approach to the "problem hernia": through a laparoscope the hernia is no longer viewed actually as a protrusion from the abdominal wall but rather the extrusion of a viscus from the peritoneal cavity. The layers that constitute the inguinal region and the lower anterior abdominal wall are dissected according to a reversed order and seen from an opposite viewpoint. Indeed, as early as 1945 Lytle wrote: "The operating surgeon knows little of the posterior wall of the inguinal canal, so well it is hidden from his view." For a safe approach to laparoscopic herniorrhaphy, it would seem appropriate to reverse the habitual order and visualize the anatomy from the inner layers, since laparoscopy provides an optimal panoramic view of the posterior surface of the abdominal wall.

Peritoneal Folds and Fossae

The deep surface of the abdominal wall above the iliopubic tract is covered by peritoneum (Fig. 1). Five peritoneal folds are visible below the umbilicus. The median umbilical ligament, which represents the obliterated remnant of the embryonic urachus, lies in the midline and extends from the fundus of the bladder to the umbilicus. The medial umbilical ligament consists of a fold of peritoneum covering the distal portion of the umbilical artery. This is usually obliterated, atrophic, and cordlike in the adult, but it is normally patent proximally. The lateral umbilical ligament consists of a fold of peritoneum around the inferior epigastric vessels together with a variable amount of fatty tissue. On either side of the midline the medial and lateral umbilical ligaments delineate three shallow fossae. The lateral fossa lies lateral to the inferior epigastric vessels. It is the site where indirect hernias pass through the internal inguinal ring. The medial fossa is defined as the space between the lateral and the medial umbilical ligament and corresponds to the site of development of direct inguinal hernias. Finally, the supravesical fossa lies between the medial and the median umbilical ligaments. The rectus abdominis muscle and its sheath confer greater strength to this area, making supravesical hernias rare. The umbilical fossae have been previously considered of no surgical importance in regard to either the etiology or the repair of groin hernias. However, a consistent relationship between inguinal herniation and the umbilical fossae has been routinely observed laparoscopically, and they are now considered important landmarks for orientation.

Preperitoneal Space

The preperitoneal space is delimited posteriorly by the peritoneum and anteriorly by the transversalis fascia (Fig. 2). It contains a variable amount of connective tissue, together with many vascular and neurological structures.

The transversalis fascia is the portion of the endoabdominal fascia that covers the internal surface of the transversus abdominis muscle. Some appendices and thicknesses of the transversalis fascia (transversalis fascia analogues) are important landmarks for the laparoscopic surgeon. The internal inguinal ring is the internal opening of the inguinal canal and is located in the lateral fossa about 1.25 cm above and slightly lateral to the middle of the inguinal ligament. It allows passage of the vas deferens, the testicular vessels and normally the genital branch of the genitofemoral nerve. It appears nearly closed when viewed laparoscopically. The transversalis fascia sling is another important analogue; it consists of a thickness of the medial border of the internal inguinal ring and has superior and inferior extensions known as the superior and inferior crura, which tend to approximate during straining, thus reinforcing the weak area of the ring. The iliopubic tract is a fascial condensation connected laterally with the iliac crest and the anterior superior iliac spine. It runs parallel to the inguinal ligament, but in a plane posterior to it, crosses the femoral vessels anteriorly while bordering the deep inguinal ring inferiorly, and finally fans out to attach to the medial portion of Cooper's ligament.

Cooper's ligament has often been modified. Regardless of its origin or exact makeup, for practical purposes the ligament is the shiny, fibrous structure covering the superior pubic ramus. The iliopectineal arch is a condensation of the transversalis fascia on the medial side of the iliac fascia. It is attached laterally to the anterior superior iliac spine and medially with the iliopectineal eminence. The iliopectineal arch is an important landmark because it divides the medial vascular compartment (lacuna vasorum) and the femoral canal from the lateral muscular compartment (lacuna musculorum).

The lower fibers of the transversus abdominis muscle fuse with the transversalis fascia and cross downward and medially to form an aponeurotic arch. This bridges over the superior margin of the internal inguinal ring before inserting at the pubic tubercle and the medial side of Cooper's ligament. It is responsible for a physiological system known as the shutter mechanism which functions in the prevention of direct and indirect herniation. It is activated when the internal oblique and the transversus abdominis muscle contract simultaneously during straining and approximate the transversus aponeurotic arch to the iliopubic tract and the inguinal ligament, thus reinforcing the posterior wall of the inguinal canal. In approximately 25% of individuals, however, the arch cannot descend enough to reach the inguinal ligament; it may be located too superiorly or simply remain poorly developed.

Hesselbach's Triangle

The inguinal triangle (Hesselbach's triangle) is another weak area of the groin. According to the original description, its boundaries were described as the inferior epigastric vessels superolaterally, the rectus sheath medially, and Cooper's ligament inferiorly. These borders have subsequently been modified with the substitution of the inguinal ligament for Cooper's ligament to allow an easier identification of the area by surgeons who use the traditional anterior approach for herniorrhaphy. For the laparoscopic procedure, however, it seems more appropriate to return to Hesselbach's original description since the inguinal ligament is not visible laparoscopically. The inferior portion of the triangle includes the weak area seen in the medial umbilical fossa where direct hernias develop; its boundaries are the aponeurotic arch superiorly and the iliopubic tract inferiorly.

Vessels of the Retroperitoneal and Preperitoneal Space

The vascular structures of the preperitoneal space (Fig. 2) are easily damaged during surgical dissection or while applying staples or sutures, often resulting in the formation of a hematoma or worse. The external iliac vessels run on the medial aspect of the psoas muscle over its investing fascia before passing under the iliopubic tract and the inguinal ligament to become the femoral vessels. The inferior epigastric vessels normally originate from the external iliacs; they run superiorly and medially toward the umbilicus from a point midway between the anterior superior iliac spine and the symphysis pubis, ascend obliquely along the medial margin of the internal inguinal ring between the transversalis fascia and the peritoneum, and finally pierce the transversalis fascia to enter the sheath of the rectus muscle. The inferior epigastric arteries usually give rise to two branches in the inguinal region: the external spermatic (cremasteric) artery and the anastomotic pubic branch. The former runs upward from its origin along the medial aspect of the internal inguinal ring and pierces the transversalis fascia to join the spermatic cord. The pubic branch courses inferiorly toward the obturator foramen, where it anastomoses with the obturator artery and sometimes gives rise to an inconstant small branch, called the anterior pubic branch, along the superior ramis of the pubis. This anastomotic ring of arteries, together with their corresponding veins, is also known as the *corona mortis* ("crown of death") because of the bleeding which occurs if it is injured while suturing or applying staples to Cooper's ligament. An obturator artery originating from the inferior epigastric or external iliac has been observed in approximately 30% of the specimens studied. The deep circumflex iliac artery and vein also originate from the external iliac vessels, then course laterally between the iliopubic tract and the iliopectineal arch to reach the space between the transversus abdominis and the internal oblique muscles, where they finally anastomose with the iliolumbar vessels.

It is important to become familiar with the deep inguinal venous circulation. The iliopubic vein courses deep to the iliopubic tract and accompanies the anterior pubic branch when this is present. It either empties directly into the inferior epigastric vein or joins the venous anastomotic pubic branch to form a common trunk that drains into the inferior epigastric vein. Another tributary of the inferior epigastric vein, the rectusial vein, runs along or embedded within the lower lateral fibers of the rectus muscle. Finally, a small collateral branch of the anastomotic pubic vein is commonly observed on the lower posterior aspect of the pubic ramus, beneath

Cooper's ligament, and has been called the retropubic vein.

Innervation

Five major nerves responsible for the innervation of the lower abdominal wall, the inguinal and genital region, the thigh and the leg are found in the preperitoneal and extraperitoneal space (Figs. 3, 4). The iliohypogastric nerve appears at the lateral margin of the psoas muscle and crosses obliquely on the quadratus lumborum, passes beneath the inferior pole of the kidney to pierce the transversus abdominis muscle, and then divides into two branches. The most important one is the hypogastric, which lies between the external and the internal oblique muscle at the level of the anterior superior iliac spine and reaches the suprapubic skin by piercing the muscular layers. It innervates the skin of the anterior abdominal wall above the pubis. The ilioinguinal nerve follows a course similar to that of the iliohypogastric but more inferior. It crosses the quadratus lumborum and the iliacus muscles before piercing the transversus abdominis and the internal oblique; it continues along the inguinal canal, over the cremasteric muscle, and finally exits through the external inguinal ring to innervate the skin of the superomedial portion of the thigh, root of the penis, pubic region, and scrotum or labium majorus. The genitofemoral nerve emerges from the fibers of the psoas muscle at the level of the lower lumbar vertebrae and crosses behind the ureter to divide into the genital and femoral branches. The genital branch is medial, traverses the iliac vessels to reach the internal inguinal ring and runs along the inguinal canal together with the spermatic cord. The genital branch of the genitofemoral nerve provides motor innervation to the cremaster muscle and sensory innervation to the skin of the penis and scrotum. The femoral branch lies usually on the lateral edge of the psoas muscle, beneath the psoas fascia, and may bifurcate before crossing the deep circumflex iliac artery to pass under the iliopubic tract. In the femoral sheath it lies lateral to the femoral artery to reach the femoral triangle and provide sensory innervation to the anteromedial surface of the upper thigh. The lateral femoral cutaneous nerve emerges from the lateral margin of the psoas muscle and crosses the iliacus muscle obliquely toward the anterior superior iliac spine. Medial to the latter, it passes below the iliopubic tract to reach the thigh. The innervated area extends from the greater trochanter to the midcalf level. The femoral nerve is the largest nerve originating from the lumbar plexus. It emerges from the inferior aspect of the psoas muscle, passes along the lateral border, and then runs between the iliacus and pectineus muscles, covered by a layer of fascia. It passes below the iliopubic tract and reaches the femoral triangle within the lacuna musculorum. Its branches innervate the skin of the lower anteromedial thigh, the medial aspect of the leg and the great toe. It also contains muscular branches that provide motor innervation to the pectineus, sartorius and quadriceps.

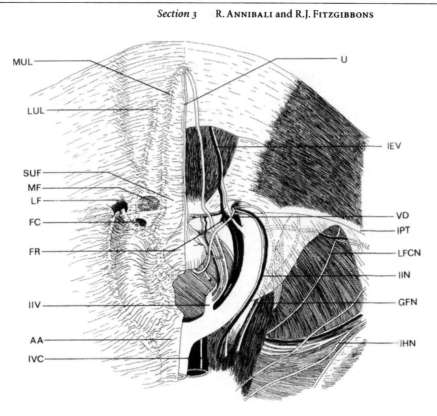

Fig. 1. The anatomy of the internal surface of the lower abdominal wall, inguinal region and lower trunk according to the laparoscopic perspective. *Left*, the peritoneum has been left intact; *right*, it has been removed to show the underlying structures. *MUL*, Medial umbilical ligament; *LUL*, Lateral umbilical ligament; *SUF*, Supravesical fossa; *MF*, Medial fossa; *LF*, Lateral fossa; *FC*, Femoral canal; *FR*, Femoral ring; *AA*, Abdominal aorta; *IVC*, Inferior vena cava; *IIA*, Internial iliac artery; *IHN*, Iliohypogastric nerve; *GFN*, Genitofemoral nerve; *IIN*, Ilioinguinal nerve; *LFCN*, Lateral femoral cutaneous nerve; *VD*, Vas deferens; *IPT*, Iliopubic tract; *IEV*, Inferior epigastric vessels; *U*, Urachus. (From Annibali et al. 1993)

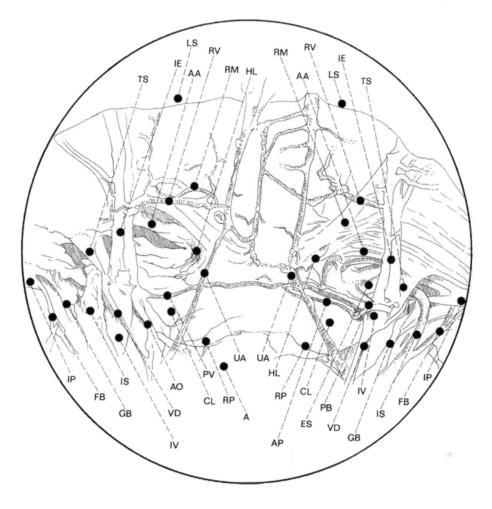

Fig. 2. Panoramic view of the deep surface of the anterior abdominal wall in a cadaver preparation to demonstrate the vessels of the preperitoneal space. *RM*, Lateral border of the rectus abdominis muscle; *LS*, linea semicircularis (of Douglas); *IE*, inferior epigastric vessels; *ES*, external spermatic vessels; *RV*, rectusial vein; *CL*, Cooper's ligament; *IP*, iliopubic tract; *UA*, umbilical arteries; *HL*, falx inguinalis (or Henle's ligament); *AA*, aponeurotic arch of the transversus abdominis muscle; *VD*, vas deferens; *IS*, internal spermatic vessels; *PB*, anastomotic pubic branch; *AP*, anterior pubic branch and iliopubic vein; *RP*, retropubic vein; *AO*, anomalous obturator artery; *GB*, genital branch of the genitofemoral nerve; *FB*, femoral branch of the genitofemoral nerve; *TS*, transversalis fascia sling. (From Annibali et al. 1994b)

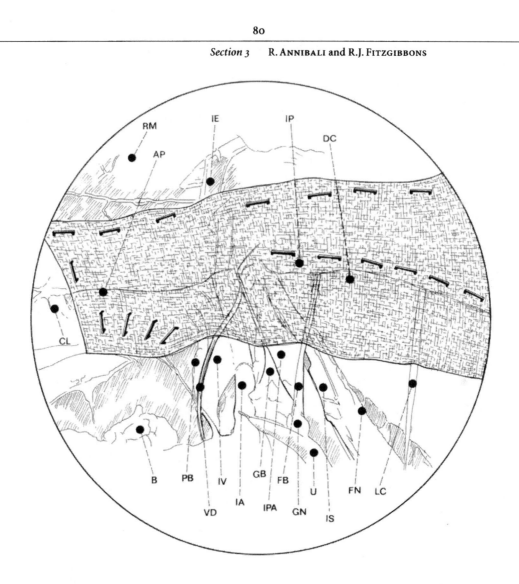

Fig. 3. Mesh positioned in the cadaver preparation to demonstrate the relationships of mesh and staples with the neurologic and vascular structures. All the six staples in the lower row, lateral to the epigastric vessels, possibly injuring to the underlying nerves though placed above the iliopubic tract. *VD*, Vas deferens; *IS*, internal spermatic (testicular) vessels; *IV*, external iliac vein; *IA*, external iliac artery; *IP*, iliopubic tract; *IE*, inferior epigastric vessels; *RM*, rectus abdominis muscle; *PB*, anastomotic pubic branch; *AP*, anterior pubic branch; *IPA*, iliopectineal arch; *CL*, Cooper's pectineal ligament; *DC*, deep circumflex iliac vessels; *GN*, genitofemoral nerve; *GB*, genital branch of the genitofemoral nerve; *FB*, femoral branch of the genitofemoral nerve; *FN*, femoral nerve; *LC*, lateral femoral cutaneous nerve; *U*, ureter; *B*, bladder (reflected posteriorly). (From Annibali et al. 1993)

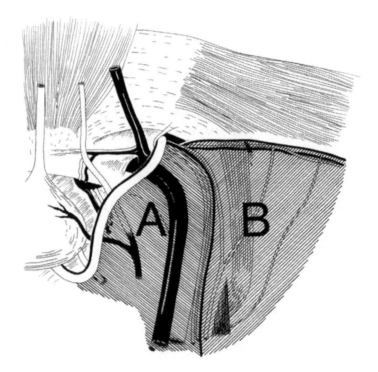

Fig. 4. Drawing showing the two critical areas for avoiding staple placement during laparoscopic hernia repair in the groin. *A*, Triangle of doom; *B*, triangle of pain

Comments

Two triangular anatomical areas within the groin have considerable importance for laparoscopic hernia repair. The first triangular area lies between the vas deferens medially and spermatic vessels laterally and is often referred to as the "triangle of doom." The external iliac vessels lie in its floor, usually hidden by the peritoneum and the transversalis fascia. Initially, to avoid injury to these important structures, it had been strongly recommended that suturing or stapling be carried out only medial to the vas deferens or lateral to the spermatic vessels.

We subsequently started some thorough anatomical studies to explain the unexpectedly high incidence of neuralgias initially reported by several authors following laparoscopic hernia repairs. The results of our investigations led us to the belief that the borders of the "dangerous area" should be extended. For laparoscopic inguinal hernia repair, in fact, the iliopubic tract is another extremely important landmark to observe if sta-

ples are to be safely applied. Lateral to the spermatic vessels and immediately below (or, in some instances, directly through) the fibers of the iliopubic tract are the genital and femoral branches of the genitofemoral nerve, the femoral nerve and the lateral femoral cutaneous nerve. Consequently, staples placed caudal to the iliopubic tract and lateral to the internal spermatic vessels can result in transient or permanent neuralgias involving one or more of the above-mentioned nerves or branches.

Also, pain in the groin or lower abdomen can be observed if the ilioinguinal or the iliohypogastric nerve is injured. Although injury of these latter nerves is less frequent during laparoscopic hernia repair than with conventional anterior inguinal herniorrhaphy (they lie in a plane superficial to the preperitoneal space), on occasion they can be compromised by staples placed deeply, especially if a vigorous bimanual technique is used to apply them. The genital branch of the genitofemoral nerve is not commonly encountered in the area in which staples are applied.

The femoral branch of the genitofemoral nerve and the lateral femoral cutaneous, on the other hand, are at higher risk of being injured during laparoscopic hernia repair since they are more superficial (they lie on the anterior surface of the psoas and iliacus muscle, respectively) and in the area where staples are usually applied to tack the inferolateral border of the mesh. The femoral nerve is medial and in a relatively deeper position; although less vulnerable, it may be injured by staples placed medially and close to the iliopectineal arch, with consequent possible sensory and/or functional consequences.

Accordingly, it seems appropriate to introduce the concept of a second dangerous triangular zone and include it beside (lateral to) the triangle of doom. This other dangerous area, which we have named "triangle of pain" for its connections with possible nerve injuries, is included between the internal spermatic vessels inferomedially and the iliopubic tract superolaterally. Staples or sutures should not be applied in the triangle of pain or the triangle of doom.

In conclusion, to prevent damage to the vessels and nerves we recommend that, lateral to the vas deferens, staples be placed only above and parallel to the iliopubic tract.

References

Annibali R (1994) Surgical anatomy of the inguinal region and lower abdominal wall from the laparoscopic perspective. In: Nyhus L, Condon RE (eds) Hernia. Lippincott, Philadelphia, pp 64–72

Annibali R, Quinn TH, Fitzgibbons RJ jr (1994a) Surgical anatomy of the inguinal region and lower abdominal wall: the laparoscopic perspective. In: Bendavid R (ed) Prostheses and abdominal wall hernias. Landes Medical, Austin, pp 82–103

Annibali R, Quinn TH, Fitzgibbons RJ jr (1994b) Avoiding nerve injury during laparoscopic hernia repair: critical areas for staple placement. In: Arregui ME, Nagan RF (eds) Inguinal hernia: advances or controversies? Radcliffe Medical, Oxford, pp 41–54

Annibali R, Fitzgibbons RJ jr, Filipi C, Litke BS, Salerno GM (1994c) Laparoscopic hernia repair. In: Green FL, Ponsky JL (eds) Endoscopic surgery. Saunders, Philadelphia, pp 352–386

Lytle W (1945) The internal inguinal ring. Br J Surg 32:441–446

McVay CB (1974) The anatomic basis for inguinal and femoral hernioplasty. Surg Gynecol Obstet 139:931–945

Nyhus LM, Bombeck TC, Klein MS (1991) Hernias. In: Sabiston DC jr (ed) Textbook of surgery. Saunders, Philadelphia, pp 1134–1147

Skandalakis JE, Gray SW, Skandalakis LJ et al (1989) Surgical anatomy of the inguinal hernia. World J Surg 13:490–498

Spaw AT, Ennis BW, Spaw LP (1991) Laparoscopic hernia repair: the anatomic basis. J Laparoendosc Surg 1 (5):269–277

15 Laparoscopic Transabdominal Preperitoneal Hernia Repair

J. Camps, N. Nguyen, D.A. Cornet, and R.J. Fitzgibbons, Jr.

Introduction

Transabdominal hernia repair is not a new concept. Many surgeons advocate the repair of hernias found incidentally during laparotomy for other conditions. Marcy (1887) and LaRoque (1932) proposed the intra-abdominal approach as a primary method for herniorrhaphy. In fact, LaRoque performed more than 1700 procedures using this technique. However, most surgeons feel that the morbidity associated with a laparotomy is too significant for repair of a primary inguinal hernia. The advent of laparoscopy has changed this, as access to the intra-abdominal space (see Chap. 14) can be accomplished with a marked decrease in perioperative discomfort.

Positioning of the Patient and Team

Figure 1 illustrates the operating set-up most commonly employed for the laparoscopic herniorrhaphy procedure. The surgeon usually stands on the opposite side of the table from the hernia, because this provides the most appropriate angle for dissection and staple placement. After inducting general anesthesia a Foley catheter is placed to ensure continuous decompression of the bladder. Although diagnostic laparoscopy is possible under local anesthesia, the considerable dissection involved in this procedure precludes its use.

Technique

Cannulae placement is depicted in Fig. 2. The initial cannula is placed in the umbilicus, which allows generalized exploration of the abdomen. The patient is then placed in the Trendelenburg position to allow the bowel to fall away from the pelvis and to allow good access to the inguinal area. Two additional cannulae are placed lateral to the rectus sheath on either side at the level of the umbilicus. All three are large cannulae (10–12 mm) as this allows free movement of the laparoscope and the stapler to any position, depending upon the patient's anatomy.

After the first (umbilical) cannula is inserted, the inguinal regions are inspected to confirm the pathology and to check the contralateral side (Fig 3). Two additional cannulae are then inserted under direct vision. The medial umbilical ligament is identified and divided if it appears to compromise exposure. Bleeding from small vessels is controlled using electrocautery. The peritoneal flap is then created by extending this incision at a distance of 2 cm above the myopectineal defect to the anterior superior iliac spine (Fig. 4). The flap is mobilized downward using sharp and blunt dissection. The inferior epigastric vessels, symphysis pubis, transversalis fascia, and cord structures are exposed. For direct hernias the sac and preperitoneal fat are reduced from the hernia orifice using gentle traction. The thinned-out transversalis fascia (the so-called pseudosac) lining the defect is left behind, if necessary separating it by sharp dissection (Fig. 5). As dissection continues inferiorly, Cooper's ligament and the iliopubic tract laterally are exposed (Fig. 6). The dissection is completed by mobilizing the cord structures away from the peritoneal flap. Indirect hernias are clearly more difficult to deal with. If the sac is small, it can be mobilized from the cord structures and reduced back into the abdomen. However, if it is large or extending into the scrotum, complete mobilization of the sac may result in an increased incidence of spermatic cord or testicular complications. In this situation the hernia is best treated by dividing the sac at the internal ring, leaving the distal sac in situ and with dissection of the proximal sac away from the cord structures.

After completely dissecting the preperitoneal space and identification of the critical anatomical structures, the repair commences. A decision must be made whether the cord structures are to be encircled with the prosthetic material or simply covered. If a direct inguinal hernia defect is quite large, extending to the internal ring, or if an indirect inguinal hernia has caused destruction of the internal ring (Nyhus type 3), we prefer to place a slit in the mesh to accommodate the cord structures. This requires additional mobilization of the cord structures posteriorly to accommodate the mesh. In other cases the mesh is simply laid over the cord structures avoiding this dissection. Most surgeons prefer the latter as this avoids dissection, which increases the incidence of cord or testicular problems. However, proponents of the former argue that this maneuver adds stability to the prosthesis and in effect creates a new internal ring. The controversy will not be settled until longer follow-up data are obtained.

Polypropylene mesh is currently the most popular mesh, but other materials are occasionally used. The size of the prosthesis used is important as many of the earlier recurrences with laparoscopic herniorrhaphy have been thought to be due to inadequate coverage of all of the potential sites of recurrent groin herniation. As an absolute minimum it is important that the size of the prosthesis be no less than 10 x 5 cm. The mesh must be sufficiently large to cover the defect and provide an extensive overlap. This allows the intra-abdominal pressure to act on an area of the patch overlying strong healthy tissue, thus tending to keep the patch in position rather than encouraging it to herniate through the defect.

The next step is to staple the prosthesis (Fig. 7). Some surgeons actually suture the prosthesis in place, but they appear to be in the minority as suturing in this area is quite difficult. Stapling is begun along the upper border of the posterior rectus sheath and transversalis fascia at least 2 cm above the defect. If a slit has been placed in the prosthesis, it is repaired around the cord. The inferior edge is stapled to the symphysis pubis and Cooper's ligament medially, and the iliopubic tract laterally. When stapling the inferior edge, care must be taken not to place staples below the level of the iliopubic tract when lateral to the internal spermatic vessels, for an inordinately high incidence of neuralgias involving the lateral cutaneous nerve of the thigh or the femoral branch of the genitofemoral nerve is then observed. A helpful maneuver in this situation is to use a bimanual technique: Staples are not placed without being able to palpate the head of the stapler through the abdominal wall with the left hand; this ensures that the surgeon is above the iliopubic tract.

Finally, the lateral edge is stapled at a point approximately 1 cm medial to the anterior superior iliac spine. During the course of staple placement, excess mesh is trimmed in situ so that the prosthesis is perfectly tailored to the preperitoneal space. The final step is to close the peritoneum with staples, thus isolating the prosthetic patch from the abdominal contents (Fig. 8). It is important not to leave gaps between the staples because bowel has been reported to slip between these gaps causing obstruction. Peritoneal closure is facilitated by reducing the pneumoperitoneum to 6 mmHg. A long-acting local anesthetic can be injected into the preperitoneal space at this stage to reduce postoperative discomfort.

Bilateral hernias can be repaired using one long transverse peritoneal incision. A single piece of mesh, at least 20 x 6 cm, can be used for both defects fashioned similar to that described by Stoppa and Warlamount (1989) for a conventional repair. However, two separate pieces of prosthetic material are preferred by most authors because it is easier to manipulate the smaller prostheses. This may avoid the theoretical complication which might be encountered if the urachus was patent and an incision made across it and not recognized.

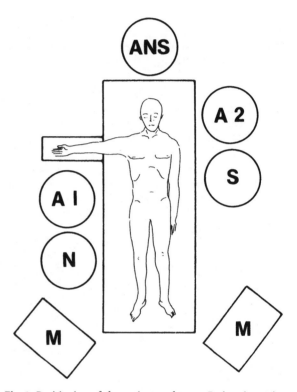

Fig. 1. Positioning of the patient and team. Patient in supine position. *ANS*, Anesthetist; *S*, surgeon; *A1, A2*, assistants; *N*, nurse; *M*, monitor

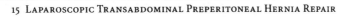

Fig. 2. Cannulae placement

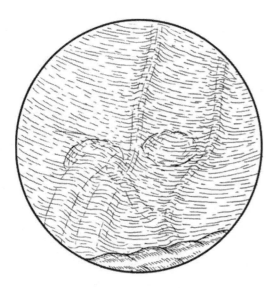

Fig. 3. Inspection of the left inguinal region

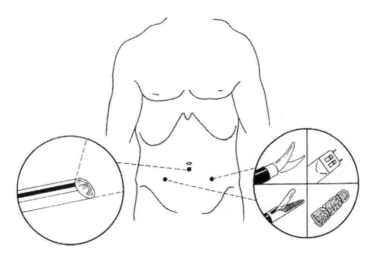

Fig. 4. Opening the peritoneum to create the peritoneal flap

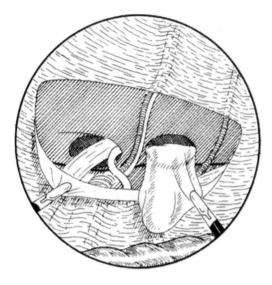

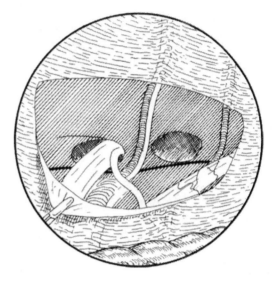

Fig. 5. Operative drawing showing reduction of the hernia sac. The transversalis fascia, or pseudosac, is depicted

Fig. 6. Appearance of the preperitoneal space after a radical dissection as performed for a laparoscopic transabdominal preperitoneal (TAPP) herniorrhaphy

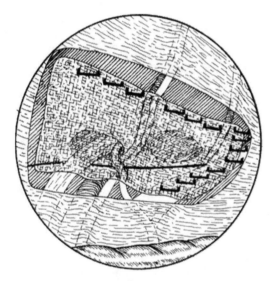

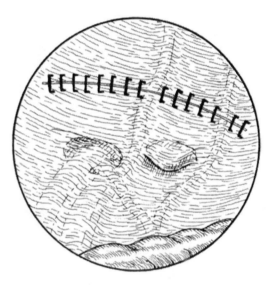

Fig. 7. Prosthesis stapled in place

Fig. 8. Closure of the peritoneum

Comments

This approach to herniorrhaphy has now been established, at least on short-term follow-up, to have an acceptably low recurrence rate and good patient acceptance. Considerable dissection is required but with experience the operating time is similar to that for a conventional herniorrhaphy.

References

Arregui EA, Navarrete J, Davis CJ et al (1993) Laparoscopic inguinal herniorrhaphy: techniques and controversies. Surg Clin North Am 73:513–527

Filipi CJ, Fitzgibbons RJ jr, Salerno GM, Hart RO (1992) Laparoscopic herniorrhaphy. Surg Clin North Am 72:1109–1124

Fitzgibbons RJ jr, Camps J, Nguyen N et al (1995) Laparoscopic inguinal herniorrhaphy results of a multi-center trial. Ann Surg 221(1):3–13

LaRoque GP (1932) The intra-abdominal method of removing inguinal and femoral hernia. Arch Surg 24:189–203

Marcy HO (1887) The cure of hernia. JAMA 8:589–592

Nyhus LM, Pollack R, Bombeck CT, Donahue PE (1988) The preperitoneal approach and prosthetic buttress repair for recurrent hernia. The evolution of a technique. Ann Surg 208:733–737

Stoppa RE, Warlamount CR (1989) The preperitoneal approach and prosthetic repair of groin hernia. In: Nyhus LM, Condon RE (eds) Hernia. Lippincott, Philadelphia, pp 199–225

16 Laparoscopic Near-Total Preperitoneal Hernia Repair

M.J. Fallas and E.H. Phillips

Introduction

Laparoscopic inguinal herniorrhaphy developed as an obvious application of the laparoscopic technique to open preperitoneal hernioplasty. The complete or near-complete preperitoneal approach avoids an incision in the peritoneum, while offering decreased postoperative pain and disability. This extraperitoneal approach, which develops the preperitoneal space without balloon dilators and without incising the peritoneum or creating peritoneal flaps, avoids one of the most serious complications of transabdominal preperitoneal (TAPP) repairs: adhesive or internal hernia bowel obstruction.

Positioning of the Patient and the Team

The patient is placed on the operating room table in the supine position (see Fig. 1). For bilateral hernias, the operating surgeon is on the side opposite the hernia being repaired. The assistant surgeon stands on the opposite side, and the surgical nurse on the patient's right side. For unilateral hernias, the operating surgeon should be on the contralateral side of the hernia.

The monitor is placed at the patient's feet. The abdomen is shaved from umbilicus to pubis and then the entire abdomen is prepared in the usual fashion.

Technique

Under general anesthesia, pneumoperitoneum is established via the Veress needle technique through an umbilical incision. A 10–11 mm or a 5-mm trocar is then inserted into the peritoneal cavity and a 30° 10 mm or 5 mm laparoscope is introduced (Fig. 2). The hernia defects are examined directly from within the peritoneal cavity. A 10 mm incision is made just superior to McBurney's point on the right side of the abdomen. This corresponds to the site of a preperitoneal fat pad commonly located in this position. A Kelly clamp is then used to bluntly dissect through the oblique muscles

under direct vision until the transversalis fascia is reached (Fig. 3). A large Mayo clamp is then used to continue the dissection until the tip of the clamp is seen through the peritoneum, the so-called "metal sign."

The Mayo clamp is then turned curve up toward the underside of the abdominal wall, advanced toward the pubis, spread, and withdrawn in the spread position, creating a pathway for a blunt-tipped 10 mm trocar, or a 10 mm trocar with a blunt probe (Fig. 4). The trocar is placed into the preperitoneal space and a blunt-tipped grasper is advanced toward the pubic symphysis. Care must be taken to assure that the grasper is advanced between the epigastric vessels and the peritoneum. A rowing motion is used to develop the preperitoneal space with the grasper. This procedure is duplicated on the left side (Fig. 5).

Carbon dioxide is then introduced into the preperitoneal space via a lateral trocar, while the intraperitoneal carbon dioxide is slowly released until the preperitoneal space is insufflated. There are two options at this point. One is to make an incision in the midline 3 cm below the umbilical incision. A Mayo clamp is used to bluntly dissect down to the peritoneum in this location. A 10 mm blunt-tipped trocar is then inserted inferiorly toward the pubis in the midline in the preperitoneal space (Fig. 6). The other option is to reinsufflate the intraperitoneal space via the umbilical trocar to 10 mmHg. The umbilical trocar is then backed out slowly until the peritoneum and fascia are visualized. The laparoscope is oriented so the 30° angle faces down. It is advanced into the preperitoneal space, and then the trocar is slid over it. This saves one trocar and one incision.

In both techniques, the laparoscope is placed in this preperitoneal midline trocar and bluntly advanced until it touches the pubic symphysis. The scope is then gently rocked from side to side, further developing this space. The laparoscope is then withdrawn, cleaned, and reinserted in the midline trocar. At this point, orientation is gained by identifying the pubic symphysis and one or both of the graspers in the preperitoneal space.

Starting in the midline, Cooper's ligament is identified and followed laterally until the contents of the femoral canal are identified. The epigastric vessels and spermatic cord are then located. If at any time during the dissection the surgeon becomes confused or has lost anatomic orientation, Cooper's ligament and the epigastric vessels should serve as a reference point. Direct hernias should be reduced until the edges of the defect are seen circumferentially. Indirect hernias, as well as large cord lipomas, should be dissected and reduced off the spermatic cord (Fig. 7). Large indirect sacs may be transected and proximally ligated with an endoloop.

After all hernias have been reduced and all potential hernia sites, including possible femoral hernias, have been inspected, the mesh is prepared. Prolene mesh is cut in an 11 x 11 cm square and a slit is made in the mesh. The slit is created by beginning at the lower border of the mesh one-third from the medial edge and cutting horizontally, stopping one-third of the distance to the lateral border (Fig. 8 a). The mesh is rolled and two chromic sutures are used to fix the mesh in a rolled position (Fig. 8 b). The mesh is then grasped through a tube reducer and inserted on the side of the hernia via the lateral 10–11 mm trocar (Fig. 9). The slit in the mesh is placed around the cord from a lateral position, regardless of the type of hernia, to add stability without stapling lateral to the epigastric vessels. Care is taken so no medial tension is placed on the cord by the mesh. The mesh is then fixed to Cooper's ligament, and the slit in the mesh is stapled closed, leaving adequate space for the spermatic cord laterally (Fig. 10 a–c). No staples need be placed lateral to the epigastric vessels; this is to avoid injury to the ilioinguinal, genitofemoral and lateral femoral cutaneous nerves (see Fig. 4, Chapter 14, page 81).

In bilaterial hernias, the contralateral mesh is placed in a similar fashion before either mesh is unfurled and tacked to the underside of the abdominal wall. After both sides have been placed, the chromic sutures are cut (Fig. 11), and the mesh is unfurled and tacked to the underside of the abdominal wall medial to the epigastric vessels with a reticulating hernia stapler (Fig. 12).

In this manner the femoral, indirect, and direct portions of the inguinal floor are covered. The laparoscope is then returned to the peritoneal cavity. Pneumoperitoneum is reestablished in the peritoneal cavity while carbon dioxide is allowed to escape from the preperitoneal trocars. The repair is inspected to see how the mesh lies, to make sure there have been no inadvertent injuries to the peritoneum, and to assess for the infrequent occurrence of reduction en masse.

Local anesthetic is injected around each trocar site and all fascial defects are closed with 0 Vicryl suture.

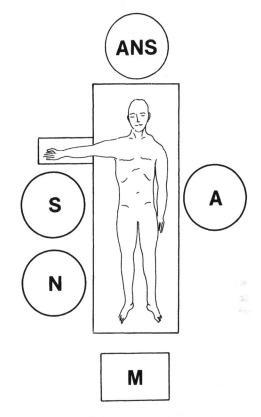

Fig. 1. Positioning of the patient and team. The patient is placed in a supine position (*ANS*, anesthetist; *S*, surgeon; *A*, assistant; *N*, nurse; *M*, monitors)

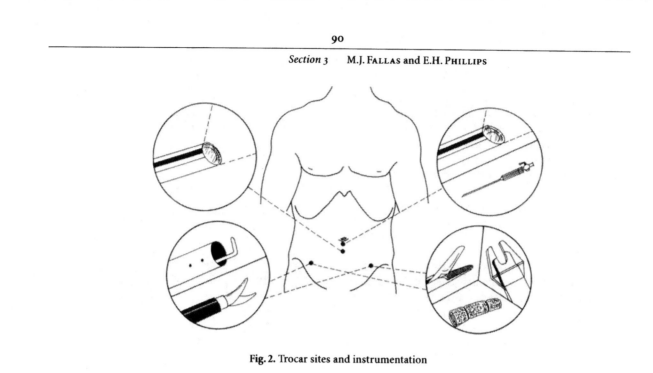

Fig. 2. Trocar sites and instrumentation

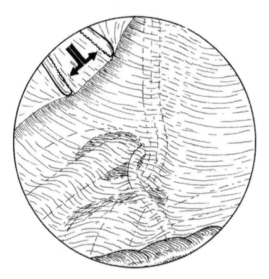

Fig. 3. Access to the preperitoneal space by means of blunt dissection

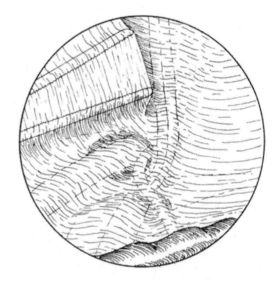

Fig. 4. A Mayo clamp is introduced into the preperitoneal space under laparoscopic guidance and a pathway is created

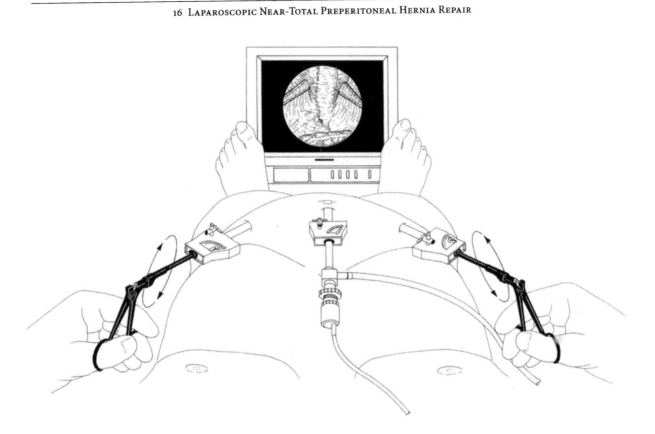

Fig. 5. Blunt trocars and graspers are introduced in the dissected preperitoneal pathway

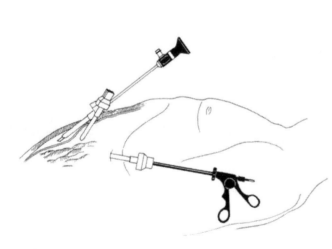

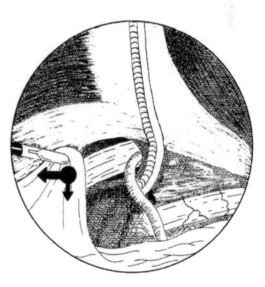

Fig. 6. After CO_2 insufflation into the preperitoneal space, a 10-11 mm trocar is inserted preperitoneally and the optic switched into this space

Fig. 7. The sac is reduced (LIH)

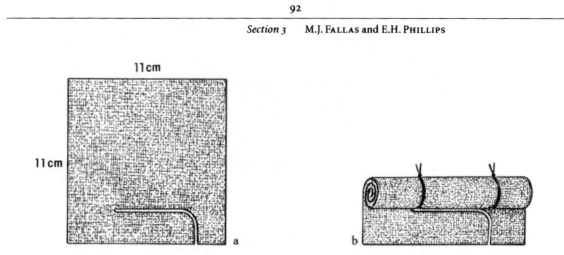

Fig. 8 a, b. Preparation of the mesh (LIH)

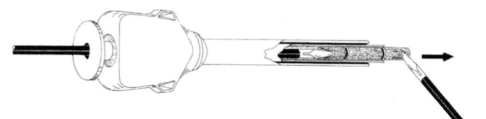
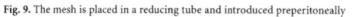

Fig. 9. The mesh is placed in a reducing tube and introduced preperitoneally

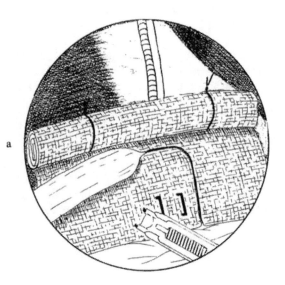

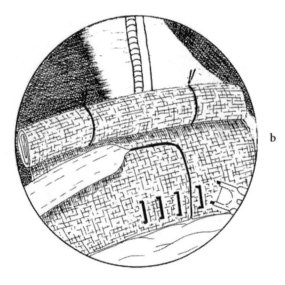

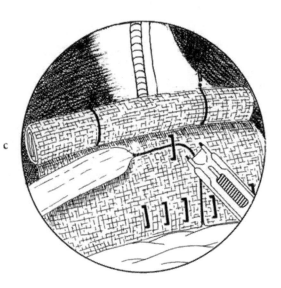

Fig. 10 a–c. The mesh is stapled to Cooper's ligament and the slit is closed (LIH)

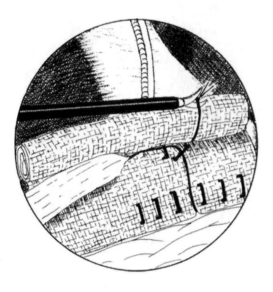

Fig. 11. Sutures are cut (LIH)

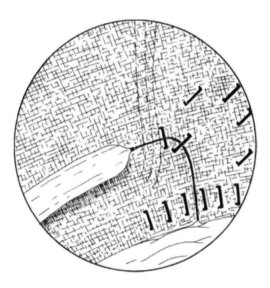

Fig. 12. The mesh is fixed to the abdominal wall (LIH)

Comments

Although there are surgeons who perform the complete preperitoneal approach without peritoneoscopy, we believe that the insertion of a 10 mm 30° angle scope at the umbilicus is helpful in the creation of the preperitoneal space and should not cause significant adhesions. The development of the preperitoneal space without incising the peritoneum is an elegant technique which can certainly be appreciated at the finish of the operation when the scope is reinserted in the peritoneal cavity and the mesh is seen lying smoothly underneath an intact, protective peritoneal lining.

References

Phillips EH, et al (1995) Incidence of complications following laparoscopic hernioplasty. Surg Endosc 9(1):16–21

Phillips EH, et al (1995) Reasons for recurrences following laparoscopic hernioplasty. Surg Endosc (in press)

McKernan JB, Laws H (1992) Laparoscopic preperitoneal prosthetic repair. Surg Rounds 15:597–608

Stoppa RE, Warlamount CR(1989) The preperitoneal approach and prosthetic repair of groin hernia. In: Nyhus LM, Condon RE (eds) Hernia. Lippincott Philadelphia, pp 199–225

Fallas MJ, Phillips EH (1994) Laparoscopic inguinal hernioplasty. Curr Opin Surg 198–202

SECTION 4

17 Thoracoscopic Heller's Myotomy

C.A. PELLEGRINI and M. SINANAN

Introduction

Achalasia of the esophagus is a disease characterized by the lack of peristalsis, the lack of adequate and complete lower esophageal sphincter relaxation, and the presence of high pressure at the lower end of the esophagus. Therapy is directed to decreasing resistance to flow through the sphincter. To a certain degree both pneumatic dilatation and Heller myotomy achieve this effect in the majority of patients, facilitating esophageal emptying. Surgical treatment, however, has an advantage over dilatation: A myotomy performed under direct vision can relieve the obstruction more precisely, more often, and with fewer complications than the blind rupture of the muscle fibers obtained with dilatation.

This chapter describes the technique of thoracoscopic extramucosal esophagomyotomy (Heller's operation), an alternative that appears to provide the same results as those obtained by the open technique but with minimal discomfort.

Preoperative Evaluation

A thorough functional and morphological evaluation of the esophagus must be carried out in all patients to characterize the degree of their disease. An upper gastrointestinal series usually shows a dilated esophagus with bird beak appearance at the distal end. This test provides invaluable information regarding location, shape (particularly useful in patients with sigmoid deformities of the esophagus), and relations of the distal esophagus. Endoscopy is important to rule out a tumor. Esophageal manometry and 24-h pH monitoring should be performed in all patients preoperatively. Manometry typically shows no peristalsis in the esophageal body, a high lower esophageal sphincter pressure, and defective relaxation of the sphincter. Pulmonary function is important to evaluate in older patients and in those with evidence of an associated chronic obstructive lung disease. Finally, antibiotics should be given preoperatively.

Positioning of the Patient and Team

For positioning of the patient and team, see Fig. 1.

Technique

After induction of general endotracheal anesthesia and double lumen tracheal intubation, a fiberoptic endoscope is positioned in the esophagus transorally. This instrument plays a key role during the thoracoscopic Heller myotomy. At the beginning of the procedure it facilitates identification of the esophagus by transillumination; subsequently it helps gauge the depth of penetration of instruments and manipulation of the esophagus. Finally, it allows an accurate assessment of the extent of the myotomy to be performed, as it is possible to gauge the degree of esophageal obstruction remaining: If the myotomy is too short, dysphagia persists; if it is too long (more than 0.5–1.0 cm into the gastric wall), gastroesophageal reflux will occur.

The patient is positioned in the right lateral decubitus (Fig. 1) and five 10- to 11-mm ports are introduced in the left chest (Fig. 2). The first is positioned at the midaxillary line, approximately at the third intercostal space. This is used for retraction of the lung upward. Next, the telescope port is placed as posteriorly as possible, usually about 4 cm behind the posterior axillary line on the sixth or seventh intercostal space. On the same intercostal space but anterior to the axillary line a port is introduced that is used for the instruments of the assistant. Finally, two additional ports for the right and left hand of the surgeon are placed in the posterior axillary line, one on the fifth and one on the seventh or eighth intercostal space. Atmospheric pressure is used in the chest, thus eliminating the need for the use of valves. It also decreases the risk of air embolus.

Exposure commences by upward retraction of the left lung, using a fan-shaped retractor. In articulating this retractor upward, it is important to put the right amount of tension on the inferior pulmonary ligament. The ligament is divided using a hook electrocautery or scissors connected to electrocautery (Fig. 3). Detachment of the ligament from the diaphragm occasionally leads to minor bleeding. Next the mediastinal pleura is divided longitudinally from the pulmonary vein all the way to the diaphragmatic crura. The esophagus is generally easily identified in the groove between the pericardium and the aorta, aided by the transillumination from the endoscope. In some patients the esophagus is displaced to the right, and manipulations with the endoscope may be necessary to bring it into view. Tilting the tip of the esophagoscope (Fig. 4) allows for the wall of the esophagus to be placed into view in the left chest. A point is then identified in the esophageal wall, and a line is marked along the esophagus (this is the myotomy line) using the heel of the electrocautery. Because of the thickness of the muscle of the esophagus, there is little risk of injuring the mucosa at this time.

As soon as this area has been marked, the myotomy must be deepened to get to and through the circular layer of muscle. This is one of the difficult maneuvers in the operation. It is carried out using a 90° angled hook (Fig. 5). The fibers are picked up individually, burning each as far away from the mucosa as possible. Once this maneuver is repeated a few times the mucosa becomes apparent. When extending the myotomy, one can use a bipolar instrument (which lessens the chance of thermal injury to the mucosa) or hook electrocautery. An electrocautery instrument with attached suction and irrigation facilitates the procedure, as it is possible to clear the field immediately and proceed to further coagulation or with the myotomy. As the myotomy is carried downward, it is important to grasp the muscular wall on the assistant's side and use it to pull the esophagus upward (Fig. 5). The surgeon may use the left hand to lower the diaphragm as far as possible, exposing the gastroesophageal junction so that the myotomy can be carried down all the way through it.

The lowest part of the myotomy represents the most delicate part of the procedure. It is also crucial to the outcome. The muscle layers are less clearly identified and the mucosa is thinner, making the risk of perforation higher. The upper part of the myotomy is usually much simpler to perform and probably less important for the result on the average patient with achalasia. On the other hand, in patients with vigorous achalasia or with nutcracker esophagus, in whom the upper extent of the myotomy is important, one can pull the hilum of the lung anteriorly, open the pleura behind it and carry out the myotomy all the way to the aortic arch.

At the completion of the myotomy, it is important to dissect the edges as far as possible, allowing the mucosa to protrude widely and exposing about 40% of its surface (Fig. 6). This avoids premature healing with stricture. This maneuver can be performed in part by gentle insufflation of the esophagus, by moving the esophagoscope laterally and/or by a combination of blunt and sharp dissection.

Finally, the lung is expanded, the chest tube is placed in position, the thoracoports are removed, and the entry sites are closed with single sutures of reabsorbable material.

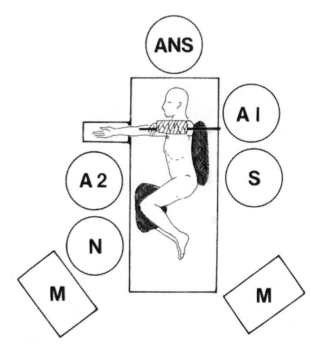

Fig. 1. Positioning of the patient and team. Patient in right lateral decubitus position. *ANS*, Anesthetist; *S*, surgeon; *A1*, *A2*, assistants; *N*, nurse; *M*, monitor

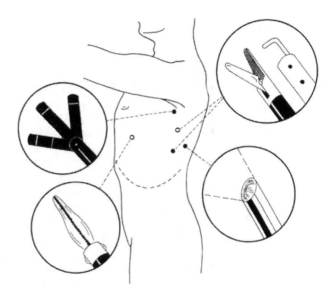

Fig. 2. Schematic representation of port placement and needed instruments

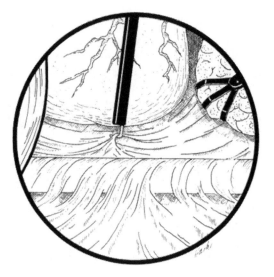

Fig. 3. The inferior pulmonary ligament and mediastinal pleura are divided below the heart and above the aorta to expose the esophagus

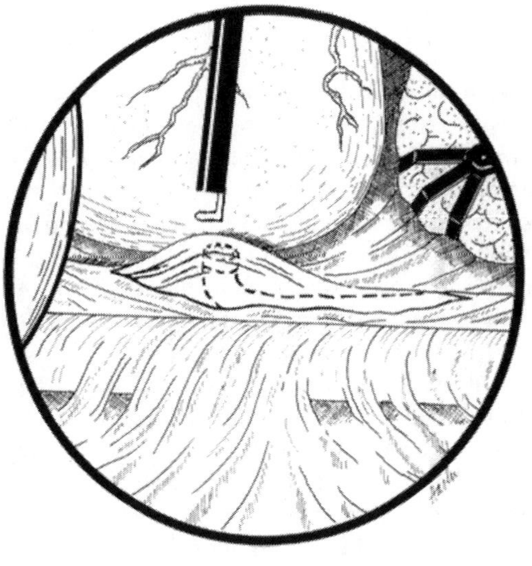

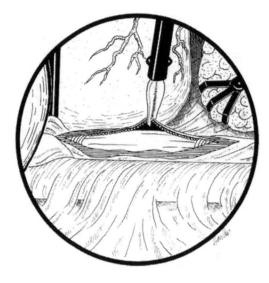

Fig. 4. The esophagus is exposed with the aid of the endoscope and the myotomy site marked with electrocautery

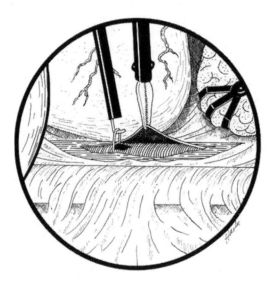

Fig. 5. The circular fibers are individually located, pulled away from the mucosa and burned

Fig. 6. The myotomy is complete

Comments

The main source of postoperative complaint is the chest tube, which is removed in 24 h if possible. Postoperative manometry should be performed whenever possible to determine the level to which resistance has been decreased. In our patients, lower esophageal sphincter pressure decreased from 33.5±7 to 14±5 mmHg. Also, 24-h pH monitoring is extremely important postoperatively, as asymptomatic reflux may occur.

Oral feedings are usually started when the patient feels well enough to tolerate them – usually on the evening of or the day after the operation. Since vomiting early after the operation may be deleterious, it is important to ask the patients how they feel before starting feedings and to recommend prudence for the first few days in the type and amount of food taken, to avoid vomiting. Patients can go home the second postoperative day and return to work within a week.

Complications and Management

The most important and most common complication is laceration of the mucosa. This has occurred in three of our patients, always in the lowermost site of the myotomy at the level of the gastroesophageal junction. The perforation is detected immediately because the esophagus is distended with air during the operation. The perforation is generally very small (1–2 mm). The hole can be closed with one or two stitches of 4-0 absorbable suture. Since the stomach is nearby, the closure may be reinforced with adjacent gastric wall tissue if needed. The first two times that this complication occurred, the chest was opened to permit repair of the mucosa. It is surprising how small a thoracostomy is needed, as the esophagus has been mobilized and the orifice is clearly visible. The hole can be closed using thoracoscopic suturing techniques.

A second possible complication is bleeding on the entry sites (which is bothersome, particularly at the level of the telescope, since blood drips down slowly along the tube and obscures the vision periodically) and on the tissues adjacent to the esophagus. It is best to control bleeding as soon as it is detected, since it tends to obscure the view substantially. On the other hand, when bleeding points are close to the mucosa, patience and gentle pressure is safer than the use of electrocautery. These bleeding points usually stop by themselves, and coagulation in this area may be dangerous, as it may lead to thermal injury to the mucosa. An unrecognized burn to the mucosa may lead to a delayed esophageal perforation. Should this occur, the perforation must be handled as any other perforation of the esophagus.

Residual dysphagia is usually caused by the persistence of a narrowing in the lower part of the esophagus. In these cases the myotomy has not been carried far enough. The endoscopic view of the obstruction allows adequate gauging of the extent of myotomy needed. In fact, the myotomy is continued until it is clear that the obstruction has disappeared.

There is an open question concerning the efficacy of adding an antireflux procedure to the esophagomyotomy. It has been shown that extending the myotomy into the gastric wall for only 0.5 cm reduces the incidence of postoperative gastroesophageal reflux to around 3%. We were, in fact, surprised that of the eight patients in whom 24-h pH monitoring was performed postoperatively, five showed evidence of abnormal reflux. However, despite the lack of peristalsis in the esophageal body, acid reflux was limited to the lower esophagus, suggesting that the volume of refluxate is very low. A longer follow-up in a larger group of patients is necessary to determine whether an antireflux procedure is needed.

References

Csendes A, Braghetto I, Henriques A, Cortes C (1989) Late results of a prospective randomized study comparing forceful dilatation and oesophagomyotomy in patients with achalasia. Gut 30:299–304

Ferguson MK (1991) Achalasia: current evaluation and therapy. Ann Thorac Surg 42:536–542

Pellegrini C, Wetter LA, Patti M et al (1992) Thoracoscopic esophagomyotomy. Initial experience with a new approach for the treatment of achalasia. Ann Surg 216:291–299

Pellegrini CA, Leichter R, Patti M, Somberg K, Ostroff J, Way LW (1993) Thoracoscopic esophageal myotomy in the treatment of achalasia. Ann Thorac Cardiovasc Surg 56:680–682

Shimi S, Nathanson LK, Cuschieri A (1991) Laparoscopic cardiomyotomy for achalasia. J R Coll Surg Edinb 36:152–154

18 Laparoscopic Heller's Myotomy

A.L. De Paula, K. Hashiba, M. Bafutto, and C.A. Machado

Introduction

Esophageal achalasia is a functional disorder characterized by the absence of peristaltic contractions in the esophageal body and failure of complete relaxation of the lower esophageal sphincter in response to swallowing. This disease is relatively frequent in some parts of the world, such as Brazil. It can be primary or idiopathic, or secondary to Chagas' disease, to pseudointestinal obstruction, to surgical trauma, or to neoplasia.

The etiology is still controversial. The main pathological finding is a decreased number or absence of ganglion cells in Auerbach's plexus. Although the etiology of neuronal lesion is unknown, the most frequent mechanisms involved are inflammatory or autoimmune disorders. These histological changes determine major pathophysiological consequences, including uncoordinated peristalsis, esophageal stasis, dilation, and elongation of the esophagus.

Typical symptoms include progressive dysphagia, regurgitation, weight loss, and chest pain. Persistent cough and aspirative pneumonia are frequent findings in more advanced cases. The diagnosis is confirmed by barium contrast radiography of the esophagus, upper digestive endoscopy and manometry.

Since the lesions are not reversible, treatment aims to relieve the main symptom (dysphagia) of the disease. The most important therapeutic options include esophageal dilation and surgical treatment. Forceful dilation produces rupture of the muscular layers of the esophagus. Subsequent dilations are frequent. The overall improvement rate is around 71%. Complications include perforation, aspiration and reflux esophagitis. The first esophageal open myotomy was performed by Heller in 1913. Zaaijer in 1923 popularized a single anterior myotomy. Although some studies favor dilation of the esophagus, the choice for surgical treatment is due to low morbidity and mortality rates, overall successful results in almost 90% of cases, and long-term remission of symptoms.

Minimally invasive surgery is a recent addition to the treatment of esophageal pathologies. It seems to apply all the benefits already demonstrated in cholecystectomy, such as efficacy, minimal postoperative pain, short hospital stay, and early return to normal activities. Esophageal myotomy can be performed with or without fundoplication, through a laparoscopic or a thoracoscopic approach (see chapter 17).

Positioning of the Patient and Team

The procedure is carried out with the patient supine, legs abducted, and reverse Trendelenburg of approximately 30° (Fig. 1). The surgeon stands between the patient's legs, with the first assistant to his right and the second to his left. The video equipment and CO_2 insufflator are placed to the left of the surgeon and the remaining equipment to the right, behind the first assistant.

Technique

A nasogastric tube is placed routinely. The pneumoperitoneum is established after the Veress needle is inserted in the midline, 3–5 cm above the umbilicus. Intra-abdominal pressure of 12 mmHg is maintained. The laparoscope, preferably 30°, is introduced through this midline trocar. The other four trocars are introduced under direct vision and positioned as shown in Fig. 2. The first step is to retract the left liver lobe upward and to the right, with the retractor being introduced through the subxiphoid trocar. Lower traction is applied on the anterior wall of the stomach with grasping forceps introduced through the left subcostal trocar. The phrenoesophageal membrane and peritoneum are divided with scissors, above the hepatic branch of the anterior vagus nerve, as shown in Fig. 3. The right crus and the anterior vagus nerve are then identified (Fig. 4). The distal esophagus is dissected for a distance of about 6 cm above the esophagogastric junction, allowing the identification of the dilated esophagus in the posterior mediastinum.

The short gastric vessels are divided routinely to an extension of approximately 6–10 cm using nonabsorbable clips (Fig. 5). After identifying the dilated esophagus, the anterior vagus nerve, and the esophagogastric junction the myotomy is carried out over the left side of the anterior aspect of the esophagus, beginning at the cardia and extending proximally for approximately 5 cm (Fig. 6). Bleeding is usually self-limited. Use of the cautery should be kept to a minimum.

The myotomy is extended onto the stomach for approximately 1–2 cm (Fig. 6). Scissors, hook, and dissectors are used during the myotomy. In some patients it is necessary to close the crura with nonabsorbable interrupted sutures. Routine partial fundoplication is performed by wrapping the anterior aspect of the gastric fundus over the myotomy with three rows of four to six stitches of nonabsorbable sutures. The first row of suture brings the gastric fundus to the posterior aspect of the esophagus (Fig. 7). The second row brings the gastric fundus to the left side edge of the esophageal myotomy (Fig. 8). The third and last row of sutures covers the exposed mucosa with the gastric fundus to the right-side edge of the myotomy (Fig. 9). In conclusion, this is a partial fundoplication of approximately 180°. In cases of perforation of the esophageal mucosa interrupted stitches of 4-0 Prolene are used.

Preoperative and intraoperative evaluation determine the best approach to be used in patients reoperated after failed surgical treatment. The most common failures are due to incomplete myotomy, in extension and in depth, and scar retraction, especially after esophageal fistula. The alternatives for surgical treatment include extension of the previous myotomy, new myotomy, and eventually esophageal resection.

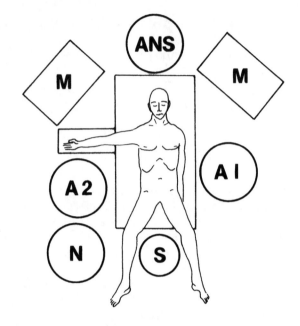

Fig. 1. Positioning of the patient and team. Patient in lithotomy position. *ANS*, Anesthetist; *S*, surgeon; *A1, A2*, assistants; *N*, nurse; *M*, monitor

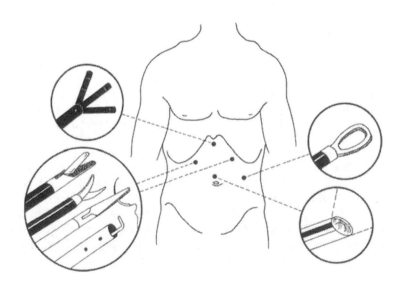

Fig. 2. Trocar sites and instrumentation

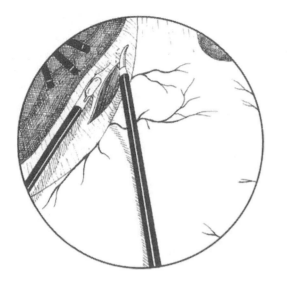

Fig. 3. Dissection of avascular plane

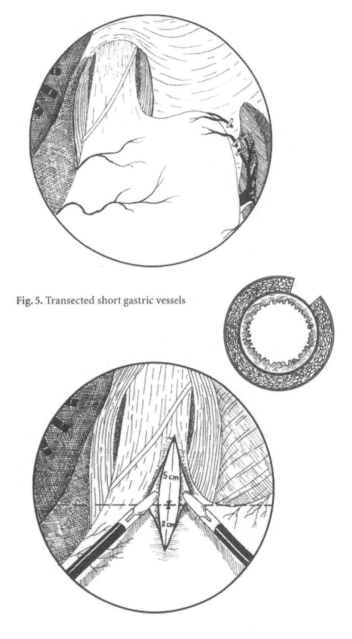

Fig. 5. Transected short gastric vessels

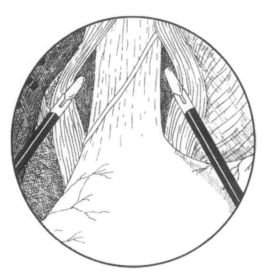

Fig. 4. Dissection of left and right crura

Fig. 6. Anterior seromyotomy

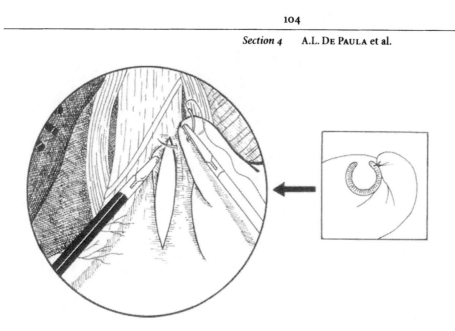

Fig. 7. First layer of gastric fundoplication

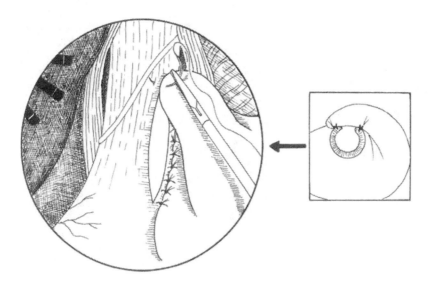

Fig. 8. Second layer of gastric fundoplication

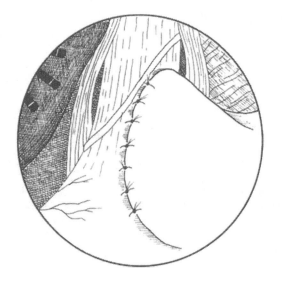

Fig. 9. Completed myotomy with fundoplication

Comments

Esophageal achalasia has been classified as incipient, nonadvanced or advanced, based on barium meal and esophageal manometry. Barium contrast radiography of the esophagus in patients with nonadvanced achalasia demonstrates esophageal dilation, narrowing of the distal esophagus, presence of anomalous contractions, maintenance of the longitudinal axis of the esophagus, and absence of gas bubble in the gastric fundus. Endoscopy revealed esophageal dilation, hyperemia, edema and thickening of the mucosa, especially in the distal esophagus. Manometric evaluation showed the absence of peristaltic contractions, high pressure in the lower esophageal sphincter and failure of complete relaxation of the lower esophageal sphincter in response to swallowing. In advanced achalasia there is a significant dilatation of the esophagus, more than 7 cm air-fluid level and loss of the longitudinal axis, i.e., sigmoid esophagus.

Laparoscopic Heller's myotomy with partial fundoplication is indicated in patients with nonadvanced esophageal achalasia and also in those with failed open or laparoscopic esophageal myotomy. Relative contraindications include patients with previous gastric resection, severe cardiopulmonary and coagulation disorders and concomitant esophageal neoplasia. Patients with sigmoid esophagus are submitted to laparoscopic transhiatal esophagectomy with cervical esophagogastroplasty.

References

Anselmino M, Hinder R, Filipi CJ, Wilson P (1993) Laparoscopic Heller cardiomyotomy and thoracoscopic long myotomy for the treatment of primary esophageal motor disorders. Surg Laparosc Endosc 3(5):437–441

Cohen S, Lipshutz W (1971) Lower oesophageal sphincter dysfunction in achalasia. Gastroenterol 61:814–820

De Paula AL, Hashiba K, Bafutto M (1995) Laparoscopic transhiatal esophagectomy. Surg Laparosc Endosc (in press)

Ellis FH, Kiser JC, Schlegal JF et al (1967) Esophagomyotomy for achalasia: experimental, clinical and manometric aspects. Ann Surg 166:645–648

Ferguson MK (1991) Achalasia: current evaluation and therapy. Ann Thorac Surg 42:536–542

Pellegrini C, Wetter A, Patti M, Leichter R, Mussan G, Mori T, Bernstein G, Way L (1992) Thoracoscopic esophagomyotomy. Initial experience with a new approach for the treatment of achalasia. Ann Surg 216:291–299

19 Thoracoscopic Resection of Esophageal Tumors

A. CUSCHIERI

Introduction

Endoscopic esophagectomy was first reported by Bueß et al. (1990) using a specially designed operating mediastinoscope which enables visually guided perivisceral dissection of the intrathoracic esophagus. This technique is the equivalent of the blunt transhiatal esophagectomy first reported by Turner and popularized by Orringer and others for both benign and malignant disease. Instead of blind mobilization the perivisceral dissection of the esophagus is carried out under visual guidance by the operating mediastinoscope inserted through a cervical exposure along the sternomastoid. Compared to the blunt transhiatal procedure, the mediastinoscopic dissection minimizes the risk of trauma to mediastinal structures, for example, azygos vein, bronchus, and recurrent laryngeal nerve, and reduces blood loss. This technique does not permit the execution of a regional lymphadenectomy and is therefore unsuitable for advanced lesions, which constitute the majority of patients in Western countries. Right thoracoscopic esophagectomy allows dissection of large thoracic esophageal tumors and regional lymphadenectomy that are equivalent in all respects to that achieved by the McKeown procedure. In addition, the dissection of the cervical esophagus is performed largely through the thoracoscopic route.

Positioning of the Patient and Team

For positioning of the patient and team, see Fig. 1.

Technique

The procedure was initially performed through the standard right posterolateral approach, but we have now changed to the prone-posterior thoracoscopic approach (Fig. 1). The operation is conducted in two stages. The thoracoscopic dissection is performed first with the patient in the prone-posterior jackknife position. Once the endoscopic stage is completed, the patient's position is changed for the second stage, which consists of gastric mobilization and cervical pull-through for proximal anastomosis in the neck. The second stage is carried out with the patient in the supine position and requires redraping. Although the second stage can be performed endoscopically, we prefer to conduct it by the open approach through a midline incision, as with the current technology, laparoscopic mobilization of the entire stomach and duodenum with preservation of the right gastroepiploic arcade adds considerably to the operating time.

A flexible endoscope is passed into the esophagus and its end placed just proximal to the upper margin of the tumor (Fig. 3). The endoscope, which is affixed by its handpiece with adhesive tape to a drip stand, is used to lift the esophagus during the dissection. We use purpose-designed curved coaxial and bayonet instruments introduced through reusable metal flexible cannulae and variable curvature shape-memory dissectors and suture/sling passers. Viewing during the operation is by means of the 10.0 mm 30° forward oblique telescope attached to the charge-coupled device camera.

The optical cannula is placed through the second intercostal space encountered below the inferior angle of the scapula (Fig. 2). The flexible operating ports are inserted through the respective intercostal spaces above and below the telescope, some 7.0 cm from the spinous processes. A 10.5- or 12.0-mm cannula is placed medially just lateral to the angle of the rib in the seventh interspace (Fig. 2).

The upper right lobe is displaced medially by a Duval grasper to display the right mediastinum, azygos vein, esophagus, and tumor (Fig. 3). A careful inspection for pleural tumor deposits is conducted. If suspicious lesions are encountered, they are excised and sent for immediate frozen-section histology. The tumor mobility and invasion of surrounding structures are then assessed.

The mediastinal pleura below the azygos vein is divided, and the vein is lifted from the underlying esophagus and root of the right lung (Fig. 4). A few small vessels require individual electrocoagulation before division. The azygos vein is retracted gently downward, and the mediastinal pleura above it is divided with the curved coaxial scissors. This incision is extended proximally to the thoracic inlet along the anterior surface of the esophagus lateral to the trachea. The fully mobilized azygos vein is ligated or stapled with the endovascular cutter (Fig. 4). Our preference is for ligature using 1-0 permanent suture mounted on a push rod and the Tayside external slip knot. The first ligature is placed medially as close to the vena cava as is possible, and the second ligature laterally near the chest wall. A large atraumatic forceps is placed on the medial end of the vein before this is divided with scissors. The grasper is released slowly and is reapplied immediately in the event of hemorrhage.

The flexible endoscope is withdrawn above the mobilized azygos vein and flexed forward with lateral rotation to expose the anteromedial wall of the gullet in the superior mediastinum. The dissection plane is between the esophagus laterally and the superior vena cava and trachea medially (Fig. 5). The right vagal trunk is identified before it gives the pulmonary branches and is divided below the origin of the recurrent laryngeal nerve. Any nodes encountered in the groove between the esophagus and lower trachea are dissected and removed separately. The lateral aspect of the proximal thoracic esophagus is esposed by forward lift and medial deflection of the gullet by the endoscope. On completion of the lateral dissection the separation of the remaining posterior attachment is aided considerably by the use of the variable curvature superelastic dissector or coaxial curved duckbill forceps.

A vascular silicon sling loaded on the 3.0-mm needle holder is introduced into the right chest and passed around the mobilized esophagus (Fig. 4). The internal end of the sling is then regrasped and exteriorized through the same stab wound in the chest wall. Traction applied to the external limbs of the sling lifts the posterior surface of the proximal thoracic esophagus from the superior mediastinum. The dissection of the cervical esophagus is also guided by the flexible endoscope. Blunt dissection (suction probe, pledget, or ultrasonic) is used to mobilize the gullet beyond the thoracic inlet distal to the tip of the endoscope. As the cervical dissection proceeds, the endoscope is withdrawn further up, and the process continued inside the root of the neck up to the level of the thyroid lobes. The dissection plane is on the prevertebral fascia posteriorly, the trachea anteriorly, and the recurrent laryngeal nerves and inferior thyroid arteries laterally.

The endoscope is advanced below the level of the azygos vein for dissection of the middle esophagus (Fig. 6). A sizeable direct arteriole which requires clipping or ligature is often encountered during separation of the esophagus from the aorta. On the medial side the tracheal bifurcation is separated from the pericardium preferably with a two-handed technique using the curved coaxial scissors and the duckbill insulated grasper. The subcarinal lymph nodes and the esophageal nodes are dissected and removed with the tumor or separately. On the medial side the esophagus is separated from the pericardium. Posteriorly the dissection is taken down to the left pleura, which is left intact unless it is involved or adherent when the affected area is cut and removed with the tumor.

The mobilization of the lower third of the esophagus poses no technical problems. The inferior pulmonary ligament is divided with scissors after electrocoagulation. Lymph nodes surrounding the esophagus are included in the dissection, which is continued until the diaphragmatic hiatus is reached.

Two underwater seal drains are inserted (apical and basal). The ports are removed under vision, and the lung is expanded. The patient is then turned to the supine position for the second stage of the operation.

The cervical and abdominal procedures are conducted synchronously by two operating teams. The carotid sheath is retracted laterally after division of the skin, platysma, investing layer of the deep cervical fascia, and omohyoid. Following division of its middle vein the thyroid lobe is lifted up, and the esophagus and at least one recurrent laryngeal nerve are identified. Very little if any further mobilization of the cervical esophagus is usually needed.

The duodenum, stomach, and abdominal esophagus are mobilized using the orthodox technique with preservation of the right gastroepiploic arcade and ligature of the left gastric artery at its origin from the celiac and with removal of the related lymph nodes. Pyloroplasty is not performed unless duodenal scarring is present. However, the right crus of the diaphragm is divided at its origin.

On completion of the esophagogastric transection the cervical esophagus is lifted into the neck wound and stapled. The end of a size 16 Ryle's tube is next anchored by transfixation to the esophagus distal to the staple line, and the gullet is transected above this level. The esophagus and tumor are then delivered through the abdominal wound. The gastric fundus is stitched to the end of the Ryle's tube, which is then used to railroad the gastric tube to the neck. The anastomosis between the cervical esophagus and the fundus is performed using a single layer all coats technique. A nasogastric tube is passed before the anterior wall of the anastomosis is completed, and its tip is placed in the intrathoracic stomach above the diaphragm. A Redivac drain leading to the anastomosis is inserted, and the cervical and abdominal wounds are closed.

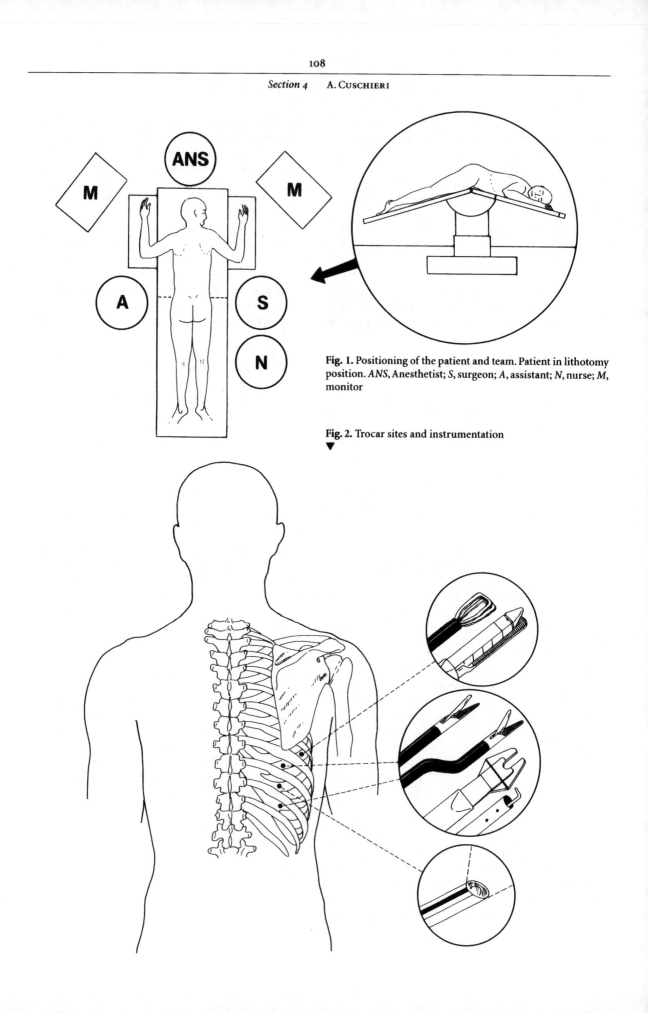

Fig. 1. Positioning of the patient and team. Patient in lithotomy position. *ANS*, Anesthetist; *S*, surgeon; *A*, assistant; *N*, nurse; *M*, monitor

Fig. 2. Trocar sites and instrumentation

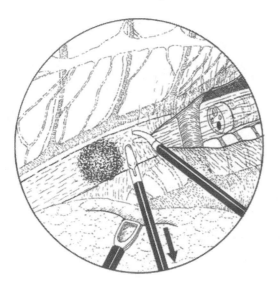

Fig. 3. Dissection of the visceral pleura

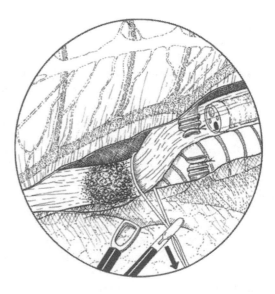

Fig. 4. Dissection and division of the azygos vein and proximal esophagus

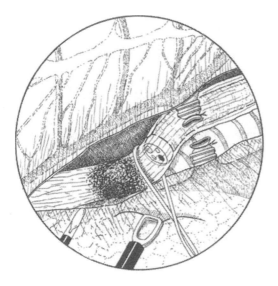

Fig. 5. The gastroscope is advanced and the middle portion of the esophagus dissected

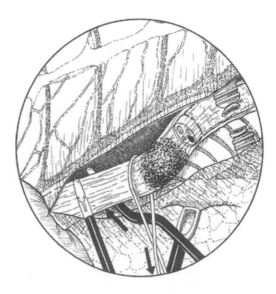

Fig. 6. Dissection of the distal portion of the esophagus

Comments

All patients undergo preoperative investigation with contrast barium series, endoscopy and biopsy, computed tomography of the chest and abdomen, and a staging laparoscopy. From the management standpoint it is important to distinguish patients with esophageal tumors (lower and middle third) from those with neoplasms involving the esophagogastric junction. This distinction is established with certainty by endoscopy and laparoscopy. In tumors confined to the esophagus the primary lesion should not be visible at laparoscopy, and the esophagogastric junction feels soft on palpation. During the laparoscopic staging particular attention is directed to the state of the left gastric and celiac lymph nodes. These can be visualized by division of the pars flaccida of the lesser omentum with retraction of the lesser curvature of the stomach downward and to the left. These nodes when enlarged should be biopsied, and if the histology confirms metastatic disease, radical node clearance down to the celiac trifurcation is necessary. Although this is possible laparoscopically, it is technically difficult and may require a small midline laparotomy.

It is our practice to perform thoracoscopic subtotal esophagectomy with gastric pull-through and cervical anastomosis for all esophageal tumors irrespective of histology (squamous or adenocarcinoma). For tumors of the esophagogastric junction we perform the endoscopic equivalent of the Lewis-Tanner operation with resection of the lower third of the esophagus and proximal stomach and intrathoracic esophagogastric anastomosis.

Results

In a consecutive series of 36 patients with esophageal cancer two were found to have hepatic deposits at laparoscopy, and six were inoperable at thoracoscopic staging. A further two patients had dense fibrous obliteration of the pleural cavity which precluded the endoscopic dissection. The first 20 procedures were conducted through the posterolateral right thoracoscopic approach, with one conversion due to aortic bleeding. The remainder have been performed through the prone-posterior jackknife route, which is now our favored approach for subtotal esophagectomy as it avoids the need for single lung anesthesia and provides excellent exposure of the esophagus and the mediastinum. The postoperative complications encountered in the series included postoperative pneumonic consolidation ($n = 3$), recurrent laryngeal palsy ($n = 2$) and one anastomotic leak. The recurrent laryngeal palsies occurred early on in the series and were probably caused by collateral damage from electrocoagulation near the thoracic inlet. No significant pulmonary complications have been observed in the patients in whom the esophagectomy was conducted by the prone-posterior jackknife approach. There were no postoperative deaths in the entire series. The median postoperative stay has been 12 days (range 9–30). The patients undergoing the endoscopic Lewis-Tanner operation ($n = 4$) for tumors of the esophagogastric junction have done remarkably well, with rapid recovery, no morbidity, and discharge from the hospital within 10 days.

References

Bueß G, Kipfmüller K, Nahrun M, Melzer A (1990) Endoskopische-mikrochirurgische dissektion des ösophagus. In: Bueß G (ed) Endoskopie. Deutscher Ärzte, Cologne, pp 358–375

Cuschieri A (1992) Endoscopic subtotal oesophagectomy for cancer through a right thoracoscopic approach. Surg Oncol 1993 2:3–11

Cuschieri A, Shimi S, Banting S (1992) Endoscopic oesophagectomy through a right thoracoscopic approach. J R Coll Surg Edinb 37:7–11

Cuschieri A (1994) Thoracoscopic subtotal oesophagectomy. Surg Endosc 2(1):21–25

Orringer MB (1987) Transthoracic versus transhiatal esophagectomy: what difference does it make? Ann Thorac Surg 44(2):116–118

Turner GC (1993) Excision of the thoracic oesophagus for carcinoma with reconstruction of an extra-thoracic gullet. Lancet II:1315–1317

20 Endoscopic Lewis-Tanner Esophagogastrectomy for Tumors of the Esophagogastric Junction

A. Cuschieri

Introduction

The procedure is conducted in two stages: (a) laparoscopic mobilization of the proximal stomach and lower esophagus and (b) thoracoscopic mobilization of the esophagus up to the level of the azygos with resection of the lower esophagus and upper stomach and an intrathoracic anastomosis. This step of the operation necessitates a small (5.0-cm) access thoracotomy.

Positioning of the Patient and Team

For positioning of the patient and team, see Fig. 1.

Technique

The patient in the lithotomy position (Fig. 1). The technique requires five ports. The optical cannula is placed to the left of the umbilicus. An upper right subcostal port is used for retraction of the liver. The two operating cannulae (flexible for curved coaxial instruments) are positioned in the left flank below the costal margin and to the right of the midline halfway between the xiphoid and the umbilicus. The fifth cannula (for an endovascular stapler) is placed in the upper part of the right lower quadrant. A 30° telescope is necessary, and the curved coaxial instruments greatly facilitate the procedure (Fig. 2).

The first step consists of identifying a lateral avascular window below the greater curvature of the stomach on the left side. This window is opened by scissors. A curved coaxial duckbill grasper is passed into the lesser sac and used to elevate the short gastric pedicle. Adhesions binding the latter to the stomach are divided. The tip of the curved coaxial grasper is used to find a more proximal avascular window. This is tented up for inspection and then perforated by the curved forceps. A second curved grasper is then passed alongside the first and the two separated to create a sufficient space for the insertion of the endovascular stapler (vascular cartridge) (Fig. 3). The stapler limbs are applied as close to the spleen as possible and then fired to secure and divide the short gastric vessels. The upper short gastric vessels, including a branch from the inferior phrenic artery, are best ligated by external slip knots. The lesser omentum is then divided from the esophagus as far as the right gastric artery. The stomach is elevated to expose the left gastric artery and vein. These are mobilized together below the nodal mass using the curved coaxial scissors and the variable curvature superelastic dissector (Storz, Tuttlingen, Germany). We prefer to ligate the left gastric vessels doubly with the Tayside slip knot using permanent suture but the endovascular cutter can be used instead (Fig. 5). The mobilization of the abdominal esophagus entails division of the peritoneal fold extending from the gullet to the diaphragm and separation of the posterior fixation of the fundus and esophagogastric junction (Fig. 6). The division of the phrenoesophageal membrane exposes the loose mediastinal areolar tissue. The mobilization of the lower esophagus is continued until the upper limit of the tumor is reached (Fig. 6).

Thoracoscopic Stage. The patient is turned to the right posterolateral or, preferably, the posterior prone jackknife position for this stage. The dissection of the thoracic esophagus from the level of the azygos is identical to that described previously (chapter 19) and uses the same access ports. On completion of the mobilization the stomach is pulled into the right chest by traction of the esophagus. A 5.0- to 6.0-cm posterior access thoracotomy is made starting at the angle of the fifth or sixth rib. After elevation of the periosteum the rib is cut at either end of the wound, and a self-retaining laminectomy-type retractor is used to distract the wound edges. A noncrushing clamp is placed on the proximal esophagus (at the level of the azygos vein).

Resection and Intrathoracic Anastomosis. The stomach is stapled obliquely from the lesser curvature toward the fundus at least 2 cm below the lower margin of the tumor. The esophagus is then divided 2 cm below the occluding clamp, and the specimen is removed through the access thoracotomy after appropriate barrier protection of the wound edges. The anastomosis can be effected by hand suture using a single layer technique with continuous posterior suture line and interrupted sutures

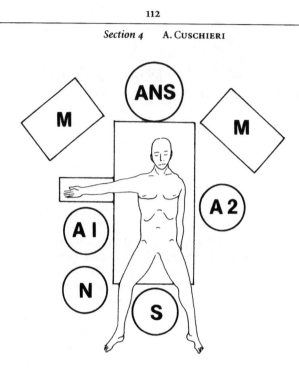

Fig. 1. Positioning of the patient and team. Patient in lithotomy position. *ANS*, Anesthetist; *S*, surgeon; *A1, A2*, assistants; *N*, nurse; *M*, monitor

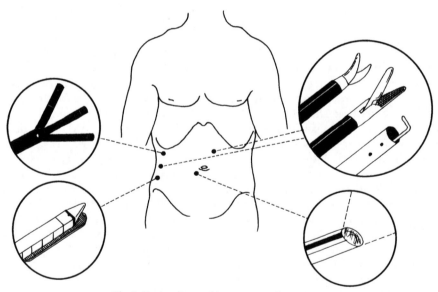

Fig. 2. Trocar sites and instrumentation

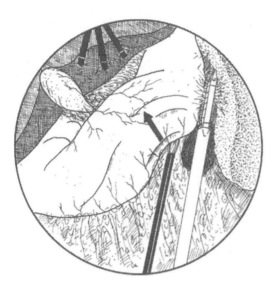

Fig. 3. Division of short gastric vessels

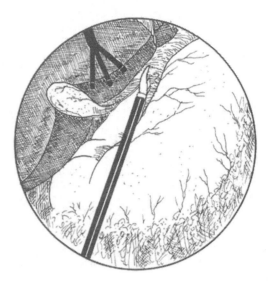

Fig. 4. Dissection of pars flaccida at the lesser curve

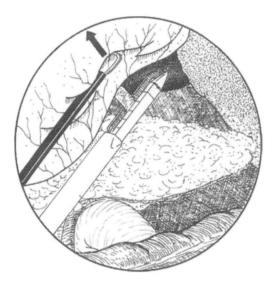

Fig. 5. Division of left gastric artery

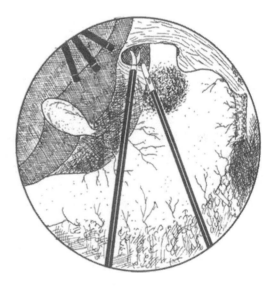

Fig. 6. Dissection of the hiatus

anteriorly. Currently we are evaluating the long flexible stapler which is introduced through the mouth and has a 27-mm stapler head.

References

Godfaden D, Orringer MB, Appelman HD, Kalish R (1986) Adenocarcinoma of the distal esophagus and gastric cardia. Comparison of transhiatal esophagectomy and thoracoabdominal esophagectomy. J Thorac Cardiovasc Surg 91:242–247

McKeown KC (1976) Total three stage oesophagectomy for cancer of the oesophagus. Br J Surg 63:259–262

Lewis I (1946) The surgical treatment of carcinoma of the oesophagus with special reference to a new operation for growths of the middle third. Br J Surg 34:18–31

Tanner NC (1947) The present position of carcinoma of the oesophagus. Postgrad Med J 23:109–139

Stewart JR, Sarr MG, Sharp KW, Efron G et al (1985) Transhiatal (blunt) esophagectomy for malignant and benign esophageal disease: clinical experience and technique. Ann Thorac Surg 40:343–348

21 Laparoscopic Nissen's Fundoplication

J.H. PETERS

Introduction

Gastroesophageal reflux is a common disease that accounts for approximately 75% of esophageal pathology. Motility abnormalities of the esophagus and stomach, including an incompetent lower esophageal sphincter, are responsible for pathologic reflux in the majority of patients. Surgical treatment offers the only chance of long-term cure. Given a precise diagnosis, careful patient selection, critical attention to detail in the perioperative period, and the meticulous performance of the appropriate antireflux procedure, long-term success can be assured in over 90% of patients.

Positioning of the Patient and Team

Failure to position the patient properly or random placement of abdominal trocars can render the procedure difficult or impossible to perform safely. The patient should be placed supine, in a modified lithotomy position, with the table elevated 30°–45° (Fig. 1). The knees should be only slightly flexed. Having the legs sharply flexed at the knees interferes with the instruments during the course of the procedure. The esophageal hiatus is a midline structure; thus the surgeon, working with both hands, is best positioned between the patient's legs, allowing the right- and left-sided instruments to approach the hiatus from the respective upper abdominal quadrants (Fig. 2). A heads-up position is used to displace the transverse colon and small bowel inferiorly, keeping them from obstructing the view of the video camera.

Technique

Five 10- to 11-mm ports are utilized. The laparoscope is placed above the umbilicus, one-third of the distance to the xiphoid process (Fig. 3). In most patients placement of the laparoscope in the umbilicus does not allow adequate visualization of the hiatal structures once dissected. Two lateral retracting ports are placed in the right and left anterior axillary lines, respectively. The right-sided liver retractor is best placed immediately subcostal in the right anterior axillary line. This allows an acute angle toward the left lateral segment of the liver and thus the ability to push the instrument toward the operating table, lifting the liver. A second retraction port is placed at the level of the umbilicus, in the left anterior axillary line. The surgeon's right- and left-handed trocars are placed in the right and left midclavicular lines, 2 in. below the costal margin. Placing the surgeon's trocars on either side of the midline allows triangulation between the camera and the instruments, avoiding the difficulty associated with the instruments being in direct line with the camera. The falciform ligament hangs low in many patients and provides a barrier around which the left-handed instrument must be manipulated. Most recently we have placed a 12-mm trocar in the left midclavicular position to allow the use of an endovascular cutter during short gastric division.

One of the most important and occasionally the most difficult elements of laparoscopic surgery is adequate retraction and exposure of the structures necessary to complete the procedure safely. Laparoscopic fundoplication begins with exposure of the esophageal hiatus. A fan retractor is placed into the right anterior axillary port and positioned to hold the left lateral segment of the liver toward the anterior abdominal wall. We prefer to utilize a table retractor to hold this instrument once properly positioned. Trauma to the liver should be meticulously avoided because subsequent bleeding obscures the field. Mobilization of the left lateral segment by division of the triangular ligament is not necessary.

A Babcock clamp is placed into the left anterior axillary port and the stomach is retracted toward the patient's feet. This maneuver exposes the esophageal hiatus (Fig. 4). Commonly a hiatal hernia does need to be reduced. An atraumatic clamp should be used and care taken not to grasp the stomach too vigorously as gastric perforations can occur.

The key to the hiatal dissection is identification of the right crus. Metzenbaum-type scissors and fine grasping forceps are preferred for dissection. In all except the most obese patients there is a very thin portion of the gastrohepatic omentum overlying the caudate lobe of the liver. Dissection is begun by incision of this portion of the gastrohepatic omentum above the hepatic branches of the vagal nerves (Fig. 5 a). A replaced left hepatic artery arising from the left gastric artery is present in up to 25% of patients and should be sought and avoided. Once the gastrohepatic omentum is opened, the outside of the right crus becomes evident. The peritoneum overlying the anterior aspect of the right crus is incised with scissors and electrocautery (Fig. 5 b). The medial portion of the right crus leading into the mediastinum is developed by blunt dissection with both instruments. At this juncture the esophagus usually becomes evident. The right crus is retracted laterally and the esophagus identified. The posterior or right vagus is identified and dissected away from the esophagus for a distance of several centimeters (Fig. 5 c). Unipolar electrocautery can injure the nerve during this dissection. The anterior or left vagus is left in place.

Meticulous hemostasis is critical. Blood and fluid tends to pool in the hiatus and is difficult to remove. Irrigation should be kept to a minimum. Care must be taken not to injure the phrenic artery and vein as they course above the hiatus. Once the right crus is identified, the dissection is carried inferiorly and laterally, exposing the medial and lateral aspects of the right crus as well as the anterior aspect of the left crus (Fig. 6 a). A blunt-tipped grasper is placed within the esophageal hiatus laterally or anteriorly to facilitate exposure. A large hiatal hernia often makes this portion of the procedure easier as it accentuates the diaphragmatic crura. At times, dissection of a large mediastinal hernia sac can be difficult.

Following dissection of the right crus attention is turned toward the angle of His and a complete dissection of the lateral aspect of the left crus and fundus of the stomach. This dissection is the key maneuver, allowing circumferential mobilization of the esophagus. Failure to do so results in difficulty encircling the esophagus, particularly if approached from the right. The lateral and anterior aspects of the left crus are dissected, followed by division of the attachments of the fundus to the diaphragm. Repositioning of the Babcock retractor toward the fundic side of the stomach facilitates retraction for this portion of the procedure.

The esophagus is mobilized by careful dissection of the anterior and posterior soft tissues within the hiatus. This can be the most difficult aspect of laparoscopic antireflux surgery, largely because the instruments are angled cephalad into the mediastinum and not toward the right or left. Circumferential dissection of the esophagus is further hampered by the limited exposure of the laparoscopic procedure. Gentle blunt dissection from both right and left is necessary. From the patient's right side the esophagus should be retracted anteriorly with the surgeon's right-hand instrument, allowing posterior dissection with the left hand, and vice versa for the left-

sided dissection (Fig. 6 b). Esophageal dissection may be particularly difficult in the presence of severe esophagitis and transmural inflammation with or without esophageal shortening. Following dissection a grasper is placed via the surgeon's left-handed port behind the esophagus and over the left crus, and a Penrose drain placed around the esophagus to facilitate crural closure and the fundoplication.

The crura are dissected inferiorly for a distance of 2–3 cm. The esophagus is held anterior and to the left and the crura approximated with three to four interrupted 0 silk sutures, staying above the aortic decussation and working anterior (Fig. 7). Because space is limited, it is necessary to use the surgeon's left-handed instrument as a retractor, facilitating placement of single bites through each crus with the surgeon's right hand. Extracorporeal knot tying using a standard knot pusher is preferred, although tying within the abdomen is perfectly appropriate (Fig. 8).

Complete fundic mobilization allows construction of a tension-free physiologic fundoplication. Removal of the liver retractor and placement of a second Babcock forceps through the right anterior axillary port facilitates retraction during division of the short gastric vessels. The gastrosplenic omentum is suspended anteroposteriorly in a clothesline fashion via both Babcock forceps and the lesser sac entered approximately one-third the distance down the greater curvature of the stomach. Short gastric vessels are sequentially dissected, doubly clipped, and divided (Fig. 9). An anterior-posterior rather than medial to lateral orientation of the vessels is preferred, with the exception of those close to the spleen. With caution and meticulous dissection the fundus can be completely mobilized in most patients.

Following complete mobilization of the fundus a Babcock clamp is placed through the surgeon's left-handed port, passed behind the esophagus, and the posterior wall of the fundus grasped (Fig. 10 a). It is then gently brought behind the esophagus to the right side (Fig. 10 b). The anterior wall of the fundus is brought anterior to the esophagus above the supporting Penrose drain. Both posterior and anterior fundic lips are manipulated to allow the fundus to envelope the esophagus without twisting. The laparoscopic visualization tends to exaggerate the size of the posterior opening that has been dissected. Consequently the space for the passage of the fundus behind the esophagus may be tighter than thought and the fundus relatively ischemic when brought around. If the right portion of the fundoplication has a bluish discoloration, the stomach should be returned to its original position and the posterior dissection enlarged. Once adequately placed, both lips of the fundoplication are released, which then frees the surgeon's left and right hand for suturing. Tension on the fundoplication should be avoided. Excess tension encourages the fundoplication to slip back to the left side when freed.

A 60-F bougie is passed to properly size the fundoplication, and it is sutured utilizing a single U-stitch of 2-0 Prolene buttressed with felt pledgets (Fig. 11). The most common error is an attempt to grasp the anterior portion of the stomach to construct the fundoplication rather than the posterior fundus. The esophagus should comfortably lie in the untwisted fundus prior to suturing. Two anchoring sutures of 3-0 silk are placed above and below the U-stitch to complete the fundoplication (Fig. 12). The abdomen is irrigated, hemostasis assured, and the bougie replaced with a nasogastric tube prior to completion of the procedure. Failure of the nasogastric tube to pass easily into the stomach indicates a potential obstruction at the cardia and should be investigated.

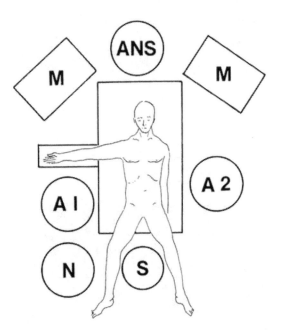

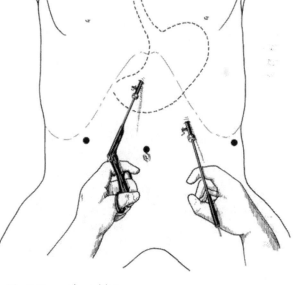

Fig. 1. Positioning of the patient and team. Patient in lithotomy position. *ANS*, Anesthetist; *S*, surgeon; *A1, A2*, assistant; *N*, nurse; *M*, monitor

Fig. 2. Surgeon's position

Fig. 3. Trocar sites and instrumentation
▼

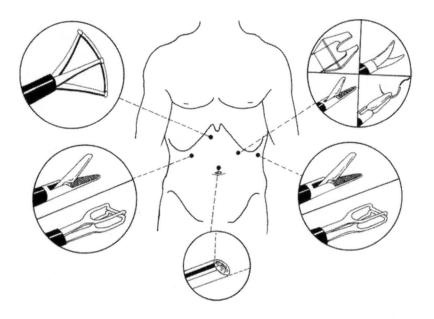

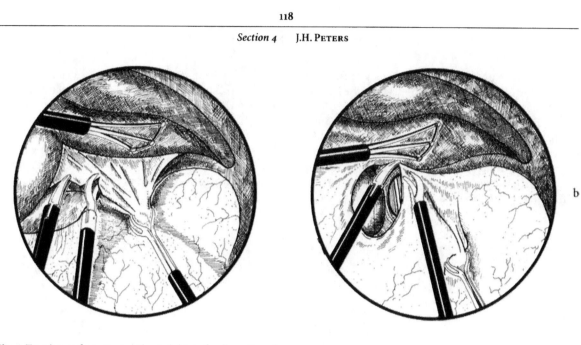

Fig. 4. Traction and countertraction to initiate the dissection of the gastroesophageal junction

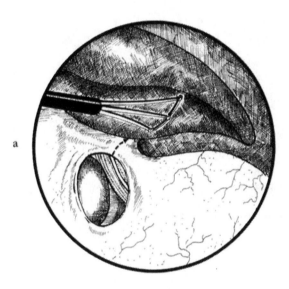

Fig. 5 a–c. Dissection of the diaphragmatic crura. The right and left crura are dissected first anteriorly and then posterior- ly with manipulation of the esophagus via the Babcock clamp on the gastroesophageal fat pad

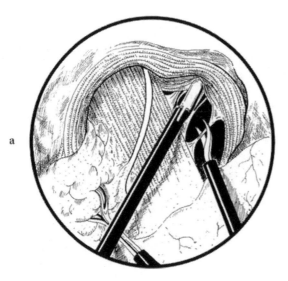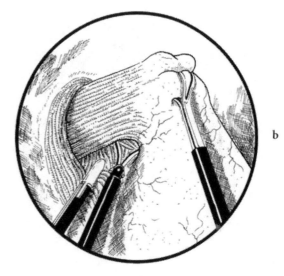

a

b

Fig. 6 a, b. Initial retraction for exposure of the esophageal hiatus. A fan retractor is placed below the left lateral segment of the liver to retract it anteriorly. A Babcock clamp is placed on the esophageal fat pad and retracted toward the patient's feet to expose the phrenoesophageal membrane

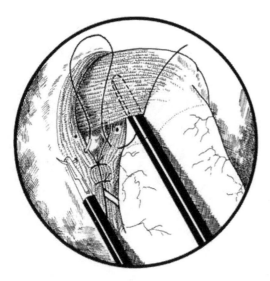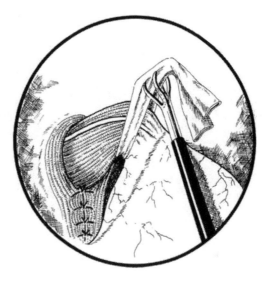

Fig. 7. Closure of the diaphragmatic crura. The esophagus is displaced anteriorly and to the left and three to four sutures of 2-0 silk are placed to approximate the crura

Fig. 8. The GE-Junction is being retracted with a Penrose drain showing the sutured hiatus

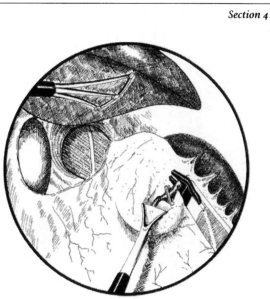

Fig. 9. Division of short gastric vessels

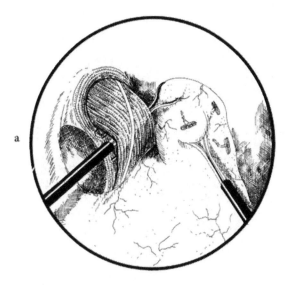

Fig. 10 a, b. Creation of the fundoplication. A Babcock clamp is placed behind the esophagus, and the posterior fundus of the stomach is grasped and brought to the right. Careful attention must be paid to grasping the posterior portion of the stomach and not the anterior wall to avoid twisting of the stomach

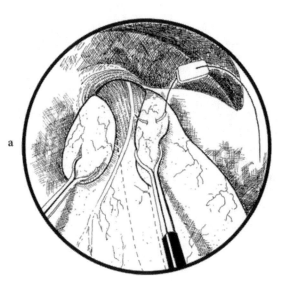

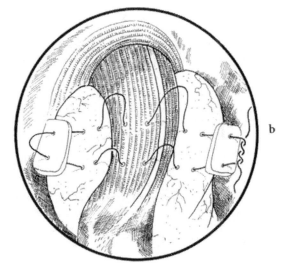

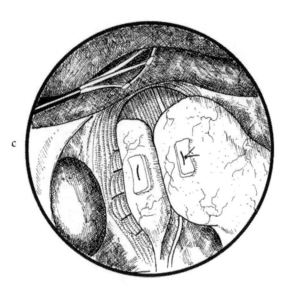

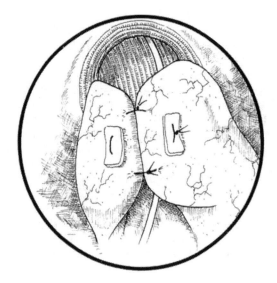

Fig. 11 a–c. Fixation of the fundoplication. The fundoplication is sutured in place with a single U-stitch of 2-0 Prolene pledgeted on the outside. A 60-F mercury-weighted bougie is passed through the gastroesophageal junction prior to fixation of the wrap to assure a floppy fundoplication

Fig. 12. Gastroesophageal junction after finishing the fundoplication

Comments

Preoperative Studies. Prior to proceeding with an antireflux procedure it is necessary to confirm that the patients' symptoms are caused by increased esophageal exposure to gastric juice secondary to a mechanically defective lower esophageal sphincter. All patients considered for surgery require esophageal function studies, i.e., 24-h esophageal pH monitoring and esophageal manometry. Esophageal function studies should be carried out if the patient has persistent symptoms or unimproved esophageal mucosal injury after 8–12 weeks of acid suppression therapy. Patients who respond to a course of medical therapy but have recurrence of symptoms within 4 weeks after cessation of therapy should also be studied since they are prone to drug dependency.

Indications for Surgery. The indications to proceed with an antireflux procedure in a patient managed as outlined above are: (a) persistent or recurrent symptoms and/or complications after 8–12 weeks of intensive acid suppression therapy, (b) increased esophageal exposure to gastric juice on 24-h esophageal pH monitoring, and (c) documentation of a mechanically defective lower esophageal sphincter on manometry. The presence of endoscopic esophagitis in a symptomatic patient with a mechanically defective lower esophageal sphincter should raise the question of surgical therapy since these patients are prone to relapse of their symptoms while on medical therapy. If the patient responds symptomatically to medical therapy, but endoscopic esophagitis persists, surgery should be performed. The reason is that these patients can still progress to develop a stricture or Barrett's esophagus while on therapy because reflux of gastric contents continues through a mechanically defective sphincter. In this situation an antireflux procedure corrects the mechanically defective sphincter, prevents formation of a stricture or Barrett's esophagus, and heals the esophagitis.

Barrett's columnar-lined esophagus is almost always associated with a severe mechanical defect of the lower esophageal sphincter. Patients with Barrett's esophagus are at risk of progression of the mucosal abnormality up the esophagus, formation of a stricture, hemorrhage from a Barrett's ulcer, and the development of an adenocarcinoma. A surgical antireflux procedure can arrest the progression of the disease, heal ulceration, and prevent restricturing.

Chronic atypical symptoms of reflux, for example, chest pain, chronic cough, recurrent pneumonias, episodes of nocturnal choking, waking up with gastric contents in the mouth, or spoilage of the bed pillow, may also indicate the need for surgical therapy.

Dysphagia, regurgitation, or chest pain on eating may also be indications for an antireflux procedure. Such symptoms are usually related to the presence of a paraesophageal hernia, intrathoracic stomach, a small hiatal hernia with a Schatzki ring, or a narrow diaphragmatic hiatus.

References

Dallegmane B (1991) Laparoscopic Nissen fundoplication: preliminary report. Surg Laparosc Endosc 1(3):138–143

DeMeester TR, Bonavina L, Albertuci M (1986) Nissen fundoplication for gastroesophageal reflux disease – evaluation of primary repair in 100 consecutive patients. Ann Surg 204:9–20

Hinder RA, Filipi CJ (1992) The technique of laparoscopic Nissen fundoplication. Surg Laparosc Endosc 2:265

Peters JH, DeMeester TR (1993) The esophagus. Schwartz. Principles of Surgery, 6th edn. Mosby, St. Louis, pp 1043–1122

Peters JH, DeMeester TR (1993) Gastroesophageal reflux. Surg Clin North Am 73:1119–1122

Bagnato VJ (1992) Laparoscopic Nissen fundoplication. Surg Laparosc Endosc 2(3):188–190

Spechler SJ, Department of Veterans Affairs Gastroesophageal Reflux Disease Study Group (1992) Comparison of medical and surgical therapy for complicated gastroesophageal reflux disease in veterans. N Engl J Med 326:786–792

SECTION 5

22 Laparoscopic Gastrostomy

Q.-Y. Duh and L.W. Way

Introduction

Laparoscopic gastrostomy is usually indicated in patients with malnutrition or potential malnutrition who have a functioning gut. Most are patients with neurologic deficit due to stroke or patients with cancer. In general, enteral feeding is preferred over parenteral feeding because it is cheaper and causes fewer complications. Gastrostomy is easier to use than jejunostomy because the catheter has a larger lumen, and the stomach is a reservoir for bolus feeding. Some patients may need gastrostomy to decompress a chronically nonfunctioning stomach. Percutaneous endoscopic gastrostomy is the preferred method for placing gastrostomy in most institutions because it is effective and safe and can be placed under local anesthesia. In about 10% of these patients, however, percutaneous endoscopic gastrostomy is not possible because of esophageal obstruction, poor transillumination, or prior major abdominal operations. These patients are candidates for laparoscopic gastrostomy.

Positioning of the Patient and Team

The patient is in the supine-reverse Trendelenburg position (Fig. 1). The surgeon stands on the right side of the patient in line with the view of the laparoscope toward the left upper quadrant of the abdomen. The monitor is placed in the direction of the patient's left shoulder. The setup is the same as that for a diagnostic laparoscopy. This includes a trocar, a 30° scope, camera, light source, and CO_2 insufflator. We use a commercial kit (18-F Flexiflo Lap G kit; Ross Laboratories, Columbus, OH) for laparoscopic gastrostomy. The patient is placed in the reverse Trendelenburg position, head up-feet down, to allow the stomach to reach lower in the abdomen and allow gravity to keep the small bowel, colon, and omentum away from the field.

Technique

Laparoscopic gastrostomy can be performed under local anesthesia and intravenous sedation. Some patients tolerate local anesthesia poorly and require general anesthesia. We routinely give a dose of a first-generation cephalosporin for prophylaxis against wound infection. The bladder should be emptied by voiding before the procedure or by placing a Foley catheter. A nasogastric or orogastric tube is useful. This helps to decompress the stomach during trocar placement and to insufflate the stomach during placement of the T-fasteners and gastrostomy catheter. Without gastric insufflation a grasper through a second port is usually required to retract the stomach.

A subumbilical port (Fig. 2) is placed either by the open technique, using a 10 mm Hasson cannula (for patients with prior abdominal operations), or by the closed technique, using a 5-mm trocar and then introducing a 5-mm 30° scope or a needle scope. A diagnostic laparoscopy is performed. The pressure of the pneumoperitoneum should be decreased to the minimal amount necessary to see the stomach, usually 5–8 mmHg. The patient has less discomfort from the pneumoperitoneum, and the anterior stomach wall is closer to the abdominal wall for placement of T-fasteners (Fig. 3) and the gastrostomy catheter. Occasionally, especially if the stomach is not insufflated, a grasper is needed to help insert the first T-fastener into the stomach lumen. A 5-mm trocar can be placed in the right upper or the left lower quadrant to accommodate the grasper (Fig. 2).

A 4 x 4 cm area is visualized on the anterior surface of the body of the stomach near the greater curvature. A T-fastener is placed in each corner of the square, and the gastrostomy is placed through the center of the square. Indenting the abdominal wall with a finger and seeing it through the laparoscope helps to define the locations on the abdominal wall where the T-fasteners and the gastrostomy catheter pass through. Insufflating the stomach at this time through the nasogastric tube facilitates the placement of the T-fasteners and the gastrostomy catheter.

The first T-fastener (Fig. 4) is placed in one corner of the 4 x 4 cm square farthest from the scope, more proximal in the stomach. Pulling gently on the nylon sutures then facilitates placement of subsequent T-fasteners. It is useful to keep open the space between the abdominal wall and the stomach so that the T-fasteners and gastrostomy catheter are placed under direct laparoscopic view (Fig. 4).

Once the anterior wall of the stomach is secured by the four T-fasteners, the gastrostomy is placed through the center of the diamond marked by the T-fasteners. A transverse 1-cm incision is made in the center of the square on the skin to accommodate the gastrostomy catheter without tension. An 18-gauge needle is inserted through the skin incision and the anterior abdominal wall into the stomach. A J-guide wire is then introduced into the lumen of the stomach through this needle (Fig. 5). The needle is withdrawn, and the stoma tract is enlarged serially with dilators of increasing diameter. An 18-F balloon catheter is finally inserted through this tract over the wire into the stomach. The balloon is inflated, and the J-wire is removed (Fig. 6). The intragastric placement of the balloon catheter is again confirmed by the bulge on the anterior stomach wall when pulling on the catheter. A contrast roentgenogram can also be performed to confirm intragastric placement.

The anterior stomach wall is then fixed to the abdominal wall by squeezing the aluminum crimps on the nylon suture, and the gastrostomy catheter is secured by the inflated balloon and a skin anchor. The pneumoperitoneum is released, and the fascia is closed for any trocar site larger than 5 mm.

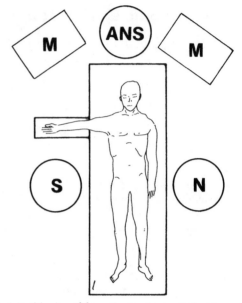

Fig. 1. Positioning of the patient and team. Patient in supine-reverse Trendelenburg position. *ANS,* Anesthetist; *S,* surgeon; *A,* assistant; *N,* nurse; *M,* monitor

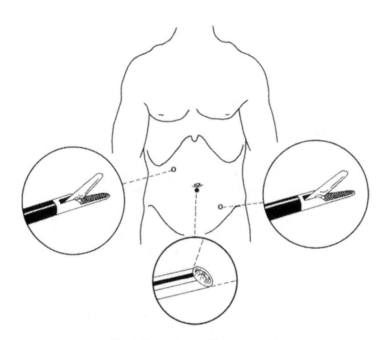

Fig. 2. Trocar sites and instrumentation

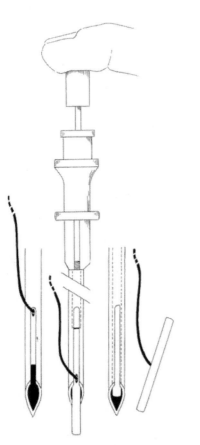

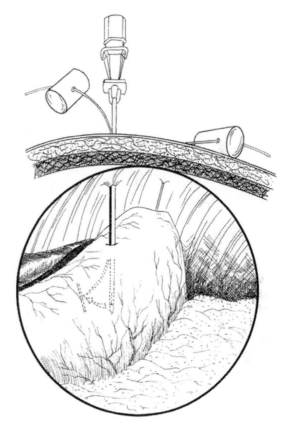

Fig. 3. The T-fastener is a 1-cm metal T-bar attached to a nylon suture. The T-bar is loaded in the tip of an 18-gauge needle and ejected by a stylet into the lumen of the stomach or jejunum. The nylon suture remains externally and is used to retract the stomach or jejunum. The T-fastener is fixed by crimping aluminum crimps onto the nylon suture against a soft bumper on the skin

Fig. 4. The first T-fastener has been placed in one corner of the 4 x 4 cm square farthest from the scope, more proximal in the stomach. The stomach is retracted gently with the nylon suture. The second T-fastener is being inserted into the stomach

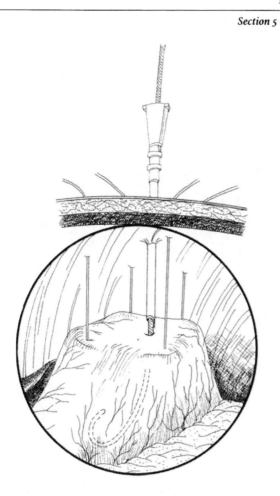

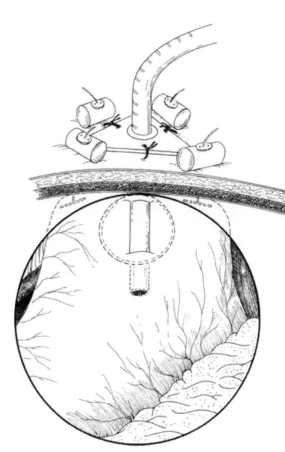

Fig. 5. The anterior wall of the stomach is secured by four T-fasteners. An 18-gauge needle is inserted through the center of this area into the stomach. A J-guide wire is then introduced into the lumen of the stomach through this needle

Fig. 6. After the tract is enlarged with serial dilators, an 18-F balloon catheter is inserted over the wire into the stomach. The balloon is inflated, and the J-wire is removed. The T-fasteners are fixed by squeezing the aluminum crimps on the nylon suture, and the gastrostomy catheter is secured by the inflated balloon and a skin anchor

Comments

The key to the successful placement of laparoscopic gastrostomy or jejunostomy is to retract and fix the stomach or the jejunum to the abdominal wall to prevent leakage. Although this can be achieved by sutures placed laparoscopically, we prefer to use T-fasteners because they are easier to place and are effective and safe. The T-fastener (Brown-Mueller) was designed to retract hollow viscera percutaneously (Fig. 3). Its design is similar to the plastic T's that keep the price tags on clothes in the stores. The T-fastener consists of a 1-cm metal T-bar attached to a nylon suture. The T-bar is loaded in a slot at the tip of an 18-gauge needle, inserted into the lumen of the stomach or the jejunum by the needle, and ejected by a stylet. The needle and stylet are withdrawn and the T-bar is left inside the lumen with the nylon suture attached. The stomach or the jejunum is retracted by pulling on the nylon suture. To fix the stomach or the jejunum to the abdominal wall by the T-fastener, a soft bumper is pushed against the skin by two aluminum crimpers that slide over the nylon suture and are immobilized by squeezing them with a needle holder. Ten days to 2 weeks after the procedure, when the stomach or the jejunum is well adhered to the abdominal wall, the nylon suture is cut at the skin level and removed, and the metal T-bar is left in the lumen to pass in the stool.

With either laparoscopic gastrostomy and jejunostomy the patient can be fed through the catheter within 24 h, usually in the morning after the procedure. We inject 30 cc saline through the catheter every 4 h to prevent clogging before feeding is started. The length of the catheter at the skin level is noted so movement of the catheter can be detected early. If the catheter is dislodged, it can usually be replaced at the bedside because the T-fasteners have fixed the bowel to the abdominal wall. If the catheter is dislodged and the stoma tract has closed, the catheter can be replaced under fluoroscopic guidance or laparoscopy can be repeated to replace the catheter.

References

Duh QY, Way LW (1993) Laparoscopic gastrostomy using T-fasteners as retractors and anchors. Surg Endosc 7:60–63

Modesto VL Harkins B, Carlton WC Jr, Martindale RG (1994) Laparoscopic gastrostomy using four-point fixation. Am J Surg 167:273–276

Murphy C et al (1992) A simple technique for laparoscopic gastrostomy. Surg Gynecol Obstet 174:424–425

23 Laparoscopic Bypass for Inoperable Cancer of the Pancreas

A. Cuschieri

Introduction

The vast majority of patients with pancreatic cancer present with advanced disease, and 90% die within 1 year of diagnosis. Staging laparoscopy provides the most useful assessment of these patients. It establishes the diagnosis and provides histological confirmation by target biopsy or fine-needle aspiration cytology. It documents hepatic secondary deposits and peritoneal seeding which are often missed by computed tomography scanning and magnetic resonance imaging. The advent of laparoscopic ultrasound scanning with high-resolution contact linear array probes has enhanced the staging potential of diagnostic laparoscopy for cancer. Vascular invasion, especially portal vein involvement, by tumor can be established by laparoscopic ultrasonography, avoiding unnecessary laparotomy in apparently localized disease. In patients with advanced inoperable disease, excellent palliation of progressive jaundice, and/or gastric outlet obstruction can be achieved by laparoscopic bypass procedures.

Positioning of the Patient and Team

For positioning of the patient and team, see Fig. 1

Technique

A cholecystocholangiogram is essential to establish adequate clearance of the entry of the cystic duct from the upper limit of the obstructing tumor. If this exceeds 1.5 cm, a cholecystojejunostomy provides adequate decompression for the duration of the patient's survival; otherwise a choledochojejunostomy is necessary. The cholecystocholangiogram is best performed by use of a Veress needle introduced percutaneously along the long axis of the distended gallbladder. The Veress needle is attached via a three-way tap to a line leading to two 50-ml syringes (one containing isotonic saline and the other sodium diatrizoate 20%–30%) and to a suction line. When the gallbladder is reached, the spring-loaded inner blunt stylet of the Veress needle is held retracted so

that the beveled cutting tip is exposed. This is then advanced through the gallbladder fundus into the lumen, when the inner blunt component is released. Confirmation of the intraluminal position of the needle is achieved by injection of a few milliliters of saline followed by aspiration. The Veress needle is then advanced further into the lumen of the gallbladder. The optimum position of the tip is near the neck of the organ. Before fluorocholangiography is commenced, the operating table is tilted head down and slightly to the right. Fluoroscopy is started with contrast injection. On average some 40–50 ml contrast is needed to fill the gallbladder before the contrast starts to opacify the cystic duct and then the biliary tract. The important information needed from the cholecystocholangiogram concerns the distance between the cystic duct insertion and the upper limit of the tumor. On completion of the cholecystocholangiogram the gallbladder is aspirated before the Veress needle is withdrawn.

A loop of jejunum approximately 50 cm from the ligament of Treitz is selected for anastomosis to the gallbladder (Fig. 3). After elevation of the transverse colon the upper jejunum is traced upward until the ligament of Treitz and the duodenojejunal junction are identified. A floppy loop some 40 cm in length is selected and its apex grasped and brought up antecolically to the gallbladder to ensure sufficient reach for a tension-free anastomosis between the two organs. The cholecystojejunostomy can be performed by hand suture or by the stapling technique.

Hand-Sutured Anastomosis

The method used consists of a single layer deep seromuscular continuous suturing technique using two sutures, one each for the posterior and anterior walls of the anastomosis. A starter loop knot (Dundee jamming loop knot) can be fashioned externally or a standard microsurgical surgeon's knot formed and tied internally to start the anastomosis. Atraumatic endoski sutures are ideal, and either Polysorb (USSC) or coated Vicryl (Ethicon, Cincinnati, OH) 3-0 is recommended.

The suturing technique involves use of the right needle holder as the active driver with the left needle holder being used to apply countertraction on the tissue to facilitate needle passage and to pick up the needle after it emerges through the tissues before transfer to the active needle holder. The individual suture bites must be inserted in a deep seromuscular fashion and be evenly spaced. Only the last suture bite is locked, and following a further passage of the needle through the two organs the suture is tied using the Aberdeen knot. Once the posterior suture line is completed (Fig. 4), the needle is left attached to the suture in case the anterior suture is too short or breaks during the performance of the final part of the anastomosis.

The seromuscular layer of the gallbladder is then incised over a distance of 3.0 cm with the electrosurgical hook knife parallel to the completed posterior suture line (Fig. 5). With the sucker in place, the mucosa is opened and the sucker tip introduced into the gallbladder lumen and the bile aspirated. The mucosal cut is then extended and the interior wall of the gallbladder inspected and irrigated thoroughly to ensure removal of all debris and blood clots. The enterotomy is fashioned to an equivalent length and with the same technique. The anterior wall of the anastomosis is closed by a continuous suture (Figs. 6, 7).

Stapled-Sutured Anastomosis

Two 3-0 stay sutures are inserted at the proposed limits of the anastomosis between the two organs (Fig. 8). A small opening sufficient to admit the limbs of an Endolinear cutter/stapler (bowel cartridge) is then made in each organ at the right extremity (Fig. 8). With the approximated organs held under stretch by tension on the right stay suture, the two limbs of the stapler are introduced through the previously formed openings in the gallbladder and jejunum as far as the hilt (Fig. 9). The stapler limbs are tilted upward before being approximated. A careful inspection is undertaken to ensure that no extraneous tissue has been caught between the two stapler limbs, and that the line of the proposed anastomosis is correct. Once this is established, the instrument is fired, disengaged, and removed (Fig. 10). The stapled anastomosis is inspected from the inside to establish its integrity and the absence of any tissue bridges. The anterior defect is closed with a running suture (Fig. 11).

Choledochojejunostomy

Choledochojejunostomy can be performed only by suturing and requires considerable experience in laparoscopic biliary surgery. It is feasible laparoscopically if a 2.5-cm section of normal common hepatic bile duct is clearly visible between the hepatic parenchyma and the upper limit of the tumor mass. Choledochojejunostomy is contraindicated if there is evidence of portal hypertension caused by tumor involvement of the portal vein. This should be suspected if the hepatoportal pedicle is surrounded by large vessels and can be confirmed by laparoscopic ultrasound examination. These patients should be managed either by open surgical segment 3 bypass or by endoscopic stenting.

The selected loop is brought up antecolically to the common hepatic duct, and a 1.5-cm opening is made on its antimesenteric border. No dissection is usually necessary of the common hepatic duct, and stay sutures are not inserted. A 1.5-cm oblique incision is made on the anterior wall of the duct, and escaping bile is aspirated. The suturing is performed with 4-0 Polysorb or coated Vicryl, and the technique consists of a single all coats layer with continuous or interrupted sutures.

Gastrojejunostomy

Gastrojejunostomy is performed in an antecolic fashion using a combined stapling-suturing technique. The ideal site of the anastomosis of the jejunal loop to the stomach is along the greater curvature at least 2.5 cm from the lesion. A loop of upper jejunum some 40–50 cm from the duodenojejunal junction is selected and marked by a serosal suture. The next step consists in the alignment of the stomach and the selected jejunal loop by the insertion of two corner deep seromuscular sutures some 6 cm apart. As traction is held on the tail of the right extremity suture, appropriate sized openings are made in the jejunum and stomach (medial to the suture) for the insertion of the limbs of the 6-cm Endolinear cutter/stapler. The two limbs of the opened stapler are introduced, respectively, into the stomach and the jejunum. Once inside the lumen of the stomach and jejunum, the stapler limbs are elevated to tent the two organs and then closed before the instrument is fired. Thereafter, the stapler heads are released and withdrawn from the anastomosis. The anterior wall of the gastrojejunostomy is then lifted up to inspect the stapled anastomotic line and to ensure that there are no mucosal bridges. The final stage of the procedure consists in the suture closure of the defect.

Double Bypass

In patients with concomitant duodenal obstruction requiring a double bypass two configurations are possible laparoscopically: continuous (Fig. 12) or split technique (Fig. 13) with entero-enteric anastomosis. We now favor the latter although it takes longer to perform. The small intestine some 80 cm from the ligament of Treitz is transected using the Endolinear cutter/stapler after the creation of a small window along the mesenteric border. The distal limb is used for the bilioenteric bypass (hand sutured) whereas the proximal loop is employed for the creation of an anterior gastrojejunostomy (stapled). An entero-enteric anastomosis is then effected using the 6-cm Endolinear cutter/stapler between the two loops, the residual defect being closed with suturing using 3-0 suture.

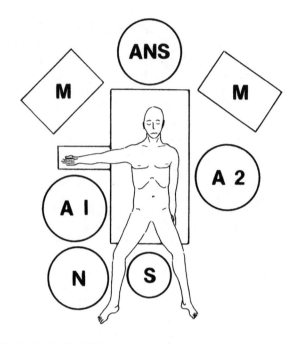

Fig. 1. Positioning of the patient and team. Patient in lithotomy position. *ANS,* Anesthetist; *S,* surgeon; *A1, A2,* assistants; *N,* nurse; *M,* monitor

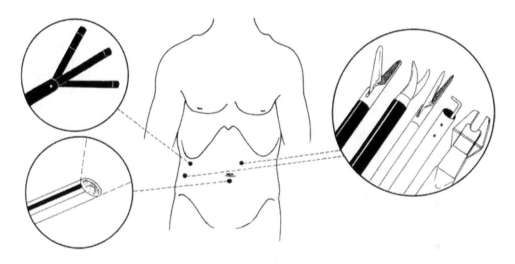

Fig. 2. Trocar sites and instrumentation

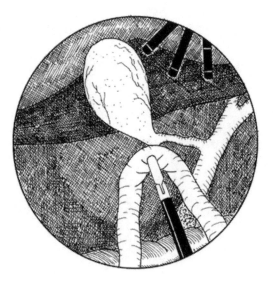

Fig. 3. A loop of small bowel is mobilized to the right upper quadrant

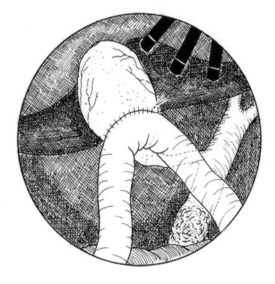

Fig. 4. The back wall of the cholecystojejunostomy has been hand sutured

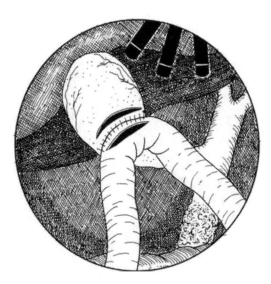

Fig. 5. The gallbladder and jejunum are incised

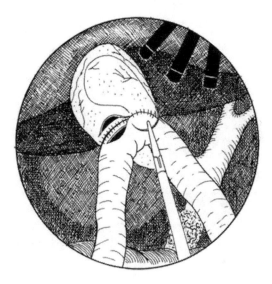

Fig. 6. The anterior wall of the cholecystojejunostomy is performed

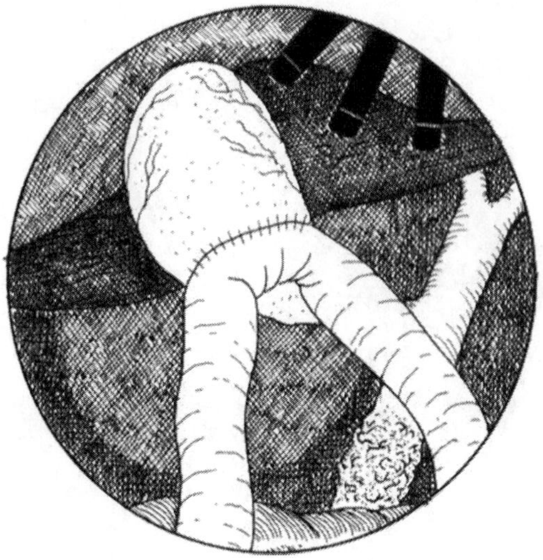

Fig. 7. The anastomosis is finished

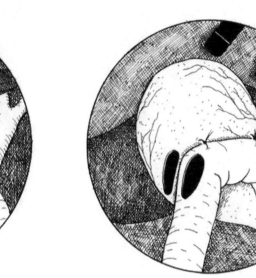

Fig. 8. Gallbladder and jejunum are held together by stay sutures, and an incision is made for the Endolinear cutter/stapler

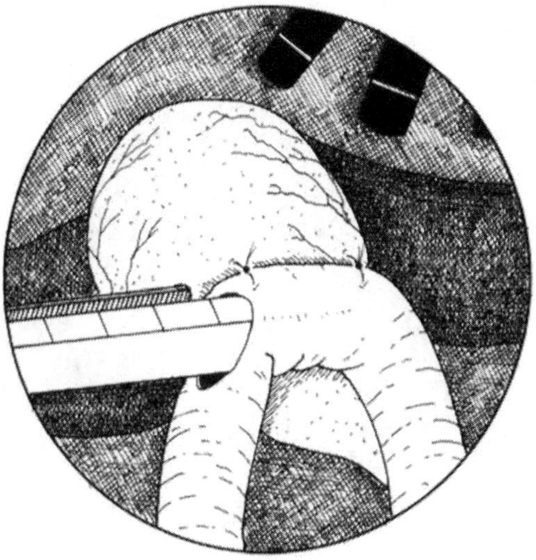

Fig. 9. The Endolinear cutter/stapler is introduced into the lumen of the gallbladder and jejunum

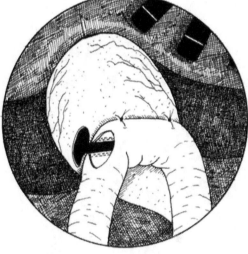

Fig. 10. The cholecystojejunostomy is partially finished

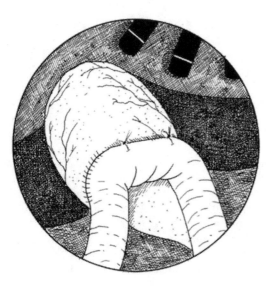

Fig. 11. The anterior defect is hand-sutured closed

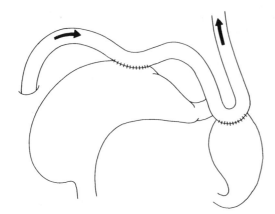

Fig. 12. Continuous gastroenteric and entero-enteric bypass

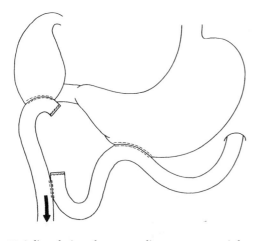

Fig. 13. Split technique for gastrocolic or entero-enteric bypass

Comments

Our experience with laparoscopic bypass procedures for these unfortunate patients has been favorable in that the need for readmission to hospital, except for terminal care, has not arisen. Moreover, there have not been any instances of cholangitis in a consecutive series of 18 patients. The relative merits of laparoscopic palliation of these patients versus endoscopic stenting awaits future comparative studies. Although to date we have adopted an all-comers policy for patients with obstructing advanced disease, it seems likely that the laparoscopic approach is best suited to patients without significant hepatic deposits or widespread peritoneal dissemination in whom survival is expected to be relatively prolonged. Another appropriate subgroup is those patients who have duodenal obstruction and require both biliary drainage and gastrojejunostomy.

References

Cuschieri A (1988) Laparoscopy for pancreatic cancer: does it benefit the patient? Eur J Surg Oncol 14:41–44

Cuschieri A (1993) Cholécysto-entérostomie per-coelioscopique: une alternative au drainage biliaire endoscopique. Acta Endosc 23:135–141

Hawsali A (1992) Laparoscopic cholecysto-jejunostomy for obstructing pancreatic cancer. J Laparoendosc 2:351–355

Ishida H, Furukawa Y, Kuroda H et al (1981) Laparoscopic observation and biopsy of the pancreas. Endoscopy 13:68–73

Nathanson LK, Shimi S, Cuschieri A (1992) Sutured laparoscopic cholecystojejunostomy evolved in an animal model. J R Coll Surg Edinb 37:215–220

Shimi S, Banting S, Cuschieri A (1991) Laparoscopy in the management of pancreatic cancer: endoscopic cholecystojejunostomy for advanced disease. Br J Surg 79:317–319

24 Laparoscopic Cystogastrostomy for Pancreatic Pseudocyst

E.H. Phillips and R.J. Rosenthal

Introduction

The development of endoscopic techniques for cysto-gastrostomy in the treatment of pancreatic pseudocysts has added treatment options when confronting this complex group of patients. However, the location of the cyst or the amount of debris in it occasionally dictates surgical drainage as catheters prove inadequate. A laparoscopic technique is presented here that allows débridement of necrotic and/or infected material while minimizing surgical trauma.

Positioning of the Patient and Team

The patient is placed on the table in lithotomy position. The surgeon stands between the legs, with assistants on the right and left sides of the patient. Two monitors should be placed at the patient's head. A third monitor may be used for the endogastric image (Fig. 1).

Technique

The operation starts with the introduction of the Veress needle at the umbilicus and creation of a pneumoperitoneum. A 10- to 11-mm trocar is introduced, and a 30° scope is used for exploration of the abdominal cavity (Fig. 2). A 5-mm and a 10-mm trocar are placed at the right and left flank of the abdomen. Two accessory 10-mm trocars are placed, one at the lowest portion of the left flank and the other under the xiphoid (Fig. 2). The anterior wall of the stomach is then opened by means of cautery (Fig. 3) and extended with the endocutter, which is partially introduced into the gastric lumen (Fig. 4). The laparoscope is then advanced through the gastrotomy into the gastric cavity (Fig. 5).

The cyst is localized by visualization of bulging in the posterior wall of the stomach. A laparoscopic needle is introduced through the back wall of the stomach, and the cyst contents are aspirated (Fig. 6). For this purpose intraoperative ultrasonography can be used for localization. When the cyst is localized, gastrotomy at the posterior wall of the stomach is performed (Fig. 7). The posterior gastrotomy is enlarged with the endocutter (Fig. 8). This step decreases the chance of bleeding from the gastric-cyst wall. The initial button of pseudocyst wall removed by cautery is sent for pathology analysis.

The fluid contents of the pseudocyst are also sent for cytology, culture, and pathological examination. Necrotic material can be retrieved with ring forceps (Fig. 9). A Penrose drain is introduced intraperitoneally and sutured to the nasogastric tube. It is then placed in the lumen of the gastrocystostomy to keep it patent (Fig. 10). This drain is removed several days later with the nasogastric tube. After the operating field is checked for hemostasis, the anterior gastric wall is closed with laparoscopic suturing or stapling technique (Fig. 11). Trocars are extracted under view to recognize any bleeding from the trocar sites, and the trocar sites are sutured closed.

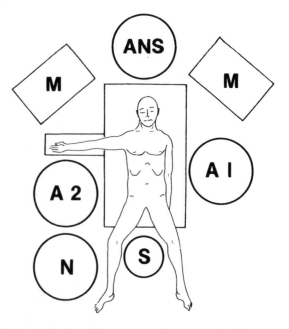

Fig. 1. Positioning of the patient and team. Patient in lithotomy position. *ANS*, Anesthetist; *S*, surgeon; *A1*, *A2*, assistant; *N*, nurse; *M*, monitor

24 Laparoscopic Cystogastrostomy for Pancreatic Pseudocyst

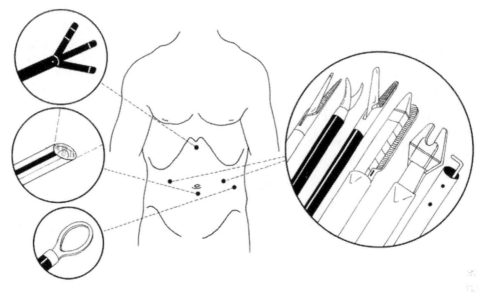

Fig. 2. Trocar sites and instrumentation

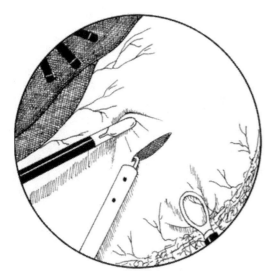

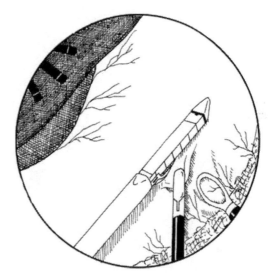

Fig. 3. Anterior wall gastrotomy

Fig. 4. Enlargement of the anterior gastrotomy with the endo-cutter

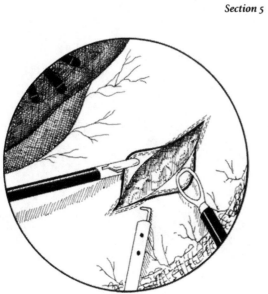

Fig. 5. View into the gastric lumen

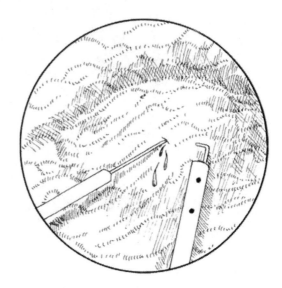

Fig. 6. Puncture of posterior gastric wall for cyst localization

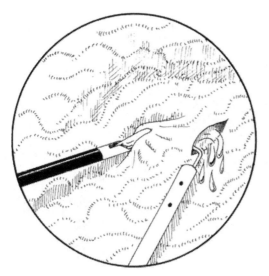

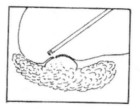

Fig. 7. Posterior wall gastrotomy

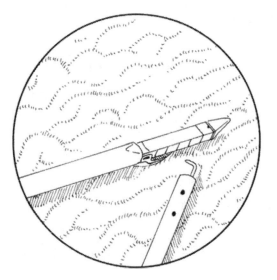

Fig. 8. Enlargement of gastrotomy and hemostasis of cystogastrostomy anastomosis

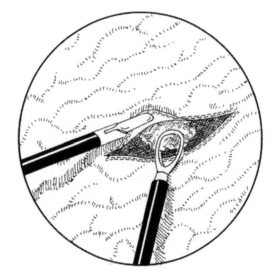

Fig. 9. Débridement of cyst contents

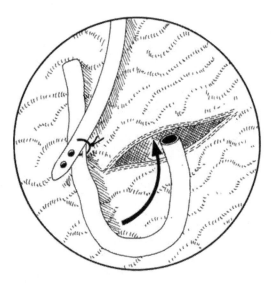

Fig. 10. Placement of Penrose drain into cyst cavity

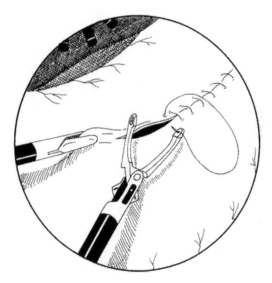

Fig. 11. Closure of anterior gastrotomy

Section 5   E. H. PHILLIPS and R.J. ROSENTHAL

Comments

An alternative technique employs radial expanding trocars to enter the stomach rather than an anterior gastrotomy. The antrum is occluded with a Penrose drain and the stomach is distended with air via the nasogastric tube. Under laparoscopic guidance a 5-mm radial expanding trocar is introduced through the abdominal wall into the distended stomach and a 5-mm 30° angle scope is then passed into the lumen. The CO_2 is attached to the endogastric trocar and two accessory 10-mm radial expanding trocars ars positioned according to the pseudocyst localization into the gastric lumen. The posterior wall of the stomach and pseudocyst cavity are entered with cautery and an endocutter can be used to enlarge the cystogastrostomy. The transgastric trocars are then removed, and the gastric sites are closed with laparoscopic suturing.

References

Buchler M, Uhl W, Beger HG (1992) Acute pancreatitis, when and how to operate. Dig Dis 10 (6):354–362

Nyhus, LM, Baker RJ (1989) Surgery of the pancreas. In: Mastery of surgery, vol II, chap IV. Little Brown, Boston

Way L (1994) Laparoscopic cystogastrostomy for pancreatic pseudocyst (abstract). SAGES, Nashville

25 Combined Laparoscopic and Endoscopic Excision of Gastric Mucosal Lesions

M. Ohgami and M. Kitajima

Introduction

The diagnosis and treatment of gastric pathology were dramatically changed with the introduction of endoscopy. Routine screening upper endoscopy permits the identification of small tumors and early cancers confined to the mucosa. Combined laparoscopic and endoscopic excision of these lesions have proven successful. It achieves exact localization and adequate excision of limited lesions of the gastric mucosa and submucosa.

Positioning of the Patient and Team

The patient is placed on the table in the lithotomy position. The surgeon stands between the legs, with assistants on the right and left sides of the patient. Two monitors should be placed at the head of the patient. A third monitor, attached to a second camera, should be used for the endogastric images. An A-V mixer can be used for a picture in picture effect (Fig. 1).

Technique

A pneumoperitoneum is created. A 5-mm or a 10- to 11-mm trocar is introduced at the umbilicus, and a 30° 5- or 10-mm scope is used to explore the abdominal cavity (Fig. 2). A 5-mm and a 10-mm trocar are placed in the right and left sides of the abdomen (Fig. 2). The antrum is occluded with an encircling Penrose drain or a clamp, and a gastroscope is introduced into the stomach for localization of the lesion (Fig. 3). After the stomach is insufflated with air, a radial expanding trocar 5 mm in diameter is introduced through the abdominal wall into the gastric lumen while observing from the laparoscope. The radial expanding device is made of a needle covered by an expanding sheath and a dilator. The needle, which is covered by the sheath, is first introduced into the gastric lumen (Fig. 4).

The balloon, which is localized at the tip of the sheath to hold the trocar in place, is inflated. The needle is removed and the dilator, covered by a rigid cannula, is introduced through the lumen of the sheath, dilating the sheath to 5 or 10-mm as required. The dilator is then removed, and the cannula is kept rigid by the sheath. The radial expanding devices provide a sealed system without air leak from the gastric lumen. A 5-mm 30° angle scope is introduced into the gastric cavity for the endoorgan view. The CO_2 is attached to the endogastric trocar, and two accessory radial expanding trocars are placed into the gastric lumen (Fig. 5). The positioning of the patient and trocars is changed according to where the tumor is localized.

The submucosal plane is first infiltrated with a 1% adrenaline solution to decrease bleeding and raise the mucosa (Fig. 6). A grasper elevates the mucosa while a bipolar scissor is used to excise the lesion (Figs. 7, 8). The specimen can be removed through a 10-mm trocar. If 5-mm trocars are used, an endoloop can be used to attach the specimen to the oral gastric tube or a polypectomy snare can be used via the gastroscope to grasp and remove the specimen through the esophagus and mouth.

After the operating field is checked for hemostasis, the radial expanding trocars are retrieved from the gastric wall but kept in the abdominal wall, and the CO2 tubing is switched back to the umbilical trocar. The gastric wall trocar defects are then closed with laparoscopic suturing. Usually only a single stitch at each site is required. Trocars in the abdominal wall are then extracted under view to identify bleeding from the trocar sites. All sites 10 mm or larger are sutured closed (Fig. 9). The mucosal defect is allowed to heal by secondary intent as a gastric ulcer would.

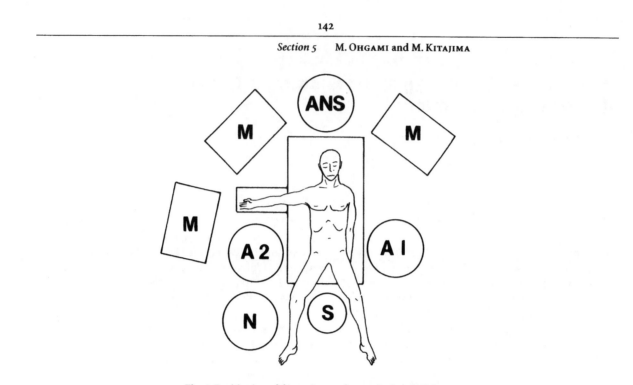

Fig. 1. Positioning of the patient and team. Patient in lithotomy position. *ANS*, Anesthetist; *S*, surgeon; *A1, A2*, assistants; *N*, nurse; *M*, monitor

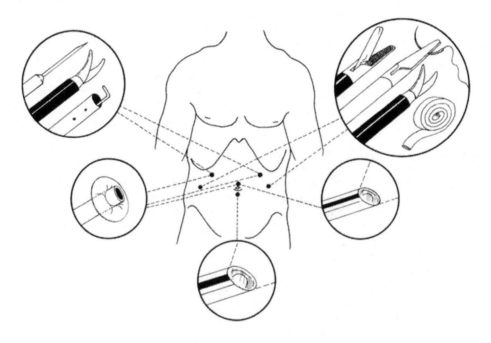

Fig. 2. Trocar sites and instrumentation

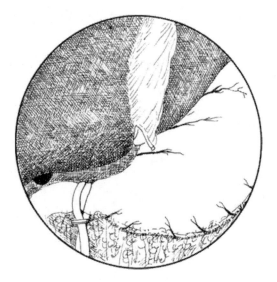

Fig. 3. The duodenum is closed with a Penrose drain

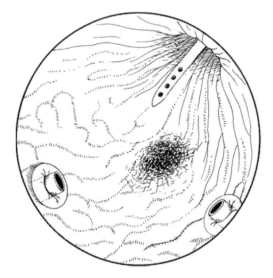

Fig. 5. View into the gastric cavity. The tumor, endotrocars, and nasogastric tube can be seen

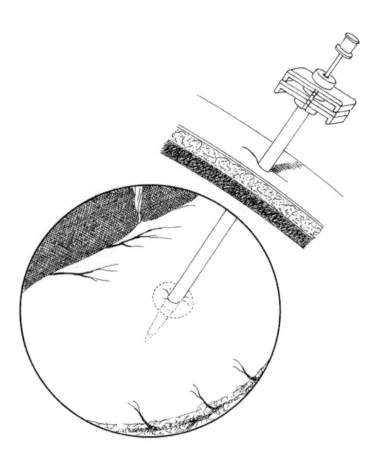

Fig. 4. Introduction of a trocar into the gastric cavity

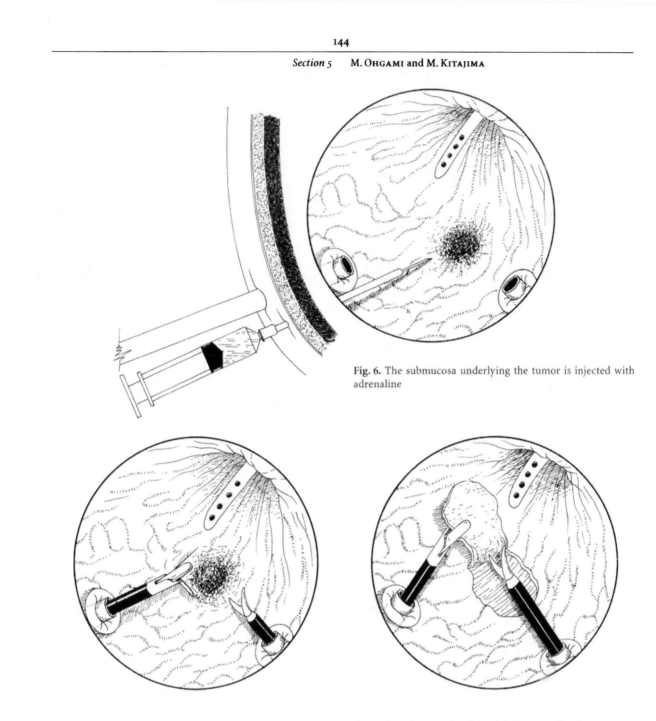

Fig. 6. The submucosa underlying the tumor is injected with adrenaline

Fig. 7. Dissection of the tumor

Fig. 8. The submucosal excision is being completed

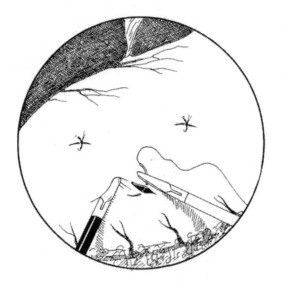

Fig. 9. After the endogastric trocars are removed, the trocar sites are sutured closed

Comments

Twenty patients with early gastric cancer have been treated with this approach or with a laparoscopic wedge resection. In a follow-up period of 1–36 months, we have had no morbidity or mortality. The gastroscopic follow-up showed no recurrences. The combined endoscopic approach offers the possibility of more precise and extensive excision of small lesions of hollow intra-abdominal organs without the need for major resections.

References

Branicki FJ, Nathanson LK (1994) Minimal access gastroduodenal surgery. Aust NZ J Surg 64 (9):589–698

Farley DR, Donoheu JH (1992) Early gastric cancer. Surg Clin North Am 72 (2):401–421

Nyhus LM, Baker RJ (1984) Mastery of surgery, vol II, chap 5 II. Little, Brown, Boston

Ohashi S (1995) Laparoscopic intraluminal surgery for early gastric cancer. Surg Endosc 9:169–171

Ohgami M, Kumai K, Xoshihide O, Wakabayashi G, Tetsuro Kubota, Kitajima M (1994) Laparoscopic wedge resection of the stomach for early gastric cancer using a lesion lifting method. Dig Surg 11:64–67

Takekoshi T, Baba V, Ota H, Kato Y, Yanagisawa A, Takagi K, Noguchi Y (1994) Endoscopic resection of early gastric carcinoma: results of a retrospective analysis of 308 cases. Endoscopy 26 (4):352–358

26 Laparoscopic Posterior Truncal Vagotomy and Anterior Seromyotomy

N. Katkhouda and J. Mouiel

Introduction

Peptic ulcer disease affects more than 4% of the Western population. The medical management of this disease, including H_2 blockers, proton pump inhibitors, and anti-helicobacter therapy, has been very successful. However, the long-term management of chronic duodenal ulcer disease has been less successful, thus subjecting these patients to long-term disability. It is in the treatment of chronic duodenal ulcer disease and its complications, such as bleeding, obstruction, and perforation, that the surgeon can have an impact using laparoscopic surgical techniques as an added therapeutic option.

Candidates for laparoscopic surgery must meet the following criteria: (a) they have failed medical treatment on H_2 blockers, proton pump inhibitors, or triple antibiotic therapy or have had recurrences after complete medical treatment; (b) they are unable to comply with medical treatment because of socioeconomic factors; and (c) they have experienced complications of peptic ulcer disease, including hemorrhage or perforation.

As in open ulcer surgery, preoperative evaluation is important, including upper endoscopy with biopsies as well as barium upper gastrointestinal series. Gastric pool studies to document basal and maximal acid output are useful, as is the determination of serum gastrin level to rule out Zollinger-Ellison syndrome.

Positioning of the Patient and Team

As in open surgery, general anesthesia is administered. A nasogastric tube and Foley catheter are inserted. The patient is placed in the modified lithotomy position and prepared and draped. The operating surgeon stands between the legs of the patient, with the nurse and first assistant on the left and the camera assistant on the right (Fig. 1).

Technique

The instruments are those used in usual laparoscopic procedures, including the 0° scope and a 30° scope for acute-angle viewing, a variety of needle holders and atraumatic graspers. Other instruments include an angulated hook coagulator, endoloops, and absorbable monofilament sutures.

Once the pneumoperitoneum is created using a Veress needle, the first trocar is placed 3 cm above and to the right of the umbilicus and is for the laparoscope. A second trocar (5 mm) is placed in the subxiphoid position and is for a grasper or irrigation device. Two lateral trocars are placed and are for atraumatic graspers. The last trocar (12 mm) is placed 3 cm above and to the left of the umbilicus and is for other instrumentation. These five trocars, once in place, form a pentagon (Fig. 2).

The procedure involves three steps: approach to the hiatal area, posterior vagotomy, and anterior vagotomy. To approach the hiatal area it is essential to identify the landmarks of this region. The first step is to retract the left lobe of the liver with a subxiphoid fan retractor. The lesser sac is entered using graspers to hold the tissue and the scissors for dissection. The dissection is continued until the right crus of the diaphragm is identified (Fig. 3). A left gastric vein may be encountered at this point and can be divided if in the way.

The two landmarks for the posterior truncal vagotomy are the caudate lobe of the liver and the right crus of the diaphragm (Fig. 4). The right crus is grasped and held to the right while the scissors open the preesophageal peritoneum area. Manipulation of the nasogastric tube is sometimes helpful to identify the position of the esophagus. The esophagus is then retracted to the left, and it is to the posterior that the right vagus nerve is easily identified by its white pearly color. Gentle traction is held on the nerve, and a 1-cm piece is transected between two clips with the segment sent to pathology.

For the anterior seromyotomy a longitudinal incision is made on the anterior gastric seromuscular layer (taking care not to incise the gastric mucosa), thus indirectly accomplishing a highly selective vagotomy of the anterior aspect of the stomach (Fig. 5). The anterior aspect of the stomach is spread out between two grasping forceps, and the line of the incision is outlined using electrocautery parallel to only 1.5 cm from the lesser curvature of the stomach. This line extends from the esophagogastric junction at the posterior aspect of the angle of His to a point 5–7 cm from the pylorus at the level of the first branch of the "crow's foot." The two distal branches of the nerve are not divided to ensure adequate pyloric innervation, and thus adequate antroduodenal motility. Three or four blood vessels can be encountered on the anterior surface of the stomach at this point and are clipped prior to performing the seromyotomy. The first assistant elevates the stomach with the grasper, and the surgeon holds the right grasper with the left hand and uses the right hand to perform the seromyotomy with the "L"-shaped hook coagulator (Probe Plus II, Ethicon Endosurgery, Cincinatti, Oh). The oblique muscles and finally the circular muscle layers of the stomach are divided. Once the electrocautery has divided the fibers, the edges of the stomach are grasped and spread apart mechanically, thus breaking the remaining deep circular fibers. The trick is to stay above the submucosal layer where most of the veins of the gastric wall run. The gastric mucosa is identified by its bluish color and is easily recognized. If an injury is suspected, air or methylene blue can be inserted into the stomach via a nasogastric tube to look for leaks, which can then be closed with sutures.

The seromyotomy is oversewn using an overlapping running suture of 3-0 Prolene via the 5-mm port (Fig. 6). It is important to note that the closure is overlapped to prevent possible nerve regeneration, although such regeneration has not been scientifically documented. Fibrin glue, if available, can also be used to seal the seromyotomy. The hiatal area and the area of the seromyotomy are examined. The abdomen is deflated, the trocars are removed, and the skin incisions closed with sutures after closure of the fascia.

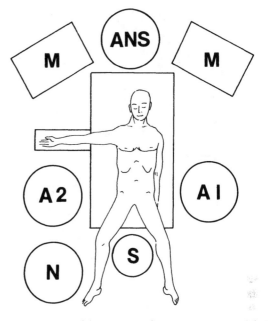

Fig. 1. Positioning of the patient and team. Patient in modified lithotomy position. *ANS*, Anesthetist; *S*, surgeon; *A1, A2*, assistants; *N*, nurse; *M*, monitor

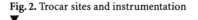

Fig. 2. Trocar sites and instrumentation
▼

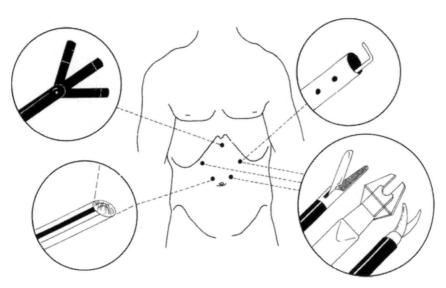

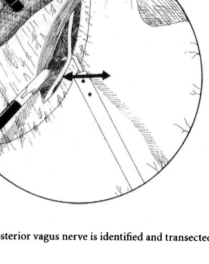

Fig. 3. Opening of avascular plane at the lesser curve of the stomach, and identification of the caudate lobe of the liver and the right crux of the diaphram

Fig. 4. The posterior vagus nerve is identified and transected

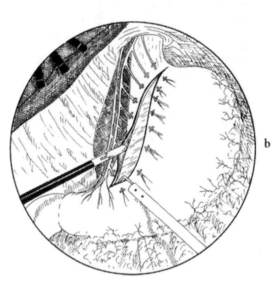

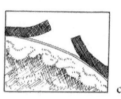

Fig. 5. a Performing the anterior seromyotomy. **b** The seromyotomy should be performed at a distance of 1 cm from the lesser curvature and should end 6 cm from the pylorus. **c** Seromuscular planes are transected. Mucosa and submucosa are intact

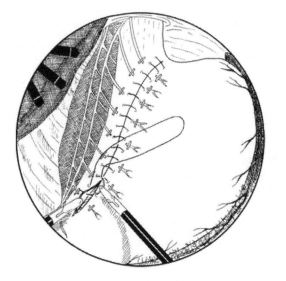

Fig. 6. The seromyotomy is closed with a running suture

Comments

Postoperative care is simple with early ambulation and resumption of oral intake 24 h postoperatively with usual discharge in 2 days. Complications occurring during this procedure include bleeding and perforation of the gastric mucosa. Bleeding can occur intraoperatively or postoperatively and usually involves gastric vessels that run across the anterior aspect of the stomach. It is best to identify and to divide these vessels prior to performing the seromyotomy. However, if hemorrhage does occur, it is essential to grasp the vessel with atraumatic forceps and to rinse the area and to precisely clip or suture the vessel. Perforation of the gastric mucosa can lead to peritonitis, and therefore the stomach should be routinely filled with methylene blue to check for leaks, which if present can be closed in an overlapping fashion. The way to avoid this complication is to be patient and meticulous when performing the seromyotomy, and stay above the submucosal layer indicated by the number of small veins running on its surface.

References

Hill GL, Barker MCJ (1978) Anterior highly selective vagotomy with posterior truncal vagotomy: a simple technique for denervating the parietal cell mass. Br J Surg 65:702–705

Hoffman J, Jensen HE, Christiansen J et al (1989) Prospective controlled vagotomy trial for duodenal ulcer. Results after 11–15 years. Ann Surg 209:40–45

Katkhouda N, Mouiel J (1993) Laparoscopic treatment of peptic ulcer disease in minimal invasive surgery. In: Hunter J, Sackier J (eds) McGraw-Hill, New York, pp 123–130

Taylor TV, MacLeod DAD, Gunn AA, MacLennan I (1982) Anterior lesser curve seromyotomy and posterior truncal vagotomy in the treatment of chronic duodenal ulcer. Lancet II:846–848

Taylor TV, Gunn AA, MacLeod DAD et al (1985) Morbidity and mortality after anterior lesser curve seromyotomy and posterior truncal vagotomy for duodenal ulcer. Br J Surg 72:950–951

27 Laparoscopic Highly Selective Vagotomy

J.G. HUNTER

Introduction

Highly selective vagotomy (HSV) was described by Griffiths and Harkin 40 years ago as an effort to provide the most physiologic ulcer operation. The goal of HSV is to provide equivalent denervation of the parietal cell mass without incurring the side effects of dumping and diarrhea occasionally seen with pyloric-destroying procedures. Several operations, such as posterior truncal vagotomy and anterior HSV or posterior truncal vagotomy and anterior lesser curvature seromyotomy, were developed as methods to achieve the same result as HSV while avoiding the tedious and time-consuming procedure of performing an HSV.

In the early 1990s, surgeons started performing vagotomy with laparoscopic access. Initially, the operations of choice were these two simplified procedures. However, as surgical skills have become more sophisticated, there has been a trend toward performance of standard HSV for the elective management of peptic ulcer disease.

The increased awareness of the role of *Helicobacter pylori* in the development of peptic ulcer disease has changed the frequency of elective surgical treatment. There is now uncontestable evidence that the majority of peptic disease may be managed with a 1-month course of antibiotics and omeprazole. Nevertheless, there are rare occurrences of truly refractory uncomplicated peptic ulcer disease. It is these cases that are best suited for laparoscopic HSV.

Positioning of the Patient and Team

Optimal performance of HSV requires a room setup very similar to laparoscopic Nissen fundoplication. The patient is placed in the supine position upon the operating table with monitors mounted as close as possible to 12 o'clock and 10 o'clock (see Fig. 1 b). Once the patient has been anesthetized and intubated, the patient's legs are spread on a modified fractured table using leg boards so as to avoid the problems of Allen stirrups. Pneumatic compression boots, Foley catheter, and an orogastric tube are placed. Initially, the surgeon stands to

the patient's right side and the first assistant to the patient's left side, with the camera operator or second assistant between the patient's legs (see Fig. 1 b).

Technique

A pneumoperitoneum is obtained through the umbilicus with a Veress needle and the abdomen is insufflated to 15 mm of mercury pressure with carbon dioxide. The primary puncture is through the left rectus sheath, 15 cm from the xiphoid, approximately 2–3 cm to the left of midline (Fig. 2). A 45°-angled scope is passed through this primary puncture and an abdominal survey is performed. A second trocar is a 10 mm trocar placed 10 cm along the left costal margin, away from the xiphoid. Through this 10 mm puncture, a blunt rod is passed which elevates the round ligament of the liver to expose the right upper abdomen. The third trocar placed is a 10 mm trocar which is passed beneath the right costal margin, 15 cm from the xiphoid. Segments 2 and 3 of the liver (left lateral) are elevated with the expandable liver retractor which is held in place with a mechanical robotic arm (Leonard Medical, Huntington Valley, PA, USA). The fourth trocar is a 5 mm trocar which is placed at the same level as the left subcostal trocar. The landmark for this trocar is internal. It is oriented so the tip will come out immediately to the right of the falciform ligament just beneath the left lobe of the liver. This allows the surgeon maximal hand spread for performance of dissection. This port will serve as the port for the surgeon's left hand. The fifth trocar is placed beneath the left costal margin, 20 cm from the xiphoid. The first assistant will use this port to provide counter traction during the surgical dissection (Fig. 2).

After all ports are placed, the surgeon moves to between the legs and the camera operator moves to the patient's right (see Fig. 1 a). Using a two-handed technique, through the two highest ports, the surgeon places an atraumatic grasper through the left port and a pair of scissors through the right port. The first assistant grasps the epiphrenic fat pad and retracts inferiorly to flatten out the phrenoesophageal ligament. The surgeon divides the phrenoesophageal ligament above the hepatic branch of the vagus coming down onto the caudate lobe. The incision is extended to the patient's left, across the left and right crura of the diaphragm. Each crus is individually dissected out in a posterior sweeping direction with the scissors using electrocautery and sharp dissection after coagulation. This reveals the esophagus between the two crura. The anterior vagus is usually apparent adherent to the anterior surface of the esophagus. The posterior vagus can be seen by gentle spreading dissection between the right crus of the diaphragm and the esophagus. Once both vagi are identified with careful dissection, the anterior vagus is separated from the esophagus and a quarter-inch Penrose drain is passed around the esophagus, excluding the vagi (Fig. 3). It is occasionally helpful to then pass a vessel loop around the anterior and posterior vagal branches so they may be retracted to the patient's right. At this point, the surgeon changes to a monopolar L-hook, bipolar scissors, or harmonic scalpel (Ultracision, Piling Weck, Smithfield, USA) to further separate the vagal trunks from the esophagus. This dissection on the esophagus must extend 6 cm from the gastroesophageal junction cephalad to ensure that all branches of anterior and posterior vagi coursing to the stomach along the esophagus have been divided.

Once 6 cm of esophagus have been skeletonized, the dissection moves inferiorly. Using a plastic ruler that has been cut down to fit through a trocar, the distance of 6 cm is measured from the pylorus along the lesser curvature. A small coagulation mark is made at this point on the stomach and the ruler is removed. This will be the start of the lesser curvature dissection. The peritoneum at this point is divided at the lesser curvature with a monopolar L-hook. The dissection along the lesser curvature progresses by use of a right angle dissector and clips, or by the use of the harmonic scalpel LCS device (Ultracision, Piling Weck, Smithfield, USA), or the use of bipolar electrosurgery (Fig. 4). Each of these three dissection modalities are equally acceptable, however the right angle and clips method is a little cumbersome as the number of instrument changes slow down the progress of the operation, and the clips tend to be dislodged.

Dissection of the anterior lesser curvature leaflet progresses cephalad and across the phrenoesophageal bundle. When a point near the gastroesophageal junction is reached, we usually go back down to the inferior aspect of dissection, pick up the posterior leaflet and enter the lesser sac through the lesser curvature. Again, staying right on the stomach, this posterior leaflet is taken down to allow complete separation of the lesser curvature from the lesser omentum (Fig. 5). At this point, we proceed to the gastroesophageal junction, retract our vagal branches to the right, retract the esophagus to the left,

and complete separation of the gastrohepatic ligament from the stomach at the gastroesophageal junction (Fig. 6). The gastroesophageal junction is often tethered to the median archowit ligament. We generally elevate the stomach off this structure to make sure all gastric branches of the posterior vagus have been divided. It is in this region that one finds the "criminal nerve of Grassi".

At this point the dissection is complete. There are several additions to the procedure that have been suggested by various authors. These include reinforcing the lesser curvature to prevent gastric perforation that has been reported with lesser curvature devascularization. But because this complication is so rare, we do not feel this is necessary unless there is discoloration or bruising. It has also been suggested that the lesser omentum be "reefed up" with a running suture to prevent nerve regrowth. We feel that this is unnecessary and may risk inadvertent injury to the nerve of Latarjet.

The additional procedure that we frequently perform is a closure of the hiatus. Often the potential for iatrogenic hiatal hernia has been created by the extensive mobilization of the gastroesophageal junction, and closure of the hiatus prevents this. It is generally unnecessary to perform a fundoplication. The side effects of this operation will double in incidence if a fundoplication is performed. The other maneuver that may be important is division of the gastroepiploic nerve, six centimeters along the greater curvature from the pylorus. We perform this by isolating the gastroepiploic vessels and using ligatures or clips to divide these vessels, 6 cm from the pylorus. After completion of the procedure, all instruments are removed under direct vision. It is rarely necessary to close any of these trocar sites as they are placed at an oblique angle through the fascia. (Editorial comment: we prefer to close all trocar sites that are 10 mm or longer).

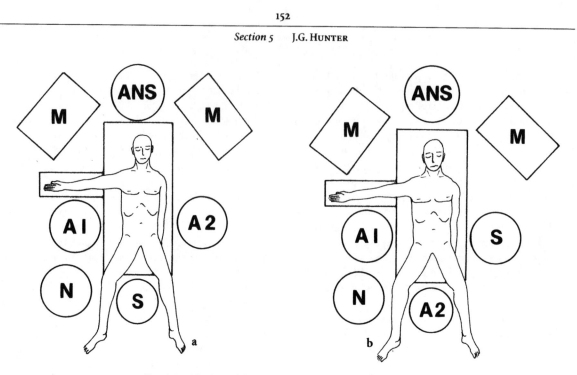

Fig. 1. Positioning of the patient and team. The patient is in a supine position (*ANS*, anesthetist; *S*, surgeon; *A1, A2*, assistant; *N*, nurse; *M*, monitor)

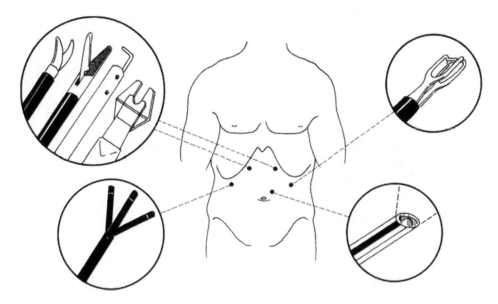

Fig. 2. Trocar sites and instruments

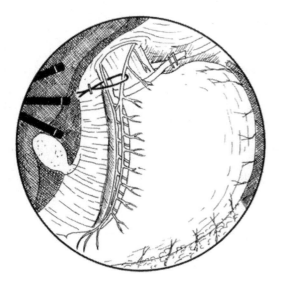

Fig. 3. Separation of the vagal trunks away from the esophagus

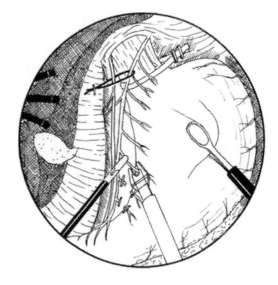

Fig. 4. Division of the anterior leaflet of the lesser sac with a grasper and clipper

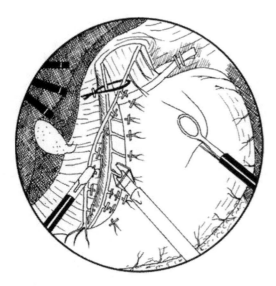

Fig. 5. Dissection of the posterior gastrohepatic omentum

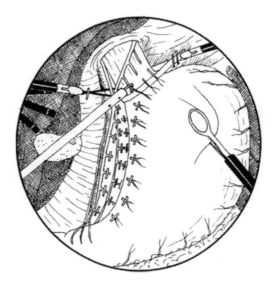

Fig. 6. Clearance of the esophagus, 6 cm above the gastroesophageal junction

Comments

No tubes are left in the patient's stomach. The Foley catheter is discontinued in the recovery room, and the compression stockings are discontinued when the patient can walk again. The patient is started on a liquid diet the morning after surgery and may progress to a soft solid diet within the first 24 h. The patient is placed on small feedings initially, as there is a propensity for delayed gastric emptying in the early postoperative period. If this occurs, it is occasionally helpful to place these patients on erythromycin or other prokinetic agents to facilitate gastric emptying during this period. It is suggested that followup studies, including determination of maximal and basal acid outputs, should only be performed to confirm the adequacy of vagotomy if these tests have also been done preoperatively. Generally, the best followup will require many years and, even with the best technique, a recurrence rate of 10%–15% can be expected.

References

Weerts JM, Dallemogue B, Jehaes C, Markiewicz S (1994) Laparoscopic gastric vagotomies. Ann Chir Ginecol 83(2):118–123

Dubois F (1994) Vagotomies – laparoscopic or thoracoscopic approach. Endosc Surg Allied Technol 2(2):100–104

Taylor TV, Bhandarkar DS (1993) Laparoscopic vagotomy: an operation for the 1990s. Annu R Coll Surg 75(6):385–386

Marciel J, Katkhouda N (1991) Laparoscopic truncal and selective vagotomy. In: Zucker KA (ed): Surgical laparoscopy. Quality Medical, St. Louis, pp 263–279

28 Laparoscopic Billroth II Gastrectomy

P. Goh and C.K. Kum

Introduction

The operation of Billroth II gastrectomy is most commonly performed through an upper abdominal midline incision. This incision leads to considerable pain to the patient and also depresses respiratory function by up to 60%. The totally intra-abdominal laparoscopic Billroth II gastrectomy offers a minimally invasive option that is remarkably less traumatic and more "patient friendly". Patients have less postoperative pain, are able to mobilize faster and thus able to leave the hospital earlier.

Positioning of the Patient and Team

Surgery is performed under general anesthesia with the patient in supine position with the legs apart level with the body. The surgeon stands between the legs with one assistant on each side (Fig. 1). Two monitors are placed over the patient's shoulders. Antibiotic coverage with a third-generation cephalosporin is given routinely at induction. A nasogastric tube and urinary catheter are inserted. The patient is tilted 20° reverse Trendelenburg.

Technique

The operation is performed through five trocar ports (Fig. 2). Except for the 10 mm subumbilical port, the rest are 12 mm. A zero degree 10 mm laparoscope attached to a three-chips camera is inserted via the umbilical port, and the abdomen is surveyed. The site of the ulcer is then identified. Occasionally, external signs of the ulcer may not be distinct, and gastroscopy is needed to ascertain the exact location.

Dissection begins on the greater curve of the stomach which is mobilized with a combination of sharp dissection and electrocautery. A convenient avascular plane in the greater omentum is selected for dissection. Large branches of the epiploic vessels are secured with clips before division. The distal two-thirds of the stomach can be mobilized this way (Fig. 3).

The proximal duodenum can be mobilized with an application of the 30 mm endovascular cutter along its inferior surface, provided it is fairly mobile. Otherwise, a combination of electrocautery and careful sharp dissection using scissors is required. Alternatively, the Ultra-cision (Piling Weck, Smithfield, USA) ultrasonic shears may be used. This instrument can cut and seal vessels up to 1 mm in size. All substantial vessels supplying this area must be secured with endoclips before division. The same technique is used to free the posterior wall of the duodenum. A window in the lesser omentum on the superior aspect of the duodenum is then created with cautery. This allows the application of an Endo GIA across the proximal duodenum (Fig. 4). The stapler transects the duodenum and seals each end of the resection margin with staples. The lesser curve is then mobilized from distal to proximal in the least vascular plane using the same technique as the greater curve dissection.

The level of gastric resection is then chosen, and a line is drawn using superficial cautery over the anterior surface of the stomach at this level. The nasogastric tube is withdrawn at this point. The transection can be done with three to four applications of 30 mm endocutters (Fig. 5). Alternatively, it can be done with two applications of the 60 mm endoscopic cutter. These longer staplers however need larger trocar ports of 15 mm or 18 mm. The stapling is usually done through the left hypochondrial port (Fig. 2). Application of subsequent staplers must be at the apex of the last stapling. The resected stomach specimen is then temporarily placed above the right lobe of the liver in a specimen bag.

The laparoscope is then swung down below the transverse colon which is lifted cephalad with a bowel grasping forceps. The duodenojejunal junction is identified and a loop of proximal jejunum is selected and brought superiorly across the transverse colon in an antecolic fashion. The loop is held against the stomach stump and the position adjusted to facilitate the creation of a gastrojejunostomy without tension or kinking. Two stay sutures are placed intracorporeal to hold the jejunum to the stomach (Fig. 6).

Cautery is used to create two small openings, one in the stomach and one in the adjacent jejunum on the right side of the proposed anastomotic line. A 30 mm endocutter is then positioned with one jaw in each of the openings (Fig. 6). The stapler is closed and fired, creating a stapled anastomosis between the stomach and the jejunal loop. This also has the effect of holding the stomach and jejunum together. The anastomosis is enlarged to 6 cm with a second firing of the stapler across the apex of the "V" of the first staple line. The staple line is then checked for hemostasis. The common small incision for the endocutter is then held up by two or three stay sutures and closed with two or three applications of the endocutter. Alternatively, the enterostomy can be closed with two layers of absorbable sutures using intracorporeal suturing techniques (Fig. 7). Although hand suturing takes slightly longer, it has a lower risk of compromising the anastomotic lumen. The Endostitch (USSC, Norwalk, USA) facilitates this step. The integrity of the anastomosis is checked by flooding the anastomotic site and introducing air into the stomach with a gastroscope. Patency of the afferent and efferent loops are also confirmed at the same time.

The resected stomach specimen is placed in a specimen bag and is extracted through an extension of the left hypochondrial port site. A spiral twisting motion is used to pull the stomach specimen through this opening. The trocar wounds are then closed in two layers and bupivacaine 1% is infiltrated around the wounds for postoperative pain relief.

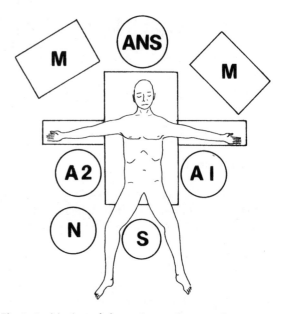

Fig. 1. Positioning of the patient and team. The patient is placed in a supine position (*ANS*, anesthetist; *S*, surgeon; *A1*, *A2*, assistant; *N*, nurse; *M*, monitor)

Postoperative Care

The patient should be able to mobilize on the first day and take fluids by the third day. Diet can usually be resumed by the fifth day. Return to home is usually within a week.

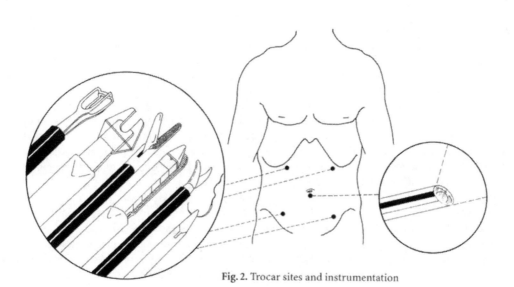

Fig. 2. Trocar sites and instrumentation

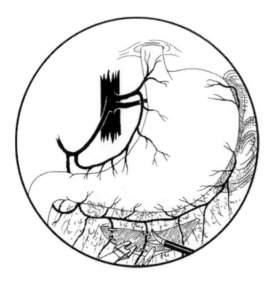

Fig. 3. Mobilization of distal two-thirds of the stomach

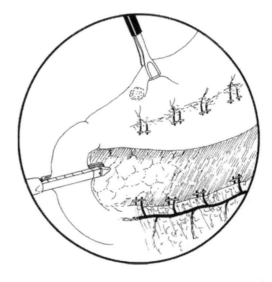

Fig. 4. Transection of the duodenum with 30 mm Endo GIA

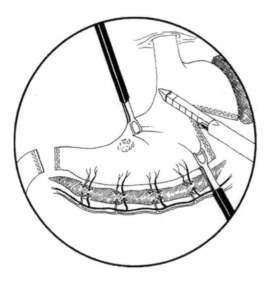

Fig. 5. Transection of the stomach with 30 or 60 mm Endo GIA

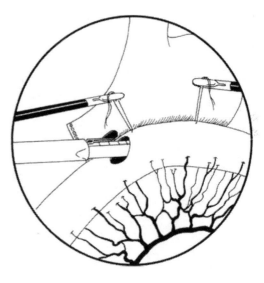

Fig. 6. A 30 mm Endo GIA positioned with one jaw in each of the openings

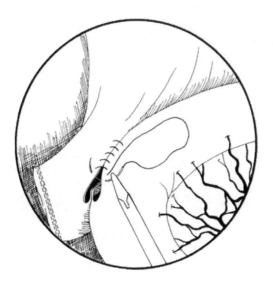

Fig. 7. Closing the enterostomy using intracorporeal suturing techniques

Comments

Unlike duodenal ulcers, surgery still has a significant role in the management of gastric ulcers. Indications for laparoscopic gastrectomy include:

1. Failure of the ulcer to heal after three months of well supervised and compliant medical treatment. Biopsy must be taken to exclude malignancy.
2. Bleeding gastric ulcer after failure of endoscopic hemostasis.
3. A perforated gastric ulcer with minimal soilage.
4. Performing this operation for carcinoma is controversial.

Relative contraindications are:

1. Patients with previous upper abdominal surgery.
2. Patients with cardiopulmonary disease as they will be subjected to prolonged CO_2 pneumoperitoneum.

References

Ellis H (1979) Billroth and the first successful gastrectomy. Contemp Surg 15:63.

Kum CK, Goh P (1992) Laparoscopic vagotomy – a new tool in the management of peptic ulcer disease. Br J Surg 79:977

Goh P, Tekant Y, Kum CK, Isaac J, Ngoi SS (1992) Totally intrabdominal laparoscopic Billroth II gastrectomy. Surg Endosc 6:160

Goh P, Kum CK (1993) Laparoscopic Billroth II gastrectomy: a review. Surg Oncol 2[Supplement 1]:13–18

29 Staging Laparoscopy for Gastric Cancer

A. Ungeheuer, S.J.M. Kraemer, H. Feussner, and J.R. Siewert

Introduction

Imaging of abdominal organs has greatly improved with the introduction of ultrasonography and computed tomography. Nevertheless, wide discrepancies between preoperative and perioperative tumor staging still occur. Accurate detection of intra-abdominal metastasis and reliable definition of local spread of the primary are of considerable importance in surgical oncology.

Diagnostic laparoscopy has become well established as an important tool to improve decision making in abdominal surgery. The so-called extended diagnostic laparoscopy (EDL) is used as part of the preoperative staging diagnostic. Laparoscopic ultrasound and intraoperative diagnostic lavage for detection of free tumor cells in the abdominal cavity are obligatory parts of the EDL. This technique has the ability to extend and improve the diagnostic spectrum in patients with abdominal tumors and patients with pathological findings of unknown identity. We perform EDL in addition to the imaging methods mentioned above.

The objectives for the use of EDL in gastric cancer are to determine the T stage of the gastric tumor with greater precision than established imaging methods can provide. Endoscopic ultrasound today provides the highest precision for preoperative estimation of T and N stage. However, its meaningfulness is limited by the range of the scanner and its means of application. Studies can be obtained in a range of up to only 2–3 cm beyond the lumen in which the endoscope is placed and along the reach or the length of the endoscope. Therefore the greatest part of the abdomen cannot be reached directly by endoscopic ultrasound.

The inclusion criterion is T3 or T4 gastric cancer according to endoluminal ultrasound. The exclusion criteria include those with suspected adhesions after prior surgeries and those with heart and lung insufficiency or other severe heart or lung problems.

Positioning of the Patient and Team

Surgeon, assistant, and scrub nurse are placed as depicted (Fig. 1). If one monitor is used, it is preferably placed above the head of the patient.

Technique

After the pneumoperitoneum has been established, the EDL begins with the introduction of an 11-mm trocar at the umbilicus (Fig. 2). A 30° 10-mm optic is then introduced into the abdominal cavity. The 30° laparoscope allows inspection of areas such as the right subphrenic space or the space of Douglas in the pelvis.

Having inserted the laparoscope, the second trocar is then placed under visual control between the lower and upper quadrant as shown. Through this trocar a retractor may be introduced to lift up the liver or other organs. Prior to any further manipulations the diagnostic laparoscopy begins with the inspection of the upper abdominal cavity. The patient is brought into a 30°–45° anti-Trendelenburg position. This brings the omentum and the small and large intestine caudad, exposing the organs of the upper abdomen.

As mentioned above, the steps of laparoscopy are always performed in the identical order, beginning with the left upper abdomen and continuing counterclockwise to the right upper abdomen and the right lower abdomen. From here one turns clockwise to the left lower quadrant, giving the omentum and the small bowel a closer look. The first inspection finishes with examination of the left lower quadrant and the organs of the pelvic space. Thus, the laparoscopic exploration follows the pattern of an "S."

The inspection is carried out to find pathological changes in the serosa and the visceral and parietal peritoneum, adhesions that may be caused by tumor spread, and bulges or lumps caused by lymph nodes or tumor masses. Local tumor spread, especially in the greater omentum, can be visualized with this method, as well as small lymph node metastasis in the omentum and smaller amounts of ascites that to date cannot be detected with the well-advanced imaging methods available. Such findings may prompt a dramatic change in the treatment course if a multimodal approach to the treatment of gastric cancer (and other tumors) is applied.

After the initial overview and prior to any further manipulation, diagnostic lavage is performed to detect any free tumor cells. Physiological saline (200 ml) is instilled into the upper abdominal cavity and aspirated with a special suction device similar to the standard suction device used in open surgery (Fig. 3).

At this point in the examination two more ports are introduced in the left upper quadrant. An 11-mm trocar is inserted cephalad and lateral from the umbilical trocar site, while the third trocar is placed just lateral from this port (Fig 2).

After the first overview, the abdominal wall and the organs of the left upper abdominal cavity are carefully inspected individually. We always begin with the inspection of the stomach. To expose the lesser curve of the stomach and the hiatus with the gastroesophageal junction, the left lobe of the liver needs to be elevated with a retractor or a blunt instrument. This allows inspection of the anterior aspect of the fundus, the corpus, and the antral part of the stomach. The lesser sac and the area of the celiac trunk can be easily inspected after dividing the gastrohepatic ligament. If the localization of the tumor necessitates a closer investigation of the gastroesophageal junction, the phrenoesophageal ligament may be partially divided. In the next step the stomach is lifted up close to the greater curve 2 in. left of the pylorus with a Babcock or Allison clamp to elevate and stretch the greater omentum. This is divided with scissors and cautery. If greater vessels are encountered, they are carefully avoided or, if necessary, clipped. This prepares a window in the greater omentum which allows direct inspection of the retrogastric space and the posterior wall of the stomach (Fig. 4). The anterior aspect of the corpus and head of the pancreas can also be inspected as well as the celiac trunk.

The spleen is examined next. By carefully pulling the left edge of the greater omentum caudally, the spleen can be visualized.

The anterior and posterior aspects of the left lobe of the liver can be examined by lifting it up with a retractor. The consistency of the liver can be tested with a blunt instrument, which also can provide first hints of liver metastasis deep within the liver parenchyma. By moving the laparoscope to the right upper abdomen the right lobe of the liver can be examined. The right subphrenic and the anterior aspect of the liver can be easily seen. With a fan retractor or a similar device the liver can be elevated and the posterior aspect partially inspected by simply turning the laparoscope axially 180°. Inspection of the gallbladder, common duct, and round ligament, pylorus, and duodenum can be easily achieved.

Now the patient is brought into a 30° Trendelenburg position. This brings the gut into the upper half of the abdominal cavity, thus exposing the pelvic organs. The abdominal wall, ileocecal junction, colon, sigmoid, and rectum can be given a closer look. The mesentery can be checked for peritoneal carcinosis.

Since peritoneal secondaries and metastasis to the ovaries (Krukenberg's tumors) play a great role in the prognosis in gastric cancer, the pelvic organs need to be inspected carefully. This can be achieved easily with blunt forceps. A small amount of ascites is frequently found, especially in women, and suctioned for histopathological investigation.

All findings are videotaped.

Following the inspection of the lower half of the abdomen the patient is brought back into the 30° anti-Trendelenburg position. The laparoscope is moved to the left 11-mm trocar and a special 10-mm flexible laparoscopic ultrasound probe is inserted into the umbilical port (Fig. 5). To avoid artifacts laparoscopic ultrasound (LUS) should be performed before any biopsies are taken. The LUS procedure is videotaped as well, using a screen divider, so that the laparoscopic picture and the ultrasound picture can be seen on the same screen at the same time. In this fashion the organs of the upper quadrants can be easily examined with LUS. The flexible head of the ultrasound probe follows the surface of the liver without problem, guaranteeing good contact to the surface and high resolution (Fig. 6 A, B). To judge the T stage of gastric carcinoma the stomach is filled with 250–300 ml saline by the anesthesiologist via the nasogastric tube, which we always have in place during any laparoscopic procedure. If necessary, an equal amount of saline may be filled into the upper abdomen to further improve the quality of the LUS picture. This trick allows checking for tumor invasion of gastric cancer into the pancreas or for enlarged lymph nodes. Especially in skinny patients tumor invasion from gastric cancer into adjacent organs is almost impossible for the radiologist to see since in these patients there is no layer of fatty tissues between the organs.

By placing the LUS probe back to the umbilical port or to a third port, which may be introduced in the right upper quadrant, the stomach and the adjacent organs can be investigated thoroughly, and any spot of the abdominal cavity may be reached with the LUS probe.

After all biopsies have been taken, another diagnostic lavage is performed, as described above. This lavage serves as a control for whether tumor cells have been spread during the surgical manipulations. To kill potentially free tumor cells we routinely rinse the abdomen at the end of the EDL with taurolidine.

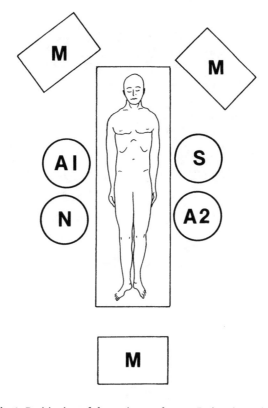

Fig. 1. Positioning of the patient and team. Patient in supine position. *ANS*, Anesthetist; *S*, surgeon; *A1, A2*, assistants; *N*, nurse; *M*, monitor

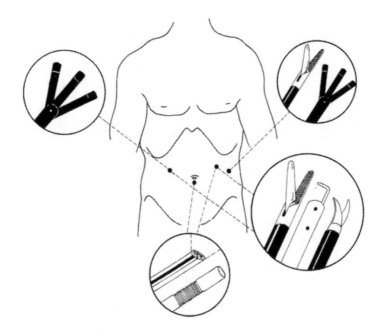

Fig. 2. Trocar sites and instrumentation

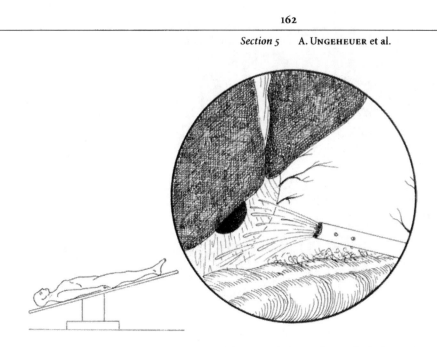

Fig. 3. Irrigation of the upper abdomen for cytological examination

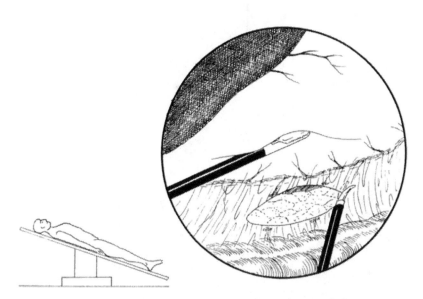

Fig. 4. Creation of a window into the lesser sac

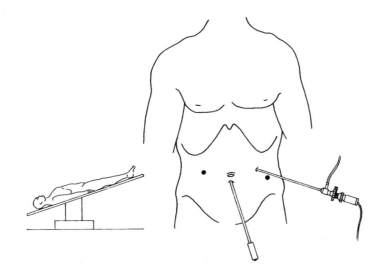

Fig. 5. The camera has been switched to a lateral port and the ultrasound probe inserted at the umbilical site

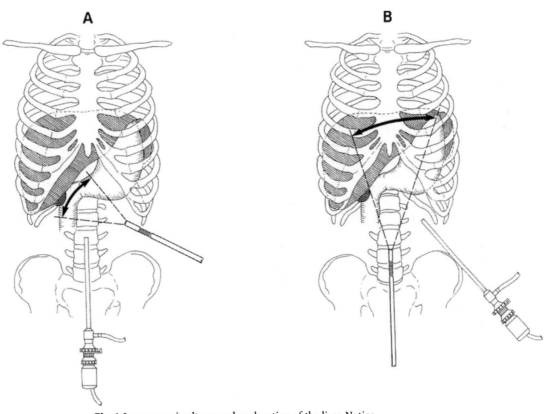

Fig. 6. Laparoscopic ultrasound exploration of the liver. Notice that the ultrasound probe and laparoscope have been switched to explore the left liver lobe

Comments

During the course of the EDL all findings are recorded, regardless of whether they are anatomical variations or tumor-related, to be compared later with the results of the other imaging methods.

To date, 170 patients with gastric cancer have been examined under this protocol with EDL. All of these patients had a T3 or T4 gastric cancer, according to the clinical staging. In 86 patients (50.6%) the clinical pre-EDL staging was confirmed by EDL, while in 80 (47.1%) the pre-EDL staging had to be revised due to the intra-operative findings. This led to a change of the therapy initially planned in 70 of the 170 patients (41.2%). LUS findings accounted for 7.1% of the changes. This number will probably increase with the development of more advanced laparoscopic ultrasound probes. Looking at the results in detail, we saw that the pre-EDL staging needed to be upgraded in 42 patients (24.7%). Here we found localized and generalized peritoneal carcinomatosis undetected by the other imaging techniques. Tumor invasion of pancreas and liver was detected in five patients (2.9%) and distant metastasis of the liver and colon in six (3.5%). A downgrading was achieved in 28 patients (16.5%).

We consider EDL a prerequisite for the determination of adequate therapy in the multimodal approach to gastric cancer. However, with the rapid development of more advanced imaging techniques or more advanced laparoscopic devices the decision for EDL will need to be reevaluated. EDL is a very invasive diagnostic procedure and entails the risks of all surgical laparoscopic procedures. Looking at the economic aspect of EDL versus classical imaging techniques, EDL can reduce overall costs only if it partially or completely replaces those established imaging procedures. Diagnostic laparoscopy and extended diagnostic laparoscopy can be an advantage for the patient only if the preoperative staging by diagnostic or extended laparoscopy provides additional information that leads to an improvement in therapy.

References

Cuschieri A (1980) Laparoscopy in general surgery and gastroenterology. Br Hosp Med 24:252–254

Feussner H (1994) Laparoskopische Exploration der Bauchhöhle. In: Kremer K, Lierse W, Platzer W, Schreiber HW, Weller S (eds) Minimal-Invasive Chirurgie. Thieme, Stuttgart (Chirurgische Operationslehre. Spezielle Anatomie, Indikationen, Technik, Komplikationen, vol 7/2)

Kriplani AK, Kapur BML (1991) Laparoscopy for pre-operative staging and assessment of operability in gastric carcinoma. Gastrointest Endosc 37:441–443

Possik RA, Franco EL, Pires DR, Wohnrath DR, Ferreira EB (1986) Sensitivity, specificity and predictive value of laparoscopy for the staging of gastric cancer and for detection of liver metastasis. Cancer 58:1–6

Warshaw AL (1991) Implications of peritoneal cytology for staging of early pancreatic cancer. Am J Surg 161 (1):26–29

Watt I, Steward I, Anderson D, Bell G, Anderson JR (1989) Laparoscopy, ultrasound and computerized tomography in cancer of the esophagus and gastric cardia: a prospective comparison for detecting intra-abdominal metastases. Br J Surg 6:1036–1039

SECTION 6

30 Laparoscopic Splenectomy

E.H. PHILLIPS and R.J. ROSENTHAL

Introduction

The importance of the spleen has been debated since the time of the ancient Greeks. From an historical point of view, its immunologic role has only recently been established. Over the past 25 years surgical extirpation for the slightest reason has been replaced by efforts to save all or some of the splenic mass, especially in children. Nevertheless, occasionally the entire spleen must be removed because of intrinsic disease, hypersplenism, or for diagnosis. The operative technique for total splenectomy is well known, and until 4 years ago had not significantly changed since the first successful splenectomy performed in 1826.

The laparoscopic revolution has clearly shown that avoidance of an upper abdominal incision for cholecystectomy and antireflux surgery significantly shortens hospital stay and decreases morbidity. Subsequently, laparoscopic techniques have been applied to splenectomy and have shown that it also decreases morbidity and mortality as well as decreasing postoperative discomfort and shortening hospital stay.

Positioning of the Patient and Team

Patients are positioned on an electric operating table on a beanbag for easier position change during surgery, left side up. This becomes an important aid when dissecting the splenorenal and the splenophrenic ligaments in obese patients or patients with enlarged spleens (Fig. 1 a, b).

Technique

Autologous blood is obtained for all elective cases. Patients should receive preoperative immunization with *Pneumovax, Haemophilus influenza*, and meningococcus vaccines. All operations are performed under general endotracheal anesthesia. Prophylactic antibiotics are given preoperatively. Preoperative splenic artery embolization is considered in obese patients, patients with AIDS, and patients with splenomegaly. A 30° viewing angle laparoscope is used for visualization.

Following the creation of the pneumoperitoneum with a Veress needle or open Hasson technique, a 10- to 11-mm trocar is placed in the umbilical area or supraumbilical area in tall patients (Fig. 2). A general inspection of the abdomen is performed with special attention to possible accessory spleens. A 5- or 10-mm trocar is placed in the subxiphoid area, and a 10- to 11-mm trocar (the operating trocar) is placed halfway between the subxiphoid and the umbilical trocar (Fig. 2). A 10- to 11-mm trocar (the lateral trocar) is placed in the left axillary line, halfway between the costal margin and the iliac crest (Fig. 2). A 12-mm trocar (the stapler trocar) is placed halfway between the umbilicus and the lateral trocar (Fig. 2). In very tall patients, when the trocar for the laparoscope is placed above the umbilicus, the left lateral trocars are moved up correspondingly.

The operation begins by ligating the splenic artery in the lesser sac. The stomach is reflected anteriorly, and the colon is retracted inferiorly with Babcock or atraumatic graspers placed via the two lateral trocars. A window in the gastrocolic omentum is opened with scissors or electrocautery (Fig. 3). The pancreas is retracted posteriorly and inferiorly with a fan retractor. The tortuous splenic artery is usually pushed up into view by this maneuver. The peritoneum is lifted with a grasper placed via the subxiphoid trocar and is divided by a scissor placed via the operating trocar. The splenic artery is then grasped, elevated, and occluded with a large endoclip (Fig. 4). The surgeon performs these tasks using two-handed technique. The left hand operates through the subxiphoid trocar and the right hand through the midline (operating) trocar.

In normal or slightly enlarged spleens attention is then paid to the colosplenic attachments (Fig. 5). These are divided sharply or with electrocautery. The spleen is grasped with a ring forceps grasper or lung clamp and elevated anteriorly and medially (with the patient positioned left side up) via the lateral trocar. The splenorenal ligament is divided with scissors and/or electrocautery hook (Fig. 6). An electrocautery hook device with suction and irrigation facilitates this dissection and is critical when bleeding is encountered. Frequent irrigation and aspiration make this instrument essential to the procedure.

The dissection is taken cephalad as far as possible. Division of the splenophrenic attachments allows the spleen to be completely elevated, exposing the hilar vessels. If splenomegaly prevents extensive mobilization, the operation is more difficult and more dangerous as the hilar vessels need to be divided first. In normal sized spleens the inferior hilar vessels are not divided until more of the retrosplenic, splenorenal, and/or splenophrenic attachments can be divided. Although some surgeons divide the hilar vessels first, this approach leaves one with fewer options if bleeding is encountered when dissecting the hilar vessels, as it is much more difficult to control the bleeding if the spleen is not already mobilized. This is especially true in the more difficult laparoscopic splenectomy. However, in the truly massive spleen this type of mobilization is impossible, and the hilar vessels require division first.

After division of as many of the posterior peritoneal attachments as possible the inferior pole vessels are divided (Fig. 7). The central vessels and the superior pole vessels are then sequentially ligated and divided. Finally, the short gastric vessels are divided (Fig. 8). The techniques of vessel ligation include endoloops (Ethicon; EndoSurgery, Cincinnati, Oh), clips, intra- and extracorporeal ties, bipolar cautery, and endovascular staplers. Ties and endovascular staplers are less likely to be disrupted by retractors than clips and are therefore preferred. The endovascular staplers are excellent but still require proper dissection of the vessels and adequate sized windows to allow safe insertion of their "jaws." Adequate dissection of the vessels should be performed in case there is bleeding from the staple lines. It is dangerous to insert the endovascular stapler blindly on the hilar vessels and to "fire" it blindly, as the device may only be cutting halfway across a splenic vein or artery. It needs to be stressed that proper dissection of hilar "windows" and application of the staplers are critical. The stapler is especially useful when dividing the short gastric vessels as they are secure even when the stomach distends.

If the spleen has already been mobilized when bleeding is encountered during the dissection of the hilar vessels, the rapid application of the endovascular stapler can quickly and securely stop the bleeding in most cases. Even a grasper can apply pressure until the field has been suctioned, and a plan for ligation of the vessel is agreed upon. If the spleen has not been mobilized, control of hemorrhage is much more difficult.

After the spleen is detached, it is placed in a Lapsac (Cook Urological, Spencer, IN), which at the present time is the strongest and safest bag (Fig. 9). If pathologic analysis is not crucial, the spleen can be morcellated manu-

ally with a ring forceps or mechanically with a tissue morcellator (Cook Urological) at the site of the 12-mm trocar (Fig. 10). If the procedure is performed for Hodgkin's disease, lymphoma, or other tumors that require careful pathologic analysis, the specimen can be removed intact via a lower abdominal incision or enlargement of the umbilical trocar site. Before the CO_2 is removed the splenic bed is reinspected for hemostasis and a decision is made regarding placement of closed suction drainage which we rarely use. Bupivacaine is then injected at each trocar site. The fascia is always closed at each 10- to 12-mm trocar site with 0 Vicryl suture.

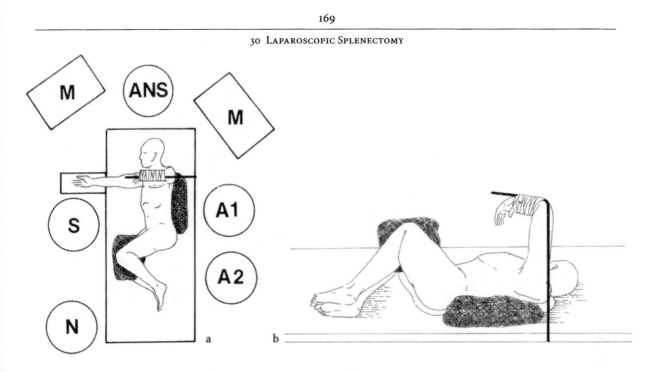

Fig. 1 a, b. Positioning of the patient and team. Patient in right lateral decubitus position. *ANS*, Anesthetist; *S*, surgeon; *A1, A2*, assistants; *N*, nurse; *M*, monitor

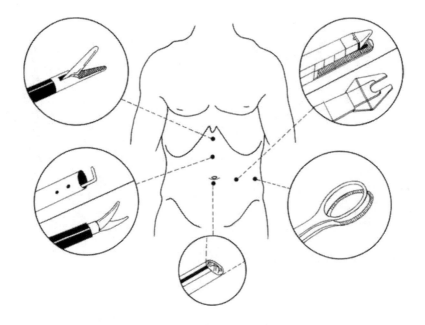

Fig. 2. Trocar sites and instrumentation

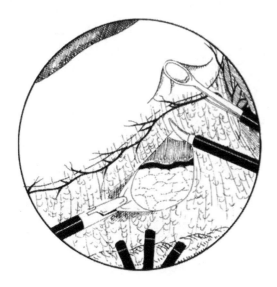

Fig. 3. Elevation of the stomach and view into the lesser sac

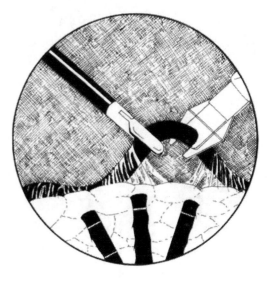

Fig. 4. The splenic artery is clipped

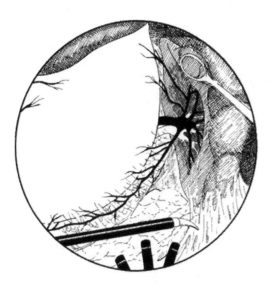

Fig. 5. Elevation of the spleen and dissection of the splenocolic ligament

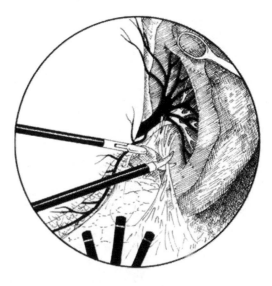

Fig. 6. Dissection of hilar and splenorenal ligaments

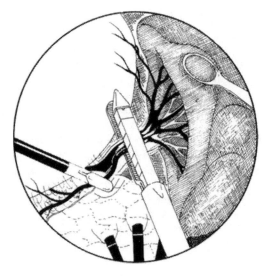

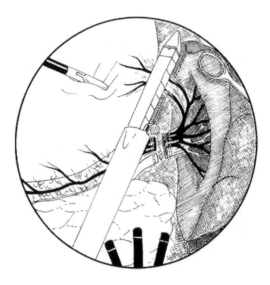

Fig. 7. Transection of spleen hilum with the endocutter

Fig. 8. Transection of short gastric vessels

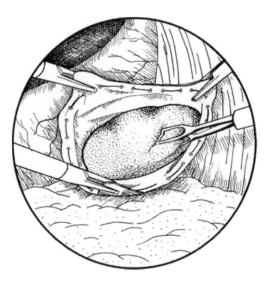

Fig. 9. Placement of specimen into bag. (Note placement of graspers holding the bag)

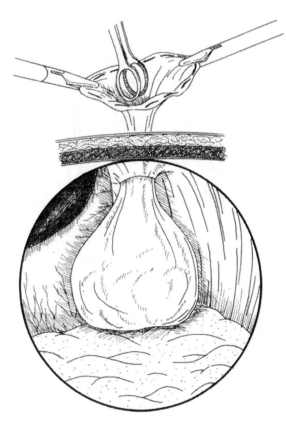

Fig. 10. Exteriorization of the bag and morcellation of the specimen

Comments

At its present stage of development laparoscopic splenectomy is best suited to the removal of normal sized spleens in the elective setting. Slightly enlarged spleens can be removed as the surgeon gains experience, and if the patient is thin and the body habitus permits. Only the most experienced surgeons can approach spleens heavier than 1000 g. The early results of laparoscopic splenectomy on enlarged spleens suggest that as experience is gained and technology advances, the more fragile patients (often on steroids) will benefit with the lower morbidity and mortality that results from the lack of an upper abdominal incision and the concomitant early ambulation that it affords.

References

Cuschieri A, Shimi S, Banting S, Vander Velpen G (1992) Technical aspects of laparoscopic splenectomy: hilar segmental devascularization and instrumentation. J R Coll Surg Edinb 37 (6):414–416

Lefor AT, Melvin WS, Bailey RW, Flowers JL (1993) Laparoscopic splenectomy in the management of immune thrombocytopenic purpura. Surgery 114 (3):613–618

Phillips EH, Carroll BJ, Fallas MJ (1994) Laparoscopic splenectomy. Surg Endosc 8:931–933

Kitano S, Kobayashi M, Sugimacho K (1994) Laparoscopic surgery for pancreatic and splenic disorders (abstract). Surg Endosc 8 (5):449

Hiatt JR, Gomes AS, Machleder HI. Massive splenomegaly (1990) Arch Surg 125:1363–1367

Tulman S, Delaitre B, Cadiere CB (1994) Laparoscopic splenectomy (abstract). Surg Endosc 8 (5):449

31 Laparoscopic Right Adrenalectomy

E.H. Phillips and R.J. Rosenthal

Introduction

Adrenalectomy can be performed transabdominally or via the flank or retroperitoneal approach. The transabdominal approach has the advantage of affording access to both adrenal glands and the other sites of potential endocrine tissue with one incision. The laparoscopic approach offers excellent exposure to both glands while avoiding the need for a large abdominal incision. The present limitations of the laparoscopic technique involve inadequate instrumentation for handling enlarged friable adrenal tumors and difficulty with exposure and dissection of tumors larger than 6 cm.

Positioning of the Patient and Team

Patients are placed on an electric operating table on a beanbag in the left lateral decubitus position (Fig. 1). The beanbag allows for easier position change during surgery and secures the patient to the operating table. The alternative position is a full left lateral position. We prefer the partial lateral position on the beanbag so that the patient can be rotated to a supine position for initial trocar insertion, then rotated to a variable lateral position depending on the requirements of the specific case. The right arm is suspended in an "airplane" sling, and the axilla is supported with a roll of towels to prevent brachial plexus injury. The positioning is critical to expose the retroperitoneal space properly in obese patients, patients with hepatomegaly, and patients with large adrenal tumors (Fig. 2).

Technique

All operations are performed under general endotracheal anesthesia. A 30° angle laparoscope is important for visualization. Autologous blood should be collected preoperatively to avoid unnecessary transfusions in the event of unexpected bleeding. Additionally, a cell saver should be in the operating room. Following creation of the pneumoperitoneum with a Veress needle or open Hasson technique a 10- to 11-mm trocar is placed in the umbilical area or supraumbilical area, depending on the body habitus (tall patients may have the optic above the umbilicus and to the side of the gland to be removed; Fig. 3). A general inspection of the abdomen is always performed. A 10- to 11-mm trocar is placed in the subxiphoid area, and a 10- to 11-mm trocar (the right hand operating trocar) is placed halfway between the subxiphoid and the umbilical trocar (Fig. 3). A 10- to 11-mm trocar (the left hand operating trocar) is placed in the patient's right axillary line or anterior axillary line, halfway between the costal margin and the iliac crest (Fig. 3). A 10- to 11-mm trocar is placed lateral to the 12-mm trocar to grasp the gland or provide exposure by elevating the liver (Fig. 3). In tall patients, when the trocar for the laparoscope is placed above the umbilicus, the right lateral trocars are moved up correspondingly.

The hepatic flexure of the colon is mobilized from its parietal attachments using sharp, then blunt dissection (Fig. 4). The colon is reflected inferiorly and medially in two locations by the assistant while the surgeon provides countertraction with a grasper. The use of an electrosurgical hook with suction and irrigation facilitates this dissection. The hook can elevate the retroperitoneal tissue of the hepatic flexure allowing safe fulguration and division while the suction can clear the smoke. The liver is retracted superiorly with a rack retractor while the colon falls inferiorly, aided by gravity and patient positioning. This maneuver enables exposure of the whole right upper retroperitoneal space in which kidney and adrenal gland are located underlying Gerota's fascia and its surrounding fatty envelope. The right adrenal gland is partially obscured in some cases by the vena cava or the liver. A decision should be made at this point about converting to an open procedure.

After division of Gerota's fascia on the upper pole of the kidney the adrenal gland should come into view. It is important in most cases to divide the central vein first, but in a practical sense dividing the adrenal arteries facilitates exposure as the vein is approached. Careful inferior and lateral retraction of the gland or adjacent tissue helps define the tissue planes while blunt dissection is initiated between the gland and the vena cava.

When dissecting the central vein of the right adrenal gland, it should be emphasized that the vein enters the vena cava on the posterior lateral aspect (not midway or anteriorly; Fig. 5). It is also important to be aware of anomalous drainage. The vein can drain into the right hepatic or renal vein. The right adrenal vein should be dissected very carefully to avoid avulsing it from the vena cava. Clips are usually sufficient for occlusion, but sometimes incontinuity ties with intracorporeal or extracorporeal knot tying technique are needed. If extracorporeal knots are employed, the suture should be lubricated with mineral oil, and a right-angled grasper should be placed posterior to the vein so that the suture runs on the grasper, not the vein (Fig. 6). An alternative technique can be employed. A clip can be placed on the gland side of the vein, and then an endoloop can be preloaded over a grasper, the vein divided, and the endoloop secured (Fig. 7). Usually an additional 5-mm trocar needs to be added for this maneuver.

After the adrenal vein is divided, the adrenal gland should be completely freed from the surrounding tissue using blunt dissection and electrocautery hook dissection. It is possible to follow the whole gland up to the cupula of the diaphragm, where any inferior phrenic vessels can be identified and divided between clips or cautery.

After the adrenal gland is completely free, it should be placed into a heavy plastic bag to avoid contamination of the abdominal cavity during extraction (Fig. 8). The adrenal bed is then copiously irrigated and hemostasis secured. The specimen can be extracted either through the umbilical trocar site or an enlarged site. All trocar sites are infiltrated with Marcaine, and the fascia is closed with sutures.

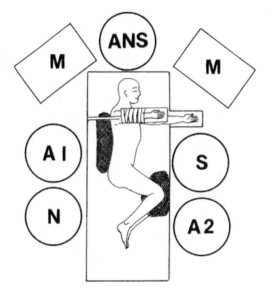

Fig. 1. Positioning of the patient and team. Patient in right lateral decubitus position. *ANS,* Anesthetist; *S,* surgeon; *A1, A2,* assistants; *N,* nurse; *M,* monitor

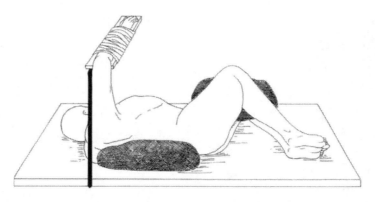

Fig. 2. Patient is placed on a bean bag in the left lateral decubitus position

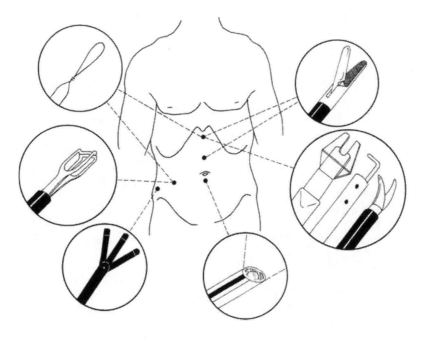

Fig. 3. Trocar sites and instrumentation

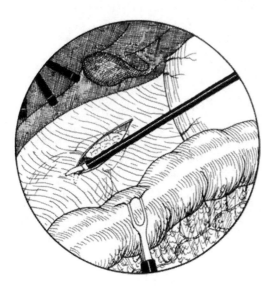

Fig. 4. Hepatocolic ligament is incised

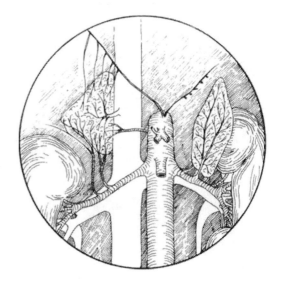

Fig. 5. Schematic view of the anatomical landmarks of the right adrenal gland

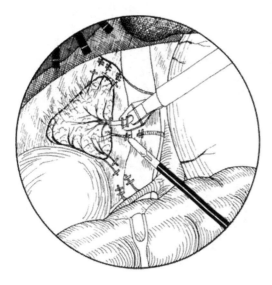

Fig. 6. The central adrenal vein is clipped

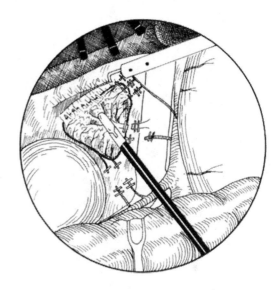

Fig. 7. Dissection of diaphragmatic adhesions of the adrenal gland

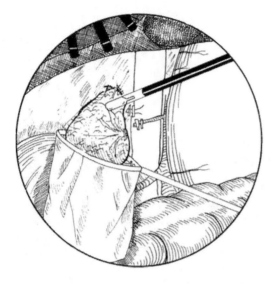

Fig. 8. The specimen is placed in a bag before extraction

Comments

The best way to grasp an adrenal gland is with an oval ring grasper, but if the gland is friable – and every tumor is – we recommend putting one or more endoloops on the mass and grasping the sutures. Performing laparoscopic adrenalectomy for cancer is controversial and certainly should not be attempted until significant experience is gained. It is very difficult to handle a malignant gland, and it is very easy to contaminate the peritoneal cavity.

References

Gagner M, Lacroix A, Pring RA, Bolte E, Albala D, Potvin C, Hamet P, Kuchel O, Querin S, Pomp A (1993) Early experience with laparoscopic approach for adrenalectomy. Surgery 114 (6):1120–1125

Go H, Takeda M, Takahashi H, Imai T, Tsutsui T, Mizusawa T, Nishiyama T, Morishita H, Nakajima Y, Sato S (1993) Laparoscopic adrenalectomy for primary aldosteronism: a new operative method. J Laparoendosc Surg 3 (5):455–459

McLeod MK (1991) Complications following adrenal surgery. J Natl Med Assoc 83:161–164

Prinz RA (1990) Mobilization of the right lobe of the liver for right adrenalectomy. Am J Surg 159:336–338

Vaughan ED jr (1991) Adrenal surgery. In: Marshall FF (ed) Atlas of urologic surgery. Saunders, Philadelphia

32 Laparoscopic Left Adrenalectomy

C. Nies and M. Rothmund

Introduction

Adrenalectomy is performed for adrenal tumors or adrenocortical hyperplasia. Except for hormone-inactive tumors that are incidentally discovered, the goal of treatment is to stop the excessive hormone production by removing the adrenal gland that bears the tumor. In rare cases, bilateral adrenalectomy may be indicated.

Adrenalectomy is a typical example of an operation, in which a small tumor is removed through a comparatively large incision. Since the patients' postoperative comfort is compromised by the incision, it is ideal to perform adrenalectomy laparoscopically.

An abdominal CT scan should be obtained preoperatively. It is very helpful to know the exact size and location of the adrenal tumor and its relationship to adjacent structures such as pancreas, kidney, and spleen.

If the operation is performed for a pheochromocytoma, an alpha blockade with phenoxybenzamin is necessary. Starting at 30 mg a day, the dosage is increased each day until the patient complains of perioral paresthesia or orthostasis. In patients with Conn's syndrome, electrolyte imbalances have to be corrected, and the blood pressure must be medically controlled. Patients with Cushing's disease or Cushing's syndrome due to a cortisol-producing adrenal tumor should receive antibiotic prophylaxis preoperatively.

Positioning of the Patient and Team

After induction of general endotracheal anesthesia, the patient is placed in lithotomy and moderate reverse Trendelenburg position (see Fig. 1). The table is tilted to the left. The position of the surgeon, the two assistants, the scrub nurse, and the monitors is shown in Fig. 1.

Technique

The first incision is made next to the umbilicus. After creation of a pneumoperitoneum, a 10 mm trocar is inserted through which a 30° laparoscope is introduced. After a brief inspection of the peritoneal cavity, three additional trocars are placed as shown in Fig. 2. In order to be able to introduce all instruments required, including the laparoscope from various angles, only 10 mm trocars are used.

First the splenic flexure of the colon has to be mobilized. The colon is gently retracted to the right and the attachments with the lateral abdominal wall and the phrenocolic ligament are divided with scissors (Fig. 3). The peritoneum lateral to the spleen is also incised up to a level above the splenic hilum. The colon is now further mobilized bluntly, so that the inferior border of the pancreas becomes visible. A retractor is introduced through the port under the left costal margin. This instrument is used to carefully retract the spleen and the tail of the pancreas cephalad and slightly to the right (Fig. 4). This gives access to the upper pole of the kidney. In lean patients, the contour of the kidney is easily seen. If this is not the case, it can be palpated with an instrument within the surrounding fat tissue.

The peritoneum is incised along the lower border of the pancreas. Gerota's fascia is then opened and the superior pole of the kidney is dissected free. It is very important to identify the upper pole of the kidney, since it serves as a landmark for locating the position of the adrenal gland. Especially in obese patients, such as those with advanced Cushing's disease, it can be very difficult to locate the adrenal gland. Again, palpation with an instrument helps to find the adrenal gland within the perirenal fat. In this phase of the operation, the preoperative CT scan also can provide important information.

Once the adrenal gland has been identified, its inferior border is carefully dissected free. The principal adrenal vein, which drains into the renal vein, is thereby inevitably encountered. It is circumferentially dissected, closed with clips and divided (Fig. 5). Particularly in patients with pheochromocytoma, it is important to perform this maneuver before the tumor itself is manipulated.

The retractor is now repositioned so that the tail of the pancreas can be retracted more cranially to expose the anterior surface of the adrenal gland. After the anterior surface has been dissected, the gland is mobilized posteriorly and medially (Fig. 6). The dissection at the medial side must be done with great care, since numerous small arterial vessels have to be clipped and divided. During this phase of the operation, it is easy to cause disturbing bleeding in the retroperitoneal fat which is sometimes difficult to control. Also, branches from the phrenic artery entering the adrenal superiorly have to be identified and controlled. A suction/irrigation electrocautery device facilitates this phase of the operation.

Once the adrenal gland has been completely mobilized, it is placed in a retrieval bag (Fig. 7). The operative field is re-inspected for hemostasis. No drain is placed. The retrieval bag is then extracted through the enlarged incision at the umbilicus. The remaining trocars are removed under vision. The fascia at each trocar site is closed with reabsorbable suture material. The skin is closed with regular skin sutures.

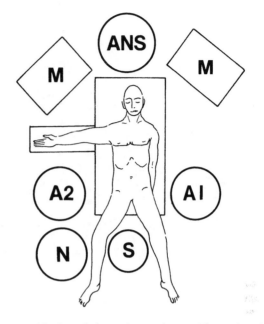

Fig. 1. Positioning of the patient and team. The patient is placed in lithotomy and moderate reverse Trendelenburg position (*ANS*, anesthetist; *S*, surgeon; *A1, A2*, assistants; *N*, nurse; *M*, monitor)

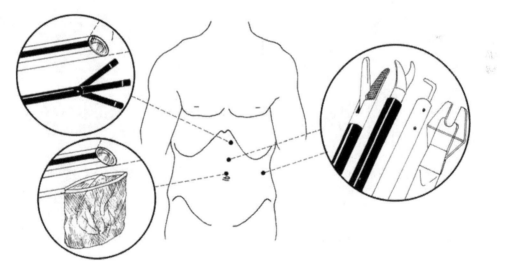

Fig. 2. Position of the trocars in laparoscopic left adrenalectomy

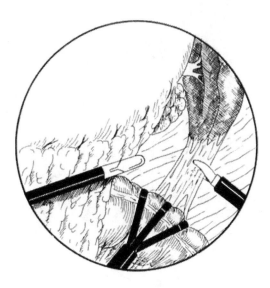

Fig. 3. Mobilization of the left colonic flexure

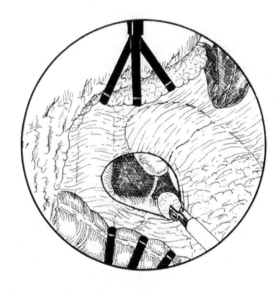

Fig. 4. Retraction of the spleen and the tail of the pancreas. The contour of the upper pole of the left kidney comes into vision

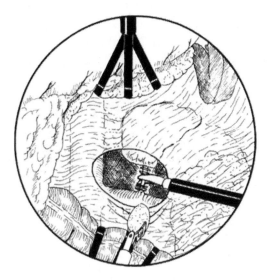

Fig. 5. Division of the main adrenal vein, which has been clipped

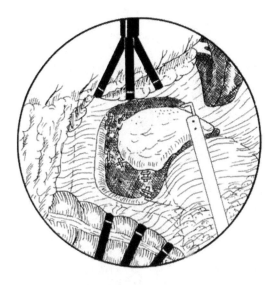

Fig. 6. Dissection at the superior and medial aspect of the adrenal gland

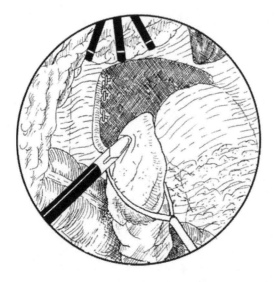

Fig. 7. The specimen is placed in a bag for extraction

Comments

Other endoscopic approaches to the left adrenal gland have been described – access through the left flank and a retroperitoneoscopic posterior approach are both possible. Supporters of these techniques claim that the time of operation is shorter than with the technique described here.

After our learning curve, our operative time averaged approximately 3 h, which is still considerably longer than our conventional posterior approach. However, the benefit of the laparoscopic procedure is reduced patient discomfort. Our patients complained of only mild pain. They were able to tolerate a full diet on the first or second postoperative day and were discharged thereafter.

The most significant surgical complication with this operation is bleeding. First, the spleen can be injured during dissection. Furthermore, the pancreas and spleen have to be retracted during the major part of the operation. Second, the adrenal gland itself is an extremely well-perfused organ. Therefore, only indirect retraction of this organ is possible. The gland itself should never be grasped and pulled, otherwise it will tear. Thirdly, the adrenal gland is nourished by numerous small arteries, which all have to be clipped and divided. Injuries to other organs (colon, pancreas) are possible, but less likely. Careful attention to technique will lead to a rewarding outcome in these interesting patients.

References

Edis AJ, Grant CS, Egdahl RH (1984) Manual of endocrine surgery. Springer, Berlin Heidelberg New York

Fernandez-Cruz, Saenz A, Benarroch G, Torres E, Astudillo E (1994) Technical aspects of adrenalectomy via operative laparoscopy. Surg Endosc 8:1348–1351

Gagner M, Lacroix A, Bolte E, Pomp A (1994) Laparoscopic adrenalectomy. The importance of a flank approach in the lateral decubitus position. Surg Endosc 8:135–138

Nies C, Bartsch D, Schafer U, Rothmund M (1993) Laparoskopische Adrenalektomie. Dtsch Med Wochenschr 118(50):1831–1836

33 Laparoscopic Resection of the Tail of the Pancreas

S.J. Shapiro and L.A. Gordon

Introduction

The pancreas is the most unforgiving abdominal organ. Its response to trauma and surgical injury mandates a cautious approach. Only recently has the laparoscopic surgeon been able to consider laparoscopic resectional therapy. Most benign tumors and cystic lesions of the tail and distal body of the pancreas should be resected with splenic preservation.

Positioning of the Patient and Team

The patient is placed in the supine position with the arms at the sides (Fig. 1). A nasogastric tube and Foley catheter are placed. One monitor is at the head of the table facing the surgeon. The other monitor faces the assistant. The surgeon stands to the patient's right. The assistant and the nurse stand on the patient's left.

Technique

After general anesthesia has been induced, a Veress needle is placed in the infraumbilical position and its position corroborated with a hanging drop test. A pneumoperitoneum is developed to 16 mmHg. A 10- to 11-mm trocar is placed in this position. A 30° angle laparoscope is then placed into the abdominal cavity and exploration carried out. The liver is evaluated, as are all peritoneal surfaces. A 10- to 11-mm trocar is then placed in the subxiphoid position. Under direct vision a 10-to 11-mm trocar is placed in the anterior axillary line approximately 6 cm below the left costal margin. Another 10- to 11-mm trocar is placed in the midclavicular line approximately 10 cm below the left costal margin. A 10- to 11-mm trocar is also placed in the right midclavicular line approximately 6 cm below the right costal margin (Fig. 2).

The splenic flexure is taken down sharply using electrocautery scissors (Fig. 3). One must be cautious with monopolar electrocautery around the colon. Using electrocautery and clips, the lesser sac is then opened, and the gastrocolic ligament is transected outside of the epiploic arch (Fig. 4). Once the entire lesser sac has been opened, two or three traction sutures of 2-0 nylon are placed through the abdominal wall, through the anterior gastric wall, retracting the stomach superiorly and anteriorly (Fig. 5).

The short gastric vessels are preserved during this operation. Using a soft balloon retractor (Advanced Surgical), the spleen is retracted superiorly and laterally, exposing the anterior surface of the pancreatic tail. The dissection then proceeds along the inferior and distal edge of the pancreas (Fig. 6). This dissection is begun with the hook coagulator to the level of the inferior mesenteric vein.

The inferior aspect of the spleen is dissected free of the retroperitoneal tissues, exposing the superior aspect of the kidney and the inferior aspect of the adrenal. The distal tail of the pancreas is held inferiorly, while the superior edge of the pancreas is dissected free of the surrounding tissues.

As the dissection proceeds medially along the superior aspect of the pancreas, several small branches of the splenic artery are clipped and transected (Fig. 7). The branches to the splenic vein are shorter and can be controlled by bipolar electrocautery and/or by metallic clips.

Once the level of the inferior mesenteric vein is reached, the umbilical trocar is replaced with a 15-mm trocar. The 60-mm endocutter is then placed through the umbilical trocar site, and the pancreatic tail is transected (Fig. 8). The distal pancreas and tumor are then placed into an isolation bag. The operative field is inspected for hemostasis.

An attempt is then made to locate the pancreatic duct. If the duct can be identified, a 3-0 silk or Prolene suture is placed, transfixing the duct, using intracorporeal tying techniques. If, during the mobilization of the superior aspect of the spleen, the splenic vessels are injured, they can be ligated using either clips or ligatures. If the short gastric vessels have been preserved, the spleen remains viable in most cases. A drain is then placed into the bed of the pancreas and brought out through the left upper quadrant. All trocar sites are closed.

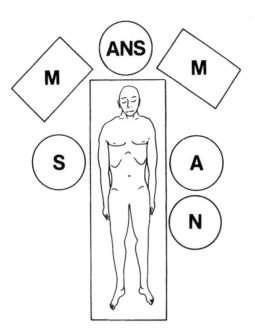

Fig. 1. Positioning of the patient and team. Patient in supine position. *ANS*, Anesthetist; *S*, surgeon; *A*, assistant; *N*, nurse; *M*, monitor

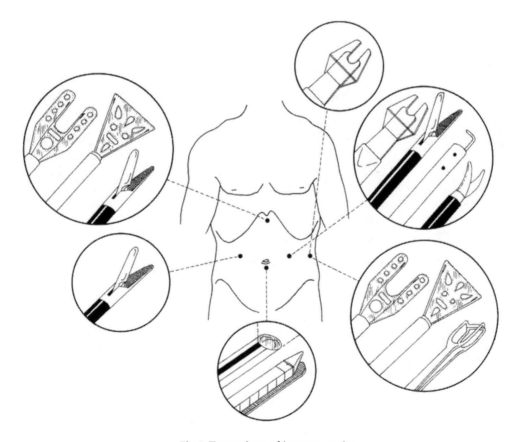

Fig. 2. Trocar sites and instrumentation

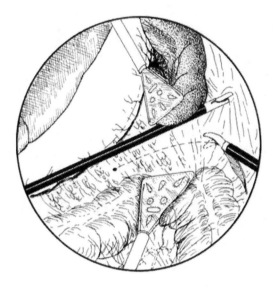

Fig. 3. The splenic flexure of the colon is mobilized

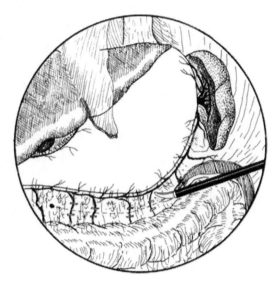

Fig. 4. The lesser sac is entered by transecting the gastrocolic ligament

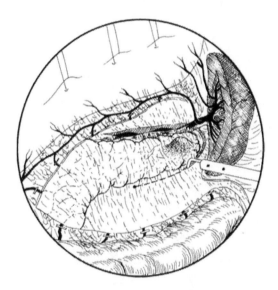

Fig. 5. Stay sutures placed on the stomach allow exposure of the pancreas

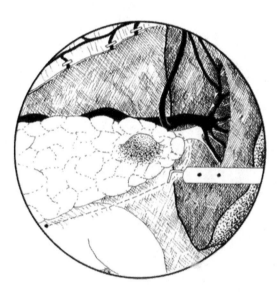

Fig. 6. The pancreatic tail is mobilized by means of electrocautery

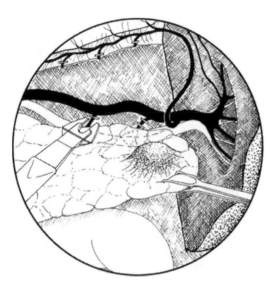

Fig. 7. Small branches of the splenic artery are clipped and transected

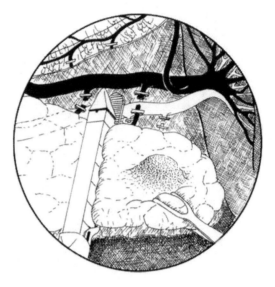

Fig. 8. The pancreatic tail is transected by means of the endo-cutter

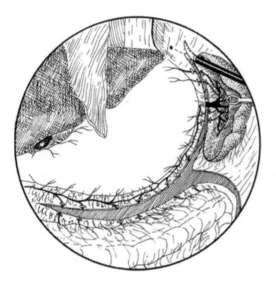

Fig. 9. In those cases where splenectomy is performed, the dissection of the gastrocolic ligament should be extended proximally

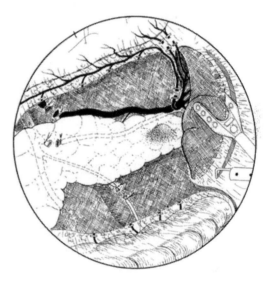

Fig. 10. View into the lesser sac after the spleen and tail of the pancreas are devascularized

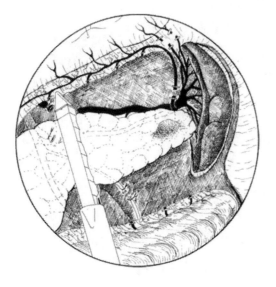

Fig. 11. Transection of the tail of the pancreas with the endo-cutter

Pancreatectomy with Splenectomy

Distal pancreatectomy involving any malignant tumor of the distal pancreas or large cystic lesion, such as a large cystadenocarcinoma or cystadenoma, should also include splenectomy.

The patient position and trocar sites are identical. In this operation, however, once the splenic flexure is taken down, the lienorenal ligament is incised, and the spleen is mobilized medially. The short gastric vessels are then serially isolated, doubly clipped, and transected. The lienophrenic ligament is incised, and the entire spleen is mobilized (Fig. 9). The spleen is then held medially, using soft balloon retractors or large atraumatic clamps. The pancreas is then dissected posteriorly in a lateral to medial direction. The dissection can proceed to the superior mesenteric vein. The inferior mesenteric vein can be isolated, ligated, and transected. The pancreas and spleen can then be mobilized to the neck of the pancreas (Fig. 10).

The major splenic vessels are ligated or clipped and transected. The pancreas is then transected as described above (Fig. 11). The entire specimen is then placed into a retrieval bag. A small incision is then made at the site of the left midclavicular trocar site. The specimen is brought out through the abdominal wall for histopathologic assessment. A drain is placed into the left upper quadrant.

Postoperatively these patients are managed without a nasogastric tube. The Foley catheter is removed within the first 24 h. Oral alimentation is begun on the first or second postoperative day. The left upper quadrant drain is removed on the third day if excessive drainage is not seen. Most of these patients can be discharged by the third postoperative day, resuming full activities by the 10th or 12th postoperative day.

References

Frantzides CT, Ludwig KA, Redlich PN (1994) Laparoscopic management of a pancreatic pseudocyst. J Laparoendosc Surg 1:55–59

Gagner M (1994) Laparoscopic pylorus-preserving pancreatoduodenectomy. Ultrasound and interventional techniques. Surg Endosc 5:408–410

Nathanson LK (1993) Laparoscopy and pancreatic cancer – biopsy, staging and bypass. Baillieres Clin Gastroenterol 7:4:941–960

Sanchez AW, Berry FSA, Garcia JC, Weber GR (1994) Laparoscopic management of a pancreatic cystadenoma. Surg Laparosc Endosc 4:304–307

Soper NJ, Brunt LM, Dunnegan DL, Meininger TA (1994) Laparoscopic distal pancreatectomy in the porcine model. Surg Endosc 8 (1):57–60

Warshaw AL, Gu ZY, Wittenberg J, Waltman AC (1990) Preoperative staging and assessment of resectability of pancreatic cancer. Arch Surg 125 (2):230–233

34 Laparoscopic Nephrectomy

R.G. Moore and L.R. Kavoussi

Introduction

The present indications for laparoscopic nephrectomy are benign renal disease necessitating surgical removal. Laparoscopic nephrectomy has also been used to treat solid renal masses less than 10 cm in diameter. Contraindications to laparoscopic nephrectomy can be divided into two categories: those to general laparoscopy and those specifically to laparoscopic nephrectomy. Laparoscopic nephrectomy is contraindicated for large renal masses (greater than 10 cm diameter), renal vein tumor thrombosis and for xanthogranulomatous pyelonephritis or multiple prior renal surgeries.

Positioning of the Patient and Team

The patient is placed in full flank position with the ipsilateral side elevated. Both arms are folded toward the head and padded with pillows. A rolled towel is placed in the axilla. Additional possible pressure points are padded, and the patient is secured to the operating table (Fig. 1). A full abdominal and flank surgical preparation is carried out, including the spine. All laparoscopic equipment is evaluated to assure proper function prior to proceeding with the operation.

Technique

All patients undergoing laparoscopic nephrectomy receive a dose of broad-spectrum parenteral antibiotics prior to the procedure. Each patient is typed and crossmatched for 2 U blood in the event of unexpected intraoperative hemorrhage. Preoperative mechanical and antibiotic bowel preparation is reserved for patients with a prior history of surgery or inflammatory bowel disease. Sequential compression devices are placed on the lower extremities to decrease the risk of deep venous thrombosis. The patient is placed under general endotracheal anesthesia. The stomach and bladder are decompressed with a nasogastric tube and Foley catheter, respectively. Two approaches for laparoscopic nephrectomy are possible: primary transperitoneal or primary retroperitoneal (see Fig. 12).

Transperitoneal Approach

When utilizing the transperitoneal route for laparoscopic nephrectomy, the pneumoperitoneum is achieved in the full flank position using a 14-gauge Veress needle. The abdominal wall is tented upward, and the needle is perpendicularly inserted lateral to the rectus muscle at the level of the umbilicus on the elevated side. Insufflation commences after confirming the intraperitoneal location of the Veress needle.

Intraperitoneal pressures are then maintained at 15 mmHg during the procedure. Two 12-mm trocars are placed in the midclavicular line, one approximately 4 cm below the level of the umbilicus and the other 2 cm below the costal margin (Fig. 2). All secondary trocars are placed under direct vision.

After trocar placement the peritoneal cavity is inspected. The procedure is initiated by incising the lateral peritoneal attachments of the colon with electrocautery scissors. The peritoneal incision should extend from the iliac vessels to the respective colonic flexure (Fig. 3). The colon should be freed from retroperitoneal attachments and reflected medially to completely expose Gerota's fascia. After reflection of the colon, an additional 12-mm trocar is placed in the anterior axillary line off the tip of the 12th rib, and another 12-mm trocar is placed 5 cm below this level. A 12-mm trocar is placed in the posterior axillary line between the two above trocars (Fig. 2).

The ureter is identified in the retroperitoneum. Gerota's fascia can be visualized by following the ureter proximally (Fig. 4). If nephrectomy is being performed for a suspected malignancy, the dissection is kept external to Gerota's fascia. The fascia is detached from adjacent tissue both anteriorly and posteriorly. Gerota's fascia may be entered when the nephrectomy is performed for benign disease.

After adequate posterior mobilization of the kidney the laparoscope is placed in the posterior axillary port. The renal vessels are located by displacing the kidney anteriorly through retraction via the lower anterior port

(Fig. 5). The renal artery is usually identified first. After sufficient mobilization the renal artery is secured with clips. Three clips are placed proximally and two distally prior to transection. The renal vein is dissected free from the surrounding perihilar tissue. Small venous branches are clipped and divided. The laparoscopic clips are usually too short to properly occlude the renal vein; therefore an endoscopic linear stapler is used to control the vein. The stapler is passed through a 12-mm port and places several rows of clips and cuts between (Fig. 6).

Residual medial attachments can be freed with blunt dissection. If lymphatic vessels are encountered they should be clipped. The upper pole of the kidney can be enucleated from Gerota's fascia when nephrectomy is performed for benign renal disease or for small middle or lower pole lesions. Radical nephrectomy (extrafascial) including removal of the adrenal gland is required when nephrectomy is performed for malignant renal disease of the upper pole. On the right the adrenal vessels are identified posteriorly by following the vena cava superiorly. These are clipped and transected (Fig. 7). The entire kidney within Gerota's fascia and the adrenal gland are then dissected free by incising the remaining medial and anterior attachments. Repositioning of the laparoscope is often required to obtain optimal visualization to complete this dissection successfully.

After the kidney is mobilized, the ureter is clipped and transected (Fig. 8). The proximal ureter is then grasped with locking Babcock forceps and displaced into the upper quadrant via the posterior axillary line port. The renal bed is irrigated with heparinized saline and inspected for hemostasis. If indicated, periaortic lymph nodes can be dissected and removed separately.

An impermeable 5 x 8 in. sac (Lapsac; Cook Urological, Spencer, IN) is introduced through the lower inferior 12-mm port and unrolled with grasping forceps. The closed end of the sac is placed in the pelvis. The laparoscope is introduced in the upper anterior port and locking graspers are placed through the three remaining ports. The Lapsac is opened by grasping tabs which are located at an equal distance about the neck of the sac, and the kidney is placed in the sac (Fig. 9). After renal entrapment is accomplished, the drawstrings are brought out a 12-mm port and the entire port is removed, taking care to bring the neck of the sac through to the external abdominal wall (Fig. 10). The kidney is morcellated using ring forceps or an electric tissue morcellator (Cook Urological; Fig. 11). The laparoscope is used to monitor the morcellation process and to prevent injury to intraperitoneal organs. After complete evacuation of the tissue the sac is withdrawn from the working space and the tissue sent for histological analysis.

If nephrectomy is performed for suspected cancer, the neck of the sac can be brought out through the pos-

terior axillary port, and a 5-cm dorsal lumbotomy incision is made to remove the specimen. This permits the kidney to be removed intact to obtain accurate histological staging.

Retroperitoneal Approach

An alternative approach for laparoscopic nephrectomy is the primary retroperitoneal route (Fig. 12). This route is applicable for small kidneys (less than 100 g) or those patients who have had multiple transabdominal procedures. The patient is positioned in the full flank position. The point of entry lies in the posterior axillary line 1 cm above the iliac crest. The Veress needle is angled slightly anteriorly (10°) and advanced until a pop is felt as the needle passes through the lumbodorsal fascia.

The tests for correct needle placement are similar to those used in the transperitoneal approach. Once proper needle placement is confirmed, the retroperitoneum is insufflated at a flow rate of 1 l/min. The initial opening pressure should be less than 10 mmHg; however, the pressures are somewhat higher (8–10 mmHg) when compared to the transperitoneal approach (< 5 mmHg). The retroperitoneal space accommodates 4–9 l carbon dioxide. A tense pneumoretroperitoneum is obtained to assist in trocar placement. Retroperitoneal working pressures are kept below 15 mmHg after initial trocar placement.

A 12-mm trocar is placed in the same location as the Veress needle. The laparoscope is then introduced via the 12-mm port to view the retroperitoneum, which can be identified by a characteristic wispy yellow fat. A balloon catheter is then fashioned from the cut middle finger of a surgical glove and sutured onto the tip of a stiff 12-F red rubber catheter (Fig. 12). Alternatively, commercially available catheters can be purchased for balloon dilatation of the retroperitoneal space. The balloon catheter is introduced through the 12-mm port into the retroperitoneum and connected to an irrigation-aspiration system (Fig. 10). The balloon is filled with 1500 ml saline.

After balloon dilatation of the retroperitoneal space both the psoas muscle and Gerota's fascia can be seen. The remaining working ports are placed under direct endoscopic vision as previously described. Nephrectomy is then performed as in the transperitoneal approach. Occasionally the retroperitoneal space is too small to accomplish renal entrapment. If this difficulty is encountered, an incision in the peritoneum is made to facilitate entrapment and morcellation of the kidney.

At the conclusion of the procedure all ports are removed under direct vision. The fascia is closed with absorbable suture on all port sites greater than 10 mm. All trocar sites are closed in the pediatric patient regardless of size.

References

Capelouto CC, Moore RG, Silverman SG, Kavoussi LR (1994) Retroperitoneoscopy; anatomic rationale for direct retroperitoneal access. J Urol 152:2008–2011

Clayman RV, McDougall EM (1992) Laparoscopic renal surgery. In: Clayman RV, McDougall EM (eds) Laparoscopic surgery. Quality Medical, St. Louis, pp 272–308

Clayman RV, Kavoussi LR, Soper NJ, Dierks SM, Meretyk S, Darcy MD, Roemer FD, Pingleton ED, Thomson PG, Long SR (1991) Laparoscopic nephrectomy: initial case report. J Urol 146:278–282

Kavoussi LR, Kerby K, Capelouto CC, McDougall E, Clayman RV (1993) Laparoscopic nephrectomy for renal neoplasms. Urology 42:603-609

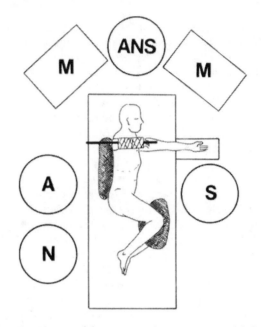

Fig. 1. Positioning of the patient and team. Patient in full flank position. *ANS*, Anesthetist; *S*, surgeon; *A*, assistant; *N*, nurse; *M*, monitor

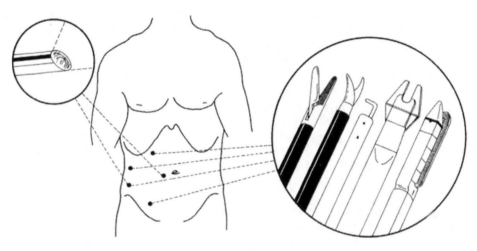

Fig. 2. Trocar sites and instrumentation

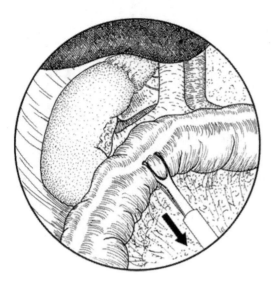

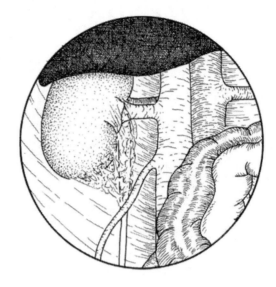

Fig. 3. The lateral peritoneal attachments of the colon have been incised from the iliac vessels to the colonic flexure

Fig. 4. Gerota's fascia can be identified by following the ureter proximally

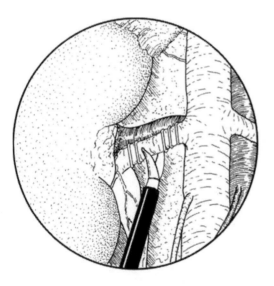

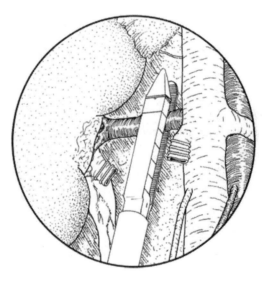

Fig. 5. The posterior view of the left renal vessels is located by displacing the kidney anteriorly

Fig. 6. Transection of renal artery and vein

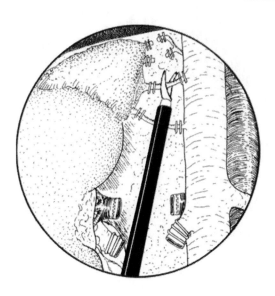

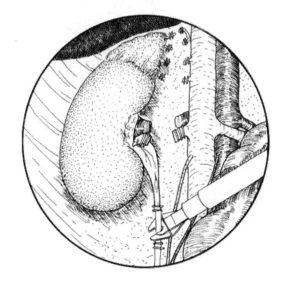

Fig. 7. The adrenal vein and arteriea are identified posteriorly by following the vena cava superiorly

Fig. 8. Clipping and transection of the ureter

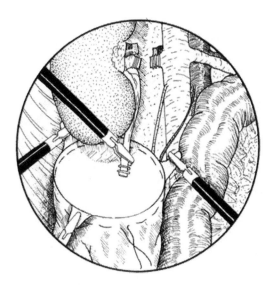

Fig. 9. Renal entrapment is accomplished

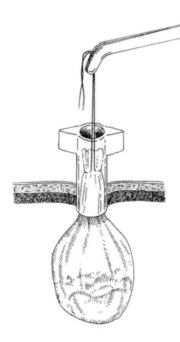

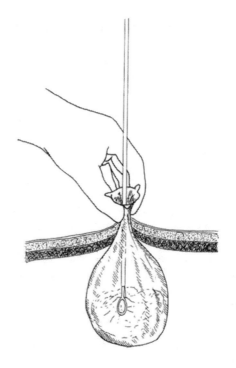

Fig. 10. The drawstrings of the renal entrapment sac are brought out a 10- to 12-mm port

Fig. 11. Renal morcellation is completed with ring forceps or an electric tissue morcellator

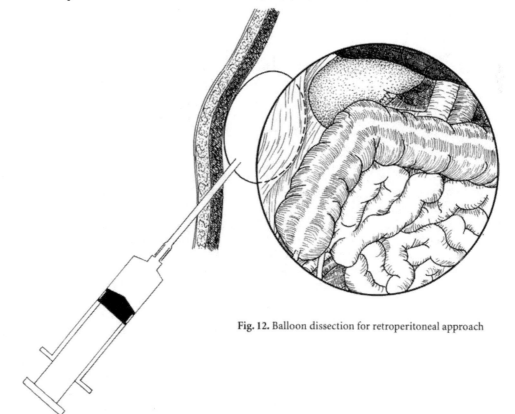

Fig. 12. Balloon dissection for retroperitoneal approach

35 Laparoscopic Pelvic Lymphadenectomy

T.J. POLASCIK, R.G. MOORE, and L.R. KAVOUSSI

Introduction

Limitations of noninvasive modalities have mandated histologic evaluation of lymph nodes in patients with pelvic urologic malignancies in whom accurate pathologic staging is needed. Pelvic lymphadenectomy is the most effective technique for evaluating metastatic spread to regional lymph nodes in prostate, bladder, and urethral carcinomas. Laparoscopic pelvic lymph node dissection (LPLND) has emerged as a minimally invasive technique that diminishes the morbidity associated with the traditional open pelvic lymphadenectomy. The laparoscopic approach to pelvic lymph node dissection was first performed by Schuessler and associates in 1989. Since their report this technique has been recognized as a safe and effective method for staging genitourinary pelvic malignancies.

Positioning of the Patient and Team

After induction of general anesthesia an indwelling urethral catheter and an oral gastric tube are placed to decompress the bladder and stomach, respectively. The patient is placed supine with both arms adducted and is secured to the table with wide cloth tape. Antiembolism stockings and pneumatic compression devices are placed for deep venous thrombosis prophylaxis. The entire abdomen and genitalia are prepared and draped, including a "turban" dressing which is applied around the penis and scrotum to prevent subcutaneous emphysema involving the genitalia. All laparoscopic equipment is tested prior to commencing. A laparotomy set should be available if an emergent celiotomy becomes necessary (Fig. 1).

Technique

The pelvic lymph nodes can be approached via a transperitoneal or an extraperitoneal technique. The latter approach is useful in patients who have undergone prior intraperitoneal surgery.

Transperitoneal LPLND

The operative table is placed in the Trendelenburg position to displace the small intestine away from the operative field. Veress needle placement is at the umbilicus.

Following achievement of an adequate pneumoperitoneum, the Veress needle is exchanged for a 10- to 11-mm trocar. The laparoscope is inserted through this port, and the abdomen is inspected for trocar or Veress needle injury. All remaining trocars are placed under direct laparoscopic vision. Depending upon the patient's body habitus and the surgeon's preference, trocar arrangement can follow either the diamond or the fan configuration (Fig. 2).

The diamond configuration utilizes a 10- to 11-mm working channel along the linea alba midway between the umbilicus and the symphysis pubis. Two 5-mm ports are placed midway between the umbilicus and the anterior superior iliac spine in both the left and right lower quadrants. These trocars are placed lateral to the rectus muscle to avoid the inferior epigastric vessels. The fan configuration positions two 5-mm ports in the lower abdomen above the internal inguinal ring in the midclavicular line. A third 5-mm port and a 10- to 11-mm working channel are placed in the midclavicular line at the level of the umbilicus on the right and left sides, respectively.

Pelvic lymph node sampling should begin on the side most likely to contain metastatic disease. The surgeon stands on the side contralateral to the area of dissection and the assistant is positioned across the table. The table is rotated laterally to elevate the operative field. Trendelenburg is increased to 30° to move the bowels cephalad and provide optimal exposure of the obturator fossa.

A survey of the pelvis reveals the urachus, medial umbilical ligament (obliterated umbilical artery), bladder, the spermatic vessels, and vas deferens as they course through the internal inguinal ring. In thin patients the iliac vessels and ureter can also be identified (Fig. 3).

To access the obturator fossa the posterior peritoneal membrane is incised lateral to the obliterated umbilical artery. The incision should begin at the level of the pubic ramus and continue posterolaterally over the external iliac artery. The vas deferens is encountered as it crosses the peritoneotomy. The vas should be coagulated and divided to facilitate access to the obturator fossa (Fig. 4).

Inspection of the obturator fossa reveals several landmarks of the dissection: the circumflex iliac artery near the femoral canal distally, the external iliac vein laterally, the obturator nerve inferiorly, and the hypogastric artery superiorly (Fig. 5). When performing LPLND for bladder, urethral, or penile carcinoma, the limits of dissection are extended to include nodes from the common, external iliac, hypogastric, presacral, and lateral sacral nodes (Fig. 6). Additionally, lymphadenectomy for penile malignancies should include adequate lymphatic tissue in the femoral canal.

The nodal packet is easiest to identify by beginning at the middle of the external iliac vein. The loose fibroareolar layer overlying the medial border of the external iliac vein is sharply incised from the vessel and teased medially. The assistant grasps the edge of the nodal packet with forceps to expose the lateral border of the dissection. As the surgeon rolls the lymphatic tissue medially, the pelvic sidewall and the pubic bone are encountered (Fig. 7). The tissue is freed distally to the circumflex iliac artery as it nears the femoral canal.

The medial border of the dissection is created by having the assistant grasp the packet and pull laterally while the surgeon retracts the umbilical ligament medially. The plane between the bladder and nodal packet should peel away easily. The pubic bone is identified distally and the apex of the obturator packet near the pubic bone is clipped and transected (Fig. 8). The obturator nerve can now be identified at the base of the packet and should be carefully preserved.

The inferior portion of the nodal packet is then retracted proximally allowing for dissection of the medial and lateral borders with simultaneous visualization of the obturator nerve (Fig. 9). The obturator artery and vein should be preserved unless excessive bleeding warrants ligation. Once the packet has been mobilized to the level of the iliac bifurcation, a 10-mm laparoscopic vein retractor can be introduced to aid in exposure. The ureter should be identified during the dissection to avoid inadvertent injury. The proximal aspect of the nodal packet is then excised with a combination of blunt and sharp dissection (Fig. 10). The packet can be removed with a 10-mm spoon-billed grasping forceps. If the amount of nodal tissue is large, the packet can be placed in a Lapsac (Cook Urological, Spencer, IN) and removed through the 10- to 11-mm lateral port.

Lymphadenectomy is completed on the opposite side in a similar fashion. Following the completion of the dissection the pneumoperitoneum is lowered to a pressure of 5 mmHg for a final inspection of hemostasis. The peritoneotomy is not closed to prevent postoperative lymphocele formation. All accessory trocar ports are se-

quentially removed under direct laparoscopic vision. The fascia of the 10- to 11-mm port sites is closed with interrupted 2-0 absorbable sutures.

Extraperitoneal LPLND

This technique may be useful in patients who have had previous intraperitoneal or pelvic surgery, or a history of a pelvic fracture.

The first step is to access the retropubic space. A small infraumbilical incision is made and bluntly dissected down to the anterior rectus fascia. Two 2-0 silk stay sutures are placed, and the fascia is sharply opened between the sutures. The preperitoneal plane is developed by finger dissection aiming toward the pubis. A 10- to 11-mm blunt-tipped Hasson trocar is then inserted without entering the peritoneal cavity. Using a combination of both carbon dioxide insufflation and blunt probe dissection, the extraperitoneal space is developed between both anterior superior iliac spines. Alternatively, a purpose-built balloon trocar (Origin Medical Systems, Laguna Hills, CA; Fig. 11) or a balloon fashioned from the middle finger of a glove and a 14-F red rubber catheter can be placed in the preperitoneal space. The remaining working trocars are then positioned in the diamond configuration. The iliac vessels and overlying lymphatic tissue are usually relatively apparent. The dissection is performed in a similar manner to the transperitoneal approach except that a posterior peritoneotomy is not necessary.

Extraperitoneal laparoscopic pelvic lymph node dissection has been shown to be similar in nodal yield to its transperitoneal counterpart. Advantages of the extraperitoneal approach include a decreased risk of hollow-viscus perforation associated with transabdominal trocar placement and dissection. Extraperitoneal laparoscopy may also diminish the risk of hypercarbia. Additionally, the need for adhesiolysis which may be required with the transperitoneal approach is obviated. However, care must be taken adequately to clip lymphatic channels during extraperitoneal LPLND to prevent postoperative lymphocele formation. Moreover, underlying structures can be injured if cautery is applied to the peritoneum.

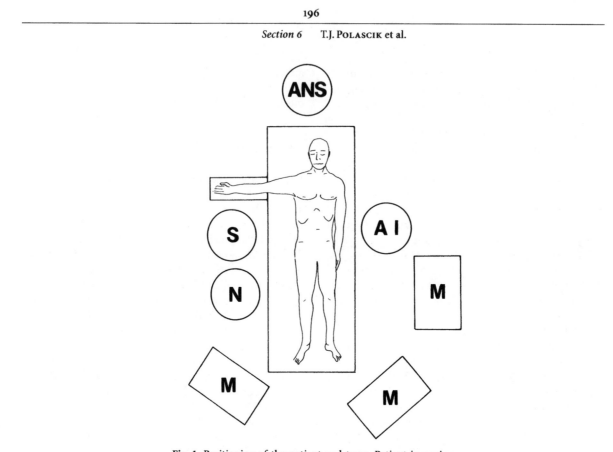

Fig. 1. Positioning of the patient and team. Patient in supine position. *ANS*, Anesthetist; *S*, surgeon; *A1*, assistant; *N*, nurse; *M*, monitor

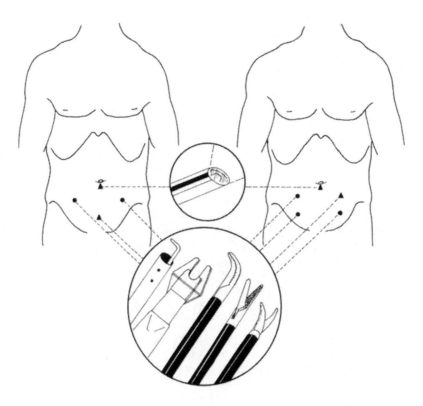

Fig. 2. Trocar configuration is illustrated. ● 10- to 12-mm trocars; ▲ 5-mm trocars

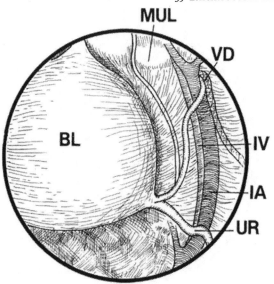

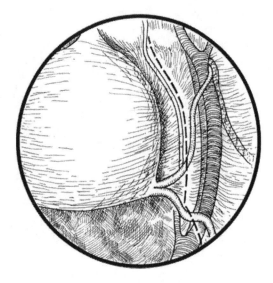

Fig. 3. Identification of the pelvic anatomic landmarks. *BL*, bladder; *MUL*, medial umbilical ligament; *VD*, vas deferens; *IV*, iliac vein; *IA*, iliac artery; *UR*, ureter

Fig. 4. Posterior peritoneotomy is made lateral to the medial umbilical ligament exposing the iliac vessels and vas deferens

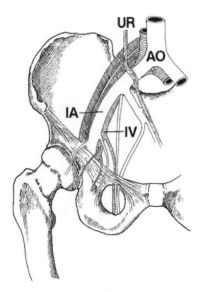

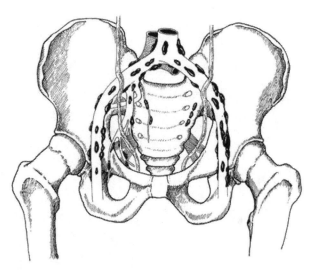

Fig. 5. Structures of the right lateral pelvic sidewall. Limits of the pelvic lymph node dissection for prostate cancer include the circumflex artery near the femoral canal distally, the external iliac vein laterally, the obturator nerve inferiorly, and the hypogastric artery superiorly. *Ao*, aorta; *UR*, ureter; *IA*, iliac artery; *IV*, iliac vein

Fig. 6. Extended limits of dissection for bladder, urethral and penile cancer: common, external iliac, hypogastric, presacral and lateral sacral nodal groups are also excised

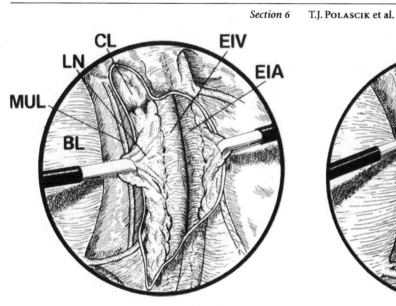

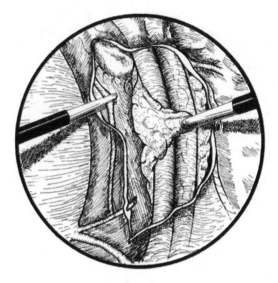

Fig. 7. The external iliac vein as the lateral border of the dissection. This is visualized by retracting the packet medially. *BL*, bladder; *MUL*, medial umbilical ligament; *CL*, Cooper's ligament; *LN*, lymphnodes; *EIV*, external iliac vein; *EIA*, external iliac artery

Fig. 8. The medial umbilical ligament is the medial border of dissection. By retracting medially and pulling the packet laterally, the pubic bone can be identified

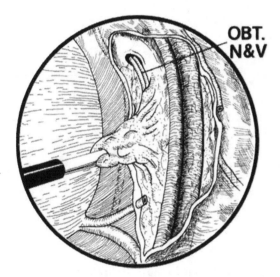

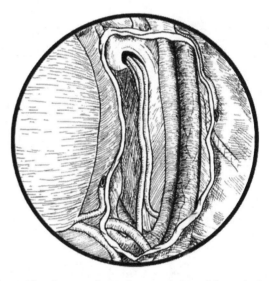

Fig. 9. Detachment of the inferior portion of the nodal package from the pubic bone identifies the obturator nerve and vessels. *OBT. N & V*, obturator nerve and vessels

Fig. 10. The obturator fossa after completion of the node dissection

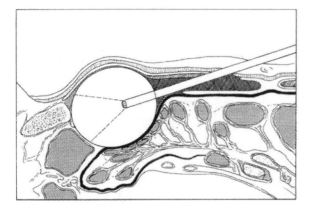

Fig. 11. Extraperitoneal balloon dilatation to create a working space

Comments

Pelvic lymphadenectomy is currently the most precise method of staging prostate cancer. At our institution, definitive local therapy is undertaken only in patients who demonstrate no evidence of metastatic disease. In surgical candidates with a low likelihood of having metastatic disease open lymphadenectomy can be performed at the time of radical prostatectomy.

Laparoscopic pelvic lymph node dissection should be utilized only in patients with prostate cancer having a high suspicion of harboring occult metastatic disease. This includes those with locally advanced disease, high grade tumors (Gleason grade 8 or greater), markedly elevated serum prostatic acid phosphatase, or prostate-specific antigen levels (> 20 ng/ml). Additionally, patients with radiographic evidence of advanced disease, including enlarged pelvic lymph nodes by computed tomography or magnetic resonance and questionable seminal vesicle invasion by the latter, may need further verification with staging lymphadenectomy. Those with negative lymph nodes who are judged to be candidates for definitive local therapy can then proceed with either radical prostatectomy or radiation therapy. For those electing surgery, LPLND can be followed by radical perineal prostatectomy either as a combined or a two-stage procedure.

Contraindications. Absolute contraindications to laparoscopy include severe cardiopulmonary disease, an uncorrectable coagulopathy, and active infection. Patients who cannot tolerate a general anesthetic should also be excluded. Relative contraindications include morbidly obese patients, those having had multiple abdominal surgeries, and individuals with a large hiatal hernia. Extensive intra-abdominal or retroperitoneal adhesions may make trocar access impossible and surgical dissection technically difficult. Large pelvic or intra-abdominal masses or a history of a pelvic fracture also favors traditional open operative techniques.

References

Ferzli G, Raboy A, Kleinerman D, Albert P (1992) Extraperitoneal endoscopic pelvic lymph node dissection vs laparoscopic lymph node dissection in the staging of prostatic and bladder carcinoma. J Laparoendosc Surg 2 (5):219–222

Kavoussi LR, Sosa E, Chandhoke P, Chodak G, Clayman RV, Hadley HR, Loughlin KR, Ruckle HC, Rukstalis D, Schuessler W, Segura J, Vancaille T, Winfield HN (1993) Complications of laparoscopic pelvic lymph node dissection. J Urol 149:322–325

Moore RG, Kavoussi LR (1993) Laparoscopic lymphadenectomy in genitourinary malignancies. Surg Oncol 2 (1):51–66

Prout GR jr, Shipley WU, Kaufman DS, Griffin PP, Heney NM (1991) Interval report of a phase I–II study utilizing multiple modalities in the treatment of invasive bladder cancer. A bladder-sparing trial. Urol Clin North Am 18:547–554

Schuessler WW, Vancaille TG, Reich H, Griffith DP (1991) Transperitoneal endosurgical lymphadenectomy in patients with localized prostate cancer. J Urol 145:988–991

Winfield HN, See WA, Donovan JF, Godet A, Farage YM, Loening SA, Williams RD (1992) Comparative effectiveness and safety of laparoscopic vs open pelvic lymph node dissection for cancer of the prostate (abstract). J Urol 147:244A

36 Laparoscopic Appendectomy

R.J. ROSENTHAL and E.H. PHILLIPS

Introduction

Laparoscopic appendectomy was the introduction of laparoscopic cholecystectomy, first described by Semm in 1983, but it was not until 1989 that this approach gained wider acceptance. Although there is still controversy about the benefits of the laparoscopic approach in the treatment of acute appendicitis, most agree that it is indicated in women of childbearing age or when the diagnosis is unclear.

Positioning of the Patient and Team

The patient is placed on an electric operating table in the supine position. The surgeon stands on the left side of the patient. Depending on the number of assistants, there are several options (see Fig. 1). A Foley catheter should be placed to decompress the bladder and the operating table rotated 15°–30° left.

Technique

An infraumbilical skin incision is made, and a pneumoperitoneum is created after inserting a Veress needle into the abdominal cavity. The Veress needle is withdrawn, and a 5- or a 10- to 11-mm trocar is placed through this incision. A laparoscope (0° or 30°) is introduced, and the abdominal cavity and its contents are carefully inspected. After localization of the appendix a 5-mm trocar is placed in the right middle or upper quadrant at the anterior axillary line. A third trocar (10 to 11 mm in diameter from the patients left side; if an endocutter is going to be used, this should be a 12 mm diameter trocar) is placed in the suprapubic region (Fig. 2). Care must be taken when inserting this trocar because of the proximity of the urinary bladder. Due to the elasticity of the peritoneum in this area a grasper introduced through the right-sided trocar should elevate the peritoneum. In cases in which the location of the appendix is retrocecal, or the appendix is fixed to other structures and cannot be elevated, a fourth trocar (5 mm in diameter) is placed in the middle between the umbilical and suprapubic ports. This allows the surgeon to work with both hands, simplifying the dissection.

Using atraumatic graspers, the cecum is reflected superiorly and medially by the first assistant's right hand as he holds the camera with his left hand (Fig. 1 a). The appendix can then be identified (Fig. 3). The tip of the appendix is grasped and elevated (Fig. 4). Using bipolar scissors and an atraumatic grasper, the peritoneum is incised and a window created in the mesenterium at the base of the appendix (Fig. 5). The appendicular artery can be coagulated with bipolar cautery and secured with clips or an endoloop (Fig. 6). This step can also be performed with an endovascular cutter.

The appendix can be excised with an endocutter, but we prefer to use pretied suture loops. One is placed at the base of the appendix. The next endoloop is placed several millimeters distal, creating a bead. The third endoloop is placed further up on the appendix. The appendix is amputated between the endoloops with scissors, not cautery, as power density is greatest where the endoloop is fashioned at the base of the appendix (Fig. 7). The specimen is placed in a bag to protect the abdominal wall from contamination during the extraction (Fig. 8). After the specimen has been extracted through the suprapubic port, suction and irrigation of the right lower quadrant should be performed. If the appendix is gangrenous or perforated there is always significant inflamation. Blunt dissection is the safest technique to identify and dissect the appendix. If the appendix is gangrenous, grasping it may cause rupture. Applying an endoloop and grasping the suture to handle the appendix is safer.

Before extracting the trocars the incisions are infiltrated with a local anesthetic to reduce postoperative discomfort. Trocars are then extracted under view to recognize bleeding from the abdominal wall incision. All 10-mm or larger trocar sites are then closed.

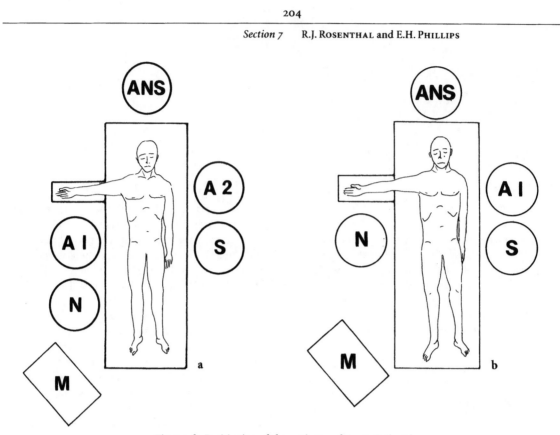

Fig. 1 a, b. Positioning of the patient and team. Patient in supine position. *ANS*, Anesthetist; *S*, surgeon; *A1, A2*, assistant; *N*, nurse; *M*, monitor

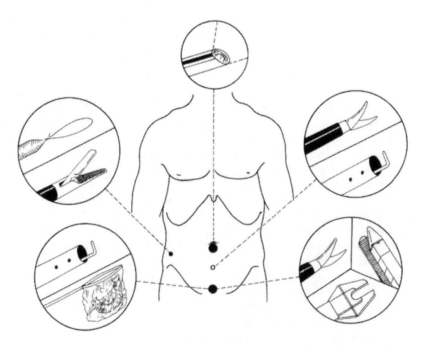

Fig. 2. Trocar sites and instrumentation

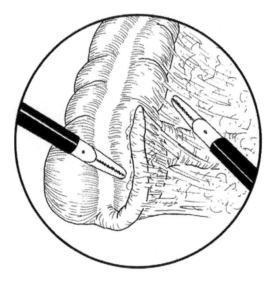

Fig. 3. Localization of the appendix

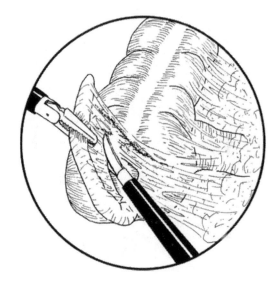

Fig. 4. Dissection of the mesenterium

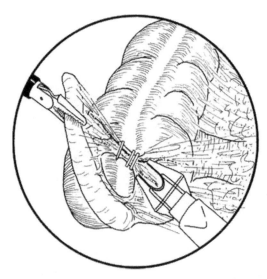

Fig. 5. Transection of appendicular artery between clips

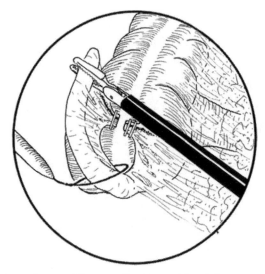

Fig. 6. Closure of the appendiceal base with endoloops

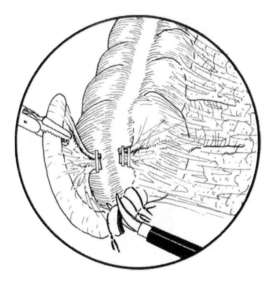

Fig. 7. Transection of appendix

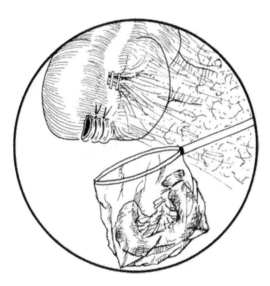

Fig. 8. Extraction of the specimen with a bag

Comments

If the appendix is normal, it is important to explore the tubes, uterus, and ovaries for diseases as well as the parietal peritoneum to rule out endometriosis. If they are normal, a perforated ulcer or diverticulum should be excluded. If the stomach, duodenum, and colon are normal, the last 2 ft small bowel must be inspected to exclude Meckel's diverticulum or regional enteritis.

References

Berryl J (1984) Appendicitis near its centenary. Ann Surg 200 (5):567–574

Deutsch A. Zelikowsky A, Reiss R (1982) Laparoscopy in the prevention of unnecessary appendectomies: a prospective study. Br J Surg 69:336–337

Frazee RC, Roberts JW, Symmonds RE, Snyder SK, Hendricks JC, Smith RW, Custer MD, Harrison JB (1994) A prospective randomized trial comparing open versus laparoscopic appendectomy. Ann Surg 219 (6):725–731

Pier A, Götz F, Bacher C (1991) Laparoscopic appendectomy in 625 cases: from innovation to routine. Surg Laparosc Endosc 1:8–13

Semm K (1983) Endoscopic appendectomy. Endoscopy 15:59–64

37 Laparoscopic Enterolysis

B. A. Salky

Introduction

Adhesions are commonly encountered during the performance of laparoscopic surgery. The ability to lyse adhesions in a safe and bloodless manner allows progression of the procedure. Conversion to open laparotomy, while reasonable, is often avoided once adhesions are divided. Therefore the ability of the laparoscopic surgeon to deal with adhesions is of paramount importance. Relatively straightforward anatomy may not be visible because of adhesions.

The character or type of adhesion present dictates the way in which it should be approached laparoscopically. This is the same as open, traditional surgery. With the exception of congenital bands, adhesions are formed by some inflammatory event. Therefore the exact state of the adhesion depends on the time when the inflammatory event occurred. The laparoscopic approach differs depending on whether the adhesions were formed recently or are older and fibrotic.

Positioning of the Patient and Team

For positioning of the patient and team, see Fig. 1

Technique

Trocar site placement depends on the location of the incision scars from previous surgery (see Chap. 3). In general the video monitor should be viewed in line with the optics of the laparoscope. For example, if the laparoscope is positioned toward the pelvis, the monitor should be at the foot of the patient (Fig. 1). The use of all 10- to 11-mm sleeves allows free movement of laparoscope and instrumentation to various ports. This gives better visualization of the proper tissue planes. The surgeon should not hesitate to put in extra trocars and sleeves if necessary for retraction. For adhesiolysis the most important instruments are atraumatic grasping forceps and sharp scissors. The author prefers disposable scissors as electrocautery quickly dulls reusable scissors. The scissors should have axial rotation as well.

Angled telescopes are invaluable when adhesions are attached to the anterior abdominal wall (Fig. 2). The abdominal wall itself limits the use of forward viewing laparoscopes. Depending on the curvature of the abdominal wall, 30° or 45° telescopes should be used.

Hemostasis is critical in laparoscopic surgery. An avascular plane exists at the point of attachment of the adhesion. The proper plane can be identified with traction and countertraction (Fig. 3). If the adhesion is attached to bowel, the dissection plane must be on the bowel. This means that the surgical tissue plane must be "opened" by retracting the bowel. This cannot be accomplished safely without the proper exposure and the use of atraumatic graspers. The use of electric energy on the bowel wall is fraught with danger. One must ensure that the scissors blade is not touching the bowel (Fig. 4), and that the transmission of thermal energy does not follow the adhesion to the bowel wall (Fig. 5). Short bursts of electric energy are safer. The tissues must not be overdesiccated. The use of a bipolar electrocautery unit should also be considered.

Adhesions in the presence of acute inflammatory disease are approached differently. It is important to find the adhesion-organ interface early in the procedure. These adhesions are thick and hemorrhagic. Electrocautery dissection is frequently needed to start the dissection. However, once the plane is developed, blunt dissection is usually more efficient. I have found the use of a blunt-tipped palpating probe or suction device to be helpful in this situation. Hydrodissection can also be of help in delineating the appropriate tissue plane in acute inflammatory disease.

Capsular tears of the liver and spleen are usually secondary to traction injuries on adhesions. These can be avoided by dividing the adhesion sharply before they are pulled upon. This is commonly seen in laparoscopic cholecystectomy. Univectored traction is required in this situation.

Filmy adhesions without vascularity are easily separated by either sharp or blunt dissection. It is good technique and a good place to "practice" sharp dissection.

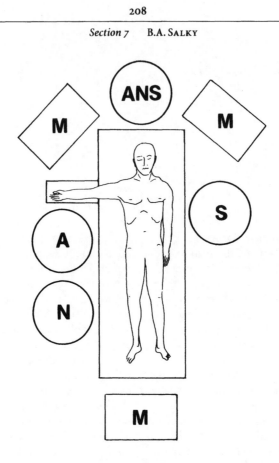

Fig. 1. Positioning of the patient and team. Patient in supine position. *ANS*, Anesthetist; *S*, surgeon; *A*, assistant; *N*, nurse; *M*, monitor

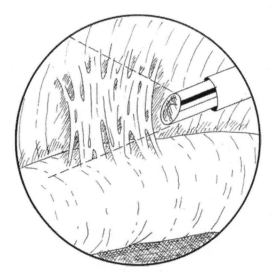

Fig. 2. Use of a 30° angle scope offers a better view

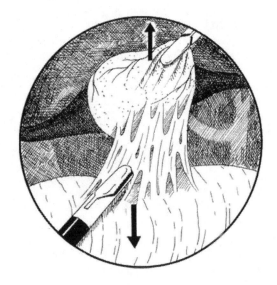

Fig. 3. Traction and countertraction are essential to identify the right plane

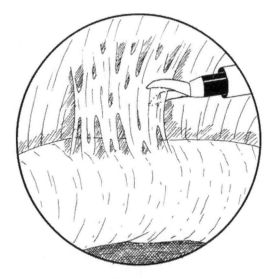

Fig. 4. Positioning of instruments when dissecting adhesions is important to avoid thermal injuries

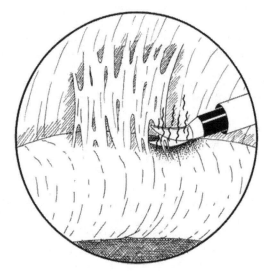

Fig. 5. Thermal injury of bowel loop due to close positioning of electrocautery instrument

Comments

The surgeon must know how to use two-handed technique. The amount of traction and countertraction should be controlled by the operating surgeon, not the assistant. This can be accomplished only with two-handed technique. Therefore at least three ports are needed, one for the video laparoscope and the other two for operating instrumentation. Even more ports are sometimes needed to view the area adequately. It is generally a good idea to use 10- to 11-mm trocars and sleeves so that the laparoscope can be inserted for views at different angles. In this way the surrounding structures can be protected. The surgeon should be very familiar with forward viewing and angled telescopes. There are some adhesions which cannot be lysed safely without the use of angled laparoscopes. The place for learning how to use these scopes is in procedures which are more commonly performed (i.e., laparoscopic cholecystectomy).

The laparoscopic surgeon encounters adhesions during routine therapeutic and diagnostic procedures, in the evaluation of chronic abdominal pain, and in acute small bowel obstruction. At present the use of laparoscopy in acute small bowel obstruction is limited. This should be attempted only by the most experienced laparoscopic surgeons. The proximal bowel is extremely friable, and perforation is a real possibility. Also, the dilatation of the obstructed bowel makes visualization of the abdominal cavity difficult. If it is attempted, the anesthetist should not use nitrous oxide gas. The diffusion of the gas into the intestinal lumen makes the bowel dilate, making visualization of proper tissue planes even more difficult.

Adhesions from previous surgery are a cause of chronic abdominal pain syndromes in a select group of patients. This is a difficult group of patients in that all have had multiple workups which have been unrewarding. The pain is typically located at one site, and it is reproducible. I prefer to use local anesthesia in this group. Multiple adhesions are generally present. The patient helps to identify which adhesion is causing the pain as the adhesion is manipulated during the performance of the laparoscopy. The use of local anesthesia in laparoscopy is well tolerated. The maintenance of a hemostatic field cannot be overemphasized when dealing with adhesions since small amounts of blood can completely obscure the operative field, making an accurate dissection plane impossible to identify. The least vascular area in an adhesion is at its point of attachment. Usually it is the parietal peritoneum or the bowel wall. Sharp scissor dissection is the preferred way to divide all but acute inflammatory adhesions.

If blood vessels require division, extreme care must be undertaken to prevent injury to adjacent intestine. If electrocautery is being used, strict adherence to electrosurgical principles must be followed. Familiarity with both monopolar and bipolar energy is a prerequisite. A certain amount of "blunt" dissection is expected, but sharp scissors dissection result in less bleeding. When using blunt dissection, the surgeon must use atraumatic technique or bowel wall injury can occur. There are some exceptions to this dictum, for example, avascular filmy adhesions.

Acute inflammatory adhesions require a slightly different approach. These are friable and hemorrhagic. It is important to stay in the proper anatomical plane here, for bleeding otherwise obscures the operative field rapidly. A combination of sharp and blunt dissection is used. Once the proper plane is identified with sharp dissection, a blunt probe is used to stay in the proper plane. This is commonly seen in acute cholecystitis, acute appendicitis, and acute diverticulitis.

References

Cuschieri A (1992) Diagnostic laparoscopy and laparoscopic adhesiolysis. In: Cuschieri A, Bueß G, Perissat J (eds) Operative manual of endoscopic surgery. Springer, Berlin Heidelberg New York, pp 180–193

Salky BA, Bauer JJ, Gelernt I, Kreel I (1985) Laparoscopy for gastrointestinal diseases. Mount Sinai J Med 52 (3):228–232

Salky BA (1990) Laparoscopy for surgeons. Igaku-Shoin, New York

38 Laparoscopic Jejunostomy

Q.-Y. Duh and L.W. Way

Introduction

Laparoscopic jejunostomy is indicated in patients with malnutrition or potential malnutrition who have a functioning gut, and in whom a gastrostomy is not possible or is contraindicated. The stomach may have been resected or used as a conduit in the chest; the patient may have gastroparesis, gastric outlet obstruction, or gastroesophageal reflux with aspiration pneumonia. Jejunostomy feeding is superior to parenteral nutrition but inferior to gastrostomy feeding. In patients whose planned laparoscopic gastrostomy is found to be difficult or impossible, laparoscopic jejunostomy becomes a good alternative; this decision can be made in the operating room. Percutaneous endoscopic jejunostomy requires first placing a gastrostomy, then converting it to a jejunostomy; this is associated with a high complication rate and is a poor alternative to laparoscopic jejunostomy.

Positioning of the Patient and Team

The patient is placed in the reverse Trendelenburg position (head up-feet down) to allow for gravity to pull the distal small bowel away from the field. The surgeon stands on the right side of the patient in line with the view of the laparoscope toward the left upper quadrant of the abdomen (Fig. 1).

Technique

Patient preparation is similar to that for laparoscopic gastrostomy. Laparoscopic jejunostomy can be performed under local anesthesia and intravenous sedation or general anesthesia. We routinely give a dose of a first-generation cephalosporin. The bladder is emptied by voiding before the procedure, or a Foley catheter is placed. A nasogastric or orogastric tube is used to insufflate the stomach and the proximal jejunum and facilitate the placement of the T-fasteners and jejunostomy catheter.

The set-up for laparoscopic jejunostomy is similar to that for laparoscopic gastrostomy. A subumbilical port is established by either the open or the closed technique (Fig. 2). A diagnostic laparoscopy is performed. The pressure of the pneumoperitoneum should be decreased to the minimal amount necessary to see the bowel, usually slightly higher than that required for a gastrostomy, 8–10 mmHg. For laparoscopic jejunostomy we use a commercial kit (10-F Flexiflo Lap J kit, Ross Laboratories, Columbus, OH). One or two atraumatic graspers are placed through 5-mm trocars in the left lower and right upper quadrants. These graspers are used to lift up the transverse colon and the omentum and to run the small bowel to identify the proximal jejunum and the ligament of Treitz.

The proximal jejunum at about 20–30 cm distal to the ligament of Treitz is identified and lifted toward the abdominal wall. The jejunostomy stoma site just over this segment of jejunum is identified by indenting the abdominal wall under laparoscopic vision (Fig. 3). A 3 x 3 cm diamond area is visualized on the antimesenteric border of the jejunum; a T-fastener (see Chap. 22) is placed in each corner of the diamond, and the jejunostomy catheter is placed through the center of the diamond. The stomach and the proximal jejunum are insufflated through the nasogastric tube to facilitate placement of the T-fasteners and the jejunostomy catheter.

The first T-fastener is placed in one corner of the 3 x 3 cm diamond that is farthest away from the scope, more proximal in the jejunum (Fig. 4). Pulling gently on the nylon suture then facilitates placement of subsequent T-fasteners. Keeping an open space between the abdominal wall and the jejunum allows direct laparoscopic viewing of the T-fasteners and the catheter during placement. Since the jejunum is more friable than the stomach, one needs to be more gentle in retracting with the T-fasteners and grasping with the atraumatic graspers.

Once the antimesenteric border of the jejunum is secured by the T-fasteners, the jejunostomy catheter is placed through the center of the diamond marked by the T-fasteners. A transverse 0.5 cm skin incision is made in the center of the diamond to accommodate the jejunostomy catheter without tension. An 18-gauge needle is inserted through the skin incision and the anterior abdominal wall into the jejunum. A J-guide wire is then introduced into the lumen of the jejunum distally through this needle (Fig. 5). The needle is withdrawn and a peel-away dilator introducer is inserted into the jejunal lumen over the wire. The wire and the stylet are removed and a 10-F straight catheter is inserted through the peel-away introducer into the jejunum. The introducer is pulled apart and removed, leaving the catheter inside the jejunum (Fig. 6).

The antimesenteric border of the jejunum is then fixed to the abdominal wall by squeezing the aluminum crimps on the nylon suture, and the jejunostomy catheter is secured to the skin by the skin anchor and sutures (Fig. 7). A contrast roentgenogram can also be performed to confirm placement inside the lumen.

References

Albrink MH, Foster J, Rosemurgy AS, Carey LC (1992) Laparoscopic feeding jejunostomy: also a simple technique. Surg Endosc 6:259–260

Duh QY, Way LW (1993) Laparoscopic jejunostomy using T-fasteners as retractors and anchors. Arch Surg 128 (1):105–108

Sangster W, Swanstrom L (1993) Laparoscopic-guided feeding jejunostomy. Surg Endosc 7:308–310

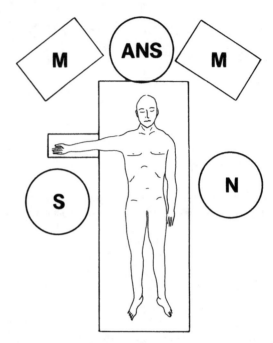

Fig. 1. Positioning of the patient and team. Patient in supine-reverse Trendelenburg position. *ANS*, Anesthetist; *S*, surgeon; *A*, assistant; *N*, nurse; *M*, monitor

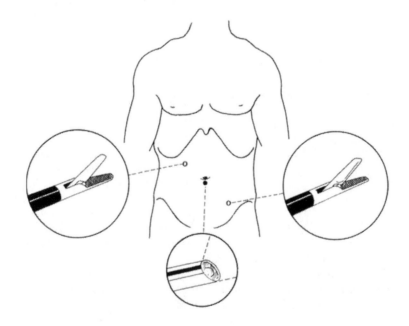

Fig. 2. Trocar sites and instrumentation

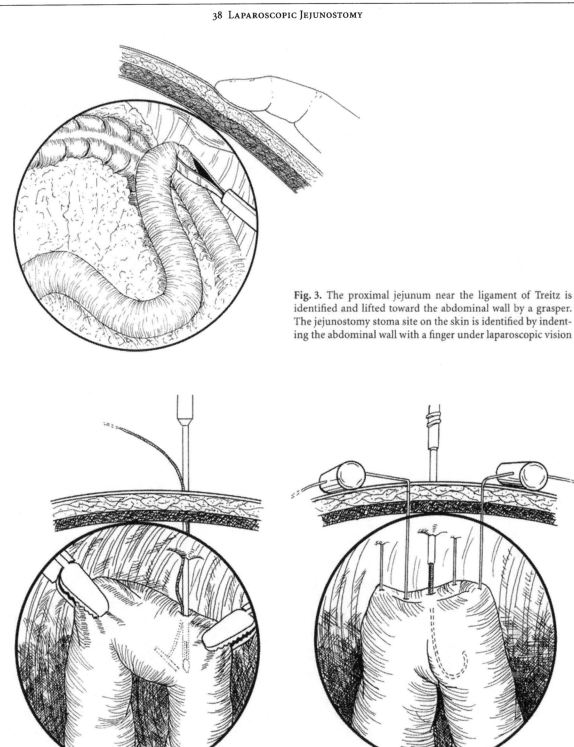

Fig. 3. The proximal jejunum near the ligament of Treitz is identified and lifted toward the abdominal wall by a grasper. The jejunostomy stoma site on the skin is identified by indenting the abdominal wall with a finger under laparoscopic vision

Fig. 4. The first T-fastener is placed in one corner of the 3´3 cm diamond visualized on the antimesenteric border of the proximal jejunum

Fig. 5. The antimesenteric border of the jejunum is secured by four T-fasteners. An 18-gauge needle is inserted through the center of the area demarcated by the T-fasteners. A J-guide wire is then introduced into the lumen of the jejunum through this needle

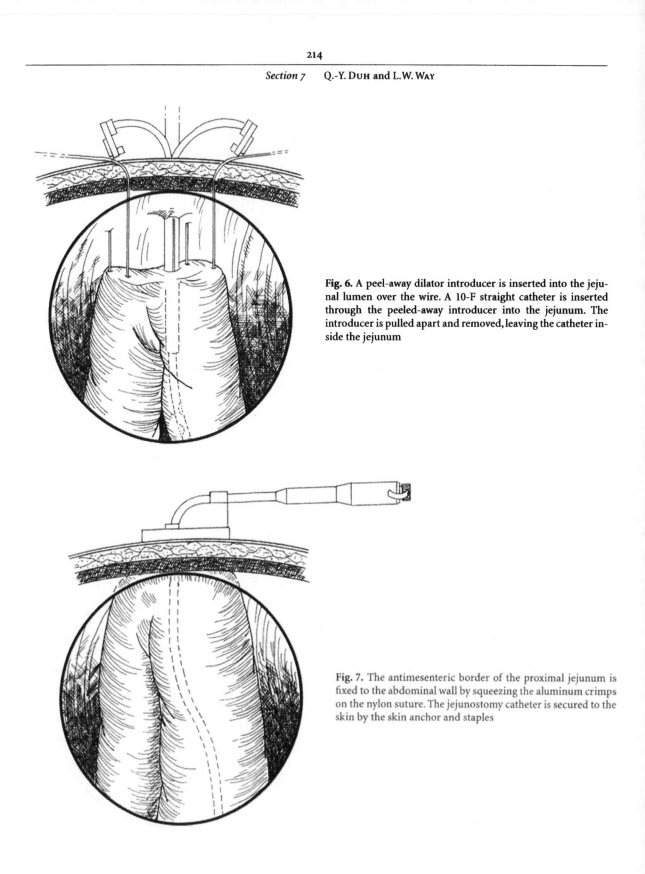

Fig. 6. A peel-away dilator introducer is inserted into the jejunal lumen over the wire. A 10-F straight catheter is inserted through the peeled-away introducer into the jejunum. The introducer is pulled apart and removed, leaving the catheter inside the jejunum

Fig. 7. The antimesenteric border of the proximal jejunum is fixed to the abdominal wall by squeezing the aluminum crimps on the nylon suture. The jejunostomy catheter is secured to the skin by the skin anchor and staples

39 Nomenclature in Laparoscopic Colon Surgery

E.H. Phillips and R.J. Rosenthal

Introduction

The following chapters in this atlas describe different laparoscopic approaches for diseases of the colon and rectum. To better understand the techniques required and the results of the different techniques, these specific terminologies are suggested.

Complete Laparoscopic Colectomy

In complete laparoscopic colectomy (Figs. 1, 2) the dissection, resection, specimen removal, and anastomosis are performed without abdominal wall incision, and trocars 30 mm or less in diameter are used. Left colon specimens can be delivered transanally, but transverse specimens and right colon specimens must be morcellated for removal. This approach is currently not adequate for some cancerous tumors as it is impossible to examine histopathologically the morcellated specimen with present pathology techniques. Surgeons who choose these techniques should possess the most advanced laparoscopic surgical skills as multiple point retraction, intracorporeal and extracorporeal suturing, and tying techniques are required.

Near-Complete Laparoscopic Colectomy

In the case of near-complete laparoscopic colectomy (Figs. 3–5) the dissection, resection, and anastomosis are performed laparoscopically, but a small incision is made to remove the specimen and/or insert the anvil of the circular stapler in the proximal bowel. After the specimen is laparoscopically resected and placed into a bag, the trocar site of the endocutter or any convenient trocar site is extended, and the specimen is removed. This situation allows the surgeon to exteriorize the proximal bowel and place the anvil extracorporeally, avoiding the intracorporeal creation of a pursestring. This technique is well suited to all benign and malignant lesions of the colon but especially resections in which the anastomosis

is within reach of the circular stapler inserted via the anus.

Resection-Facilitated Laparoscopic Colectomy

With resection-facilitated laparoscopic colectomy (Fig. 6) the dissection and resection of the colon segment are performed laparoscopically. The resected specimen is placed in a bag. An enlarged trocar site or a dedicated abdominal wall incision is used to take out the specimen. The distal and proximal colon segments are exteriorized, and the anastomosis is performed extracorporeally.

Dissection-Facilitated Laparoscopic Colon Resection

The procedure of dissection-facilitated laparoscopic colon resection (Fig. 7) consists of only mobilization of the colon segment to be removed and anastomosis. Only the parietocolic attachments are dissected under laparoscopic guidance. After the mobilization is achieved, an abdominal wall incision is made, and the colon and mesenterium are exteriorized. The resection and anastomosis are performed extracorporeally. The bowel is then replaced back into the peritoneal cavity. although the laparoscopic approach seems minimal, it allows a precise inspection of the abdominal cavity and mobilization of the flexures that would otherwise require a larger laparotomy. This technique is useful in right colon resections or even left colon resections in which the anastomosis is above the pelvic brim.

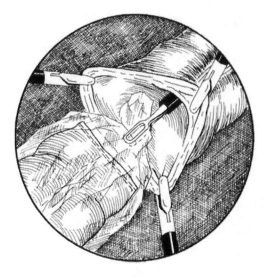

Fig. 1. Specimen is delivered transanally

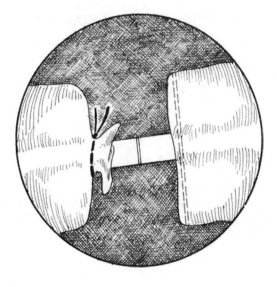

Fig. 2. Intracorporeal anastomosis

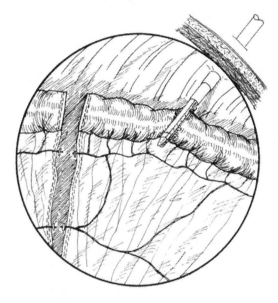

Fig. 3. Intracorporeal resection

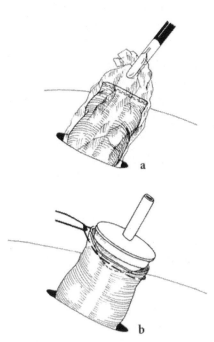

Fig. 4. a Specimen is removed through an enlarged trocar site incision. **b** Extracorporeal insertion of the anvil of the circular stapler into the proximal bowel

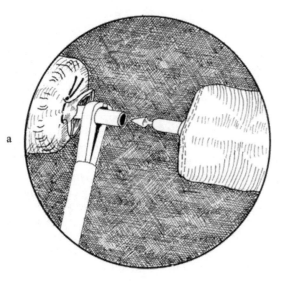

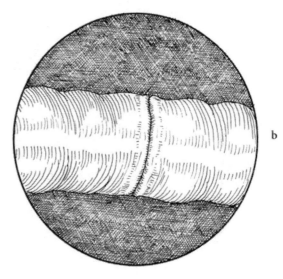

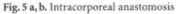

Fig. 5 a, b. Intracorporeal anastomosis

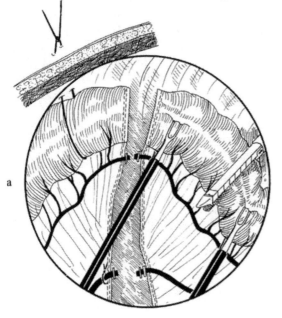

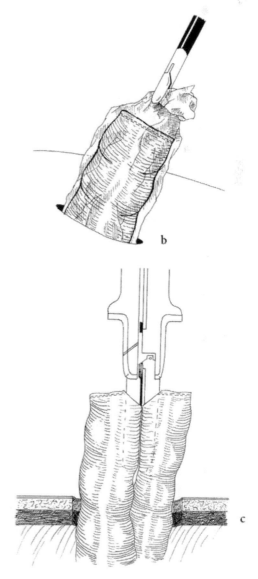

Fig. 6. a Intracorporeal dissection and resection of the colon. b Enlarged trocar site incision for specimen delivery. c Colon segments exteriorized and the anastomosis is performed extra-corporeally

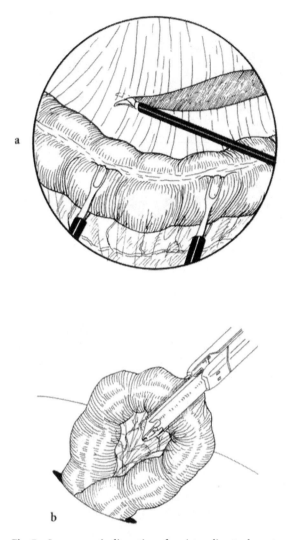

Comments

The portion of the colon to be removed dictates the best technique to use and the difficulty of the operation. The other factor to be considered in choosing a laparoscopic technique for colon resection is the pathology being operated on. When operating for benign colon disease, less mesentery requires resection, and the specimen can be partially morcellated for removal. When operating for cancer, careful attention to technique is needed. To achieve a large number of mesenteric lymph nodes in the specimen does not mean that the surgical criteria for an oncological operation are being followed. After the tumor is identified, the surgeon and assistants should pay attention that the clamps do not grasp the bowel in an area where the lesion is located. Because of the inability to palpate the bowel intraoperative colonoscopy should be used to precisely determine the appropriate resection margins. Finally, after an adequate excision of the mesentery the transected bowel with closed lumina should be placed in a bag in order to avoid seeding of tumor cells. To safely and successfully perform these complex laparoscopic procedures, special training and ongoing familiarity with the evolving endoscopic instrumentation are required of all team members.

Fig. 7. a Laparoscopic dissection of parietocolic attachments. **b** Extracorporeal dissection, resection and anastomosis

40 Dissection and Resection Facilitated Laparoscopic Right Hemicolectomy

D. Rosenthal and R. Ramos

Introduction

Laparoscopically facilitated right colectomies for benign or malignant disease can minimize the incision size and the trauma to the patient. A suitable patient is a one who after a comprehensive preoperative evaluation appears to have a lesion not involving neighboring organs, not invading the abdominal parietes, and not associated with interintestinal fistulas or abscesses. A careful history, a thorough physical examination, barium contrast studies, and enhanced computed tomography in selected patients should provide the surgeon with enough information to decide whether a patient is a suitable candidate for laparoscopic surgery.

Positioning of the Patient and Team

For positioning of the patient and team, see Fig. 1

Technique

The patient is placed in the supine position over a beanbag (Olympus VAC-PAC). The patient's legs, wrapped in sequential compression stockings, are placed in low-lying stirrups with the thighs minimally flexed. The surgeon stands on the patient's left side with the camera operator. The assistant stands on the right side of the patient. Video monitors are conveniently placed on either side of the operating table (Fig. 1). The peritoneum is grasped with fine clamps and a 10- to 11-mm blunt-tipped Endopath is placed in the supraumbilical site and secured using the two Vicryl strands. Carbon dioxide is insufflated into the peritoneal cavity. The 30° angle viewing periscope is introduced through the trocar and the peritoneal cavity and liver are carefully examined.

The right colon lesion is carefully inspected and its laparoscopic resectability assessed. If the adhesions can be easily and expeditiously taken down, additional 10- to 11-mm trocars are placed. For a right colon resection trocars are placed in the left and right lower quadrant,

and a third trocar is placed just to the left of the midline in the epigastrium (Fig. 2).

With the beanbag deflated the table is now acutely rotated sideways so as to have the right side of the patient higher than the left. For the surgeon this maneuver brings the right gutter into full view. With laparoscopic Babcock clamps placed in the supraumbilical and left lower quadrant the assistant carefully pulls the colon medially. The surgeon places his scissors connected to an electrocoagulation unit through the right lower quadrant trocar and divides the peritoneum lateral to the colon (Fig. 3). Congenital or acquired peritoneal adhesions bounding the terminal ileum down must be divided. As the peritoneal division progresses the colon is further reflected medially. With further mobilization, the right ureter is exposed. Additional proximal mobilization of the colon exposes the second portion of the duodenum (Fig. 4).

The instruments are now repositioned so that the scissors go through the epigastric and the Babcocks through the lower quadrant ports (Fig. 4). This new arrangement allows the assistant to pull the hepatic flexure medially and caudally, placing the peritoneal attachments of the hepatic flexure under tension. The hepatic flexure is taken down using scissors and electrocoagulation. Some vessels in the peritoneum holding down the hepatic flexure at times require clipping.

Attention is now turned to the mesentery of the right colon, which is placed under tension by pulling the colon laterally (Fig. 5). The ileocolic artery can generally be identified, the leaves of the mesentery on either sides of the vessels are divided, clips are placed on the artery which is then divided, and its proximal end is additionally secured with an endoloop (Ethicon, Cincinnati, OH). The right colic artery is handled in a similar fashion once the right colon and the terminal ileum have been mobilized and the ileocolic, and right colic artery are divided. The site for the abdominal wall incision should be selected laparoscopically directly over the transverse colon site of proposed transection and anastomosis. A transverse oblique incision approximately 5 cm long is usually needed (Fig. 6). The rectus muscle is divided along its fibers, and the peritoneum is entered. The edges of the incision are protected from contamination. The mobilized bowel is delivered through the incision. The terminal ileum is divided using a gastrointestinal stapler. The proximal portion of the transverse colon is now freed from its attachments to the greater omentum, and the branches of the middle colic artery destined to that segment are clamped, divided, and tied. The colon and terminal ileum are then divided using a linear stapler.

A functional end-to-end ileotransverse colostomy is now constructed using stapling instruments. The hemostasis of the staple lines is controlled with running 3-0 Vicryl stitches. The mesenteric defect is closed. The bowel is replaced in the peritoneal cavity, and the transverse incision is closed in layers.

The abdomen is again insufflated with carbon dioxide, the peritoneal cavity is checked for hemostasis, and the operative site is thoroughly irrigated with saline. All the intraperitoneal irrigation fluids are carefully aspirated. No drains are used. The trocars are removed in turn under direct vision. When operating for cancer, the trocar tracts are copiously irrigated with sterile water. The trocar site fascial defects are sutured closed to prevent hernias.

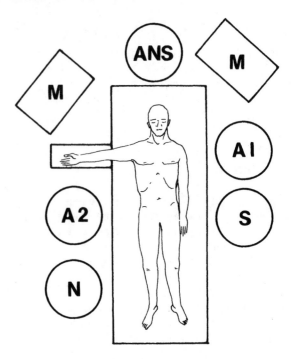

Fig. 1. Positioning of patient and team. Patient in supine position. *ANS*, Anesthetist; *S*, surgeon; *A1, A2*, assistants; *N*, nurse; *M*, monitor

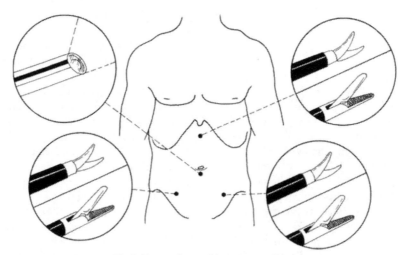

Fig. 2. Trocar sites and instrumentation

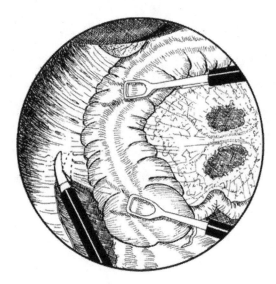

Fig. 3. Dissection of parietocolic attachments

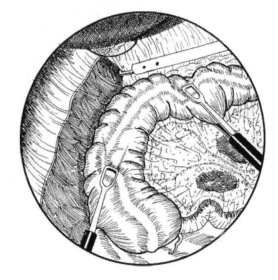

Fig. 4. Mobilization of hepatic flexure

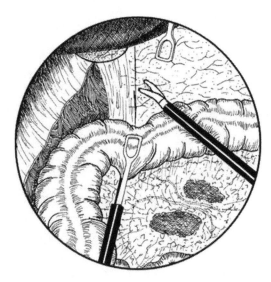

Fig. 5. Gastrocolic ligament dissection

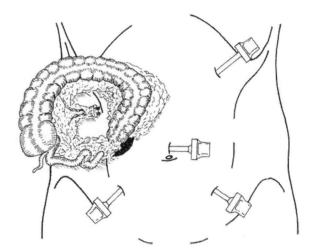

Fig. 6. Exteriorization of right hemicolon for resection and anastomosis

Comments

Technical aspects include the following:

- The patient should be securely positioned on the operating table so that marked axial tilting and rotation of the table can be safely executed.
- Antithromboembolic calf wraps should be used to counter the deleterious effect of the pneumoperitoneum on the inferior vena cava blood flow.
- Trocars of 10–11 mm should be used so that any one of them can be used to admit the camera.
- Trocar extrusion and replacement wastes time and can increase CO_2 absorption through the abdominal wall layers dissected by attempts at replacing the trocar in the peritoneal cavity. This can be avoided by using stability threads or by the use of silk stitches passed through the skin and looped around the trocar flanges to prevent the extrusion of the trocars during surgery.
- When using clamps to pull on the colon, it is preferable to grasp the colon appendices epiploicae rather than the bowel wall itself.
- Vessels up to 2 mm in diameter can be safely clipped.
- Vessels over 2 mm in diameter are best tied using extracorporeal ties. As an alternative, the vessels can be held with bulldog clamps (Solos-Bircher) passed through the trocars, then divided and tied with endoloops.
- Endovascular cutters/staplers can also be employed.
- When dividing a vessel over 2 mm in size, its division should always be made in stages, fearing the eventuality that a partially controlled vessel may retract in the mesentery.
- Staged division of a major vessel with repeat application of clips is expeditious, yet not as safe as the hemostatic techniques described above.

References

Beart RW (1994) Laparoscopic colectomy: status of the art. Dis Colon Rectum 37 (2):47–49

Franklin ME (1992) Laparoscopic colon resections. Surg Laparosc Endosc 2 (2):183–190

Jacobs M, Verdeja JC (1991) Minimally invasive colon resection. Surg Laparosc Endosc 1 (3):144–150

Phillips EH, Franklin M, Carroll BJ, Fallas MJ, Ramos R, Rosenthal D (1992) Laparoscopic colectomy. Ann Surg 216 (6):703–707

Wexner SD, Johansen OB (1992) Laparoscopic bowel resection: advantages and limitations. Ann Intern Med 24 (2):105–110

41 Laparoscopic Transverse Colectomy

M.A. Liberman and E.H. Phillips

Introduction

Near-complete laparoscopic transverse colectomy is the most technically challenging laparoscopic colectomy. On the other hand, a dissection-facilitated transverse colectomy is the most commonly employed technique. This involves delivering the bowel through a midline or transverse incision for resection and anastomosis, after mobilization of the bowel is guided laparoscopically. This often entails mobilization of both the hepatic and splenic flexures and requires a stapled or hand-sewn anastomosis.

There are no absolute contraindications to laparoscopic transverse colectomy; however, patients with multiple previous intra-abdominal procedures, those with bowel obstruction and/or marked bowel dilation, and those with a large mass contiguous with other intra-abdominal organs may be inappropriate candidates.

An adequate preoperative evaluation includes a thorough history and physical examination, appropriate blood tests, chest X-ray, abdominal computed tomography scan to fully evaluate the liver (in selected patients), and barium enema or colonoscopy. If the lesion is small, preoperative colonoscopy is needed to localize the lesion by marking the colon adjacent to it with india ink. Intraoperative colonoscopy is also an option for localization of the lesion and should be available in all cases, as the india ink is not always visible. When intraoperative colonoscopy is performed, the terminal ileum or proximal bowel must be occluded with a clamp or Penrose drain to prevent insufflation of the small bowel.

The patient must receive a thorough mechanical bowel preparation the day before surgery along with oral and/or intravenous antibiotics.

Positioning of the Patient and Team

The patient should be placed on an electric table and positioned in a supine, modified lithotomy position. The surgeon stands between the patient's legs with assistants to the patient's left and right. Two video monitors are utilized, one by each of the patient's shoulders (Fig. 1). Sequential compression stockings should be placed and functioning prior to the induction of anesthesia. The patient should receive preoperative intravenous antibiotics. An oral gastric tube and bladder drainage catheter are placed.

Technique

Dissection

Preemptive local anesthesia with 1% Xylocaine mixed 50 : 50 with 0.5% Marcaine is utilized prior to insertion of all trocars. A subumbilical skin puncture is made and a Veress needle is inserted. A pneumoperitoneum is created followed by placement of a 10- to 11-mm trocar in the left lower quadrant, just lateral to the rectus muscle. The Veress needle can be removed at the umbilical site without incident. A 30° angle 10-mm laparoscope is introduced through the trocar sleeve and into the peritoneal cavity for initial exploration. The transverse colon is closely examined, as are the liver and other adjacent organs. Laparoscopic ultrasonography of the liver is performed if available. Resectability is determined, and a decision is made whether to proceed laparoscopically.

If so, a 10- to 11-mm trocar is placed in the midline between the pubis and the umbilicus, and the laparoscope is moved to this position. Additional 10- to 11-mm trocars are placed in the right lower quadrant, lateral to the rectus muscle, as well as in the right and left upper quadrants, parallel to the two lower quadrant trocars (Fig. 2). All ports should be 10–11 mm.

Dissection of Gastrocolic Omentum

The surgeon controls the instruments inserted through the two lower ports. The patient is placed in reverse Trendelenburg position and tilted left or right as needed. The operation is begun after identifying the proximal and distal margins of resection. These points should be marked with cautery, clips, or suture on the colon. If a sleeve resection of the transverse colon is planned, a window is made in the gastrocolic omentum (Fig. 3) with the electrocautery hook or scissors (just distal to the gastroepiploic arcade for a suspected carcinoma). After the lesser sac has been entered, the dissection is continued along the avascular plane with a combination of electrocautery, bipolar scissors, electrocautery hook suction device, Endoclips (Ethicon, Cincinnati, OH), or endovascular cutters. Bipolar electrocautery prevents injuring the adjacent colon or stomach from unintended thermal injury. The endpoints of this portion of the dissection are visualization of the second portion of the duodenum on the right and the splenic flexure on the left.

Dissection of Hepatic Flexure

To dissect the hepatic flexure the table is rotated such that the patient remains in reverse Trendelenburg with the right side up. The surgeon may elect to move to the left side of the table or may stay positioned between the patient's legs. The surgeon moves the laparoscope to the left lower quadrant port, and the assistant retracts the ascending colon medially with atraumatic graspers via both upper ports. This enables the surgeon to provide his own countertraction with a grasper in the lower midline port, and three-point tension is provided (Fig. 4). This is especially important when dissecting the hepatic and/or splenic flexures. The surgeon is now able to divide the lateral postfetal adhesions of the colon using electrocautery scissors placed through the right lower quadrant port. Occasional small vessels in the lateral peritoneal attachments may require clips, sutures, pretied suture loops, or bipolar or unipolar cautery. Care is taken to identify the right ureter.

Dissection proceeds from the ascending colon to the hepatic flexure. The retroperitoneal portion of the duodenum is the next important landmark to identify. It is visualized with medial mobilization of the right mesocolon (Fig. 5). Vessels are often encountered during dissection of the hepatic flexure, and these should be cauterized with a bipolar instrument or clipped. It is important to avoid unipolar cautery or mechanical injury to the duodenum or colon. The dissection then proceeds further distally until the endpoint of the dissection is reached. This endpoint should be approximately 6 cm distal to the planned resection margin. This enables the colon to be lifted easily through an abdominal wall incision for an extracorporeal anastomosis.

Dissection of Splenic Flexure

To dissect the splenic flexure, the patient should be tilted left side up. With the laparoscope in the right lower quadrant port, the left colon is retracted medially in two points by the assistant via the upper ports. The surgeon provides countertraction with an atraumatic grasper inserted via the lower midline port and then divides the lateral peritoneal attachments with electrocautery scissors inserted via the right or left lower quadrant port (Fig. 6). The superficial splenocolic attachments are divided first with cautery or clips. Then the dissection is initiated at the mid-descending colon and proceeds proximally. Medial and/or inferior traction on the colon must be gentle when taking down the splenic flexure, as vigorous traction may cause a tear in the splenic capsule. Similar care is taken with the left ureter as was taken with the right, especially if the dissection includes the sigmoid colon.

After both the hepatic and splenic flexures are mobilized, the laparoscope is returned to the lower midline port. The transverse colon is now retracted superiorly or inferiorly, whichever exposes the middle colic vessels as they emerge from beneath the pancreas and cross over the retroperitoneal duodenum (Fig. 7). Depending upon the extent of the resection (extended right hemicolectomy, extended left hemicolectomy, true transverse colectomy) and the reason for the resection (large benign sessile polyp or carcinoma), it may not be necessary to divide the middle colic artery before it branches. With the right colon retracted medially, the ileocolic artery can be identified and in a similar fashion the left colic artery is identified with the left colon retracted.

Resection and Anastomosis

Dissection-Facilitated

A decision must be made as to the technique used for dividing the bowel and mesentery as well as creating the anastomosis. A dissection-facilitated resection entails laparoscopically guided mobilization of the bowel, division of the bowel and mesentery extracorporeally, and an extracorporeal anastomosis. This is the easiest technique and can be performed the most rapidly. The site for the abdominal wall incision is usually decided based on the location of the distal margin of resection. This is because the distal bowel is tethered by its blood supply, and the proximal bowel can usually be mobilized more readily. This is not always the case, and thus the abdominal wall incision is best made over the nonmobile margin of bowel. The size of the incision is based on the size of the tumor, mesentery, or bowel wall thickness. The site of the abdominal wall incision is usually the left lower quadrant for an extended left hemicolectomy, upper midline or left upper quadrant for an extended right hemicolectomy or occasionally at the umbilicus for a sleeve resection.

The necessary portion of colon is delivered and resected. The mesentery is reapproximated prior to fashioning the anastomosis because if the blood supply to the distal ends of the bowel is accidentally injured during closure of the mesentery, leading to bowel ischemia, the ischemic portion can be resected without having to redo the anastomosis. Either a hand-sewn, inserted biodegradable anastomotic device or stapled functional end-to-end anastomosis is created extracorporeally. The bowel is then returned to the abdomen and the incision closed.

Resection-Facilitated

In a resection-facilitated procedure there is division of the mesocolon and bowel intracorporeally, but the anastomosis is performed extracorporeally. The bowel should be divided proximally and distally with an endovascular cutter. Whether performing a true transverse colectomy, extended right colectomy, or extended left colectomy, the mesentery containing small unnamed vessels may be divided with electrocautery, clips, endoloops (Ethicon) or endovascular cutters. This is usually best performed by the assistant retracting the ascending or descending colon medially and anteriorly from the upper ports while the surgeon divides the mesocolon from one of the lower ports. The transverse colon is best retracted cephalad and anteriorly by the assistant via the upper ports while the surgeon divides the mesocolon from one of the lower ports. If necessary, the colon may be suspended by 0 nylon suture on a Keith needle passed through the skin and abdominal wall, and then the mesentery, and then again through the abdominal wall and tied.

The ileocolic, middle colic and left colic arteries must be isolated and individually divided. A window is made on either side of the artery, and a clip is placed on the distal artery. An endoloop can be introduced into the abdomen, a grasper is placed through the loop, and the proximal portion of the artery is grasped. The artery is then divided and the endoloop secured below the grasper on the proximal artery. A second clip may be placed on the proximal artery. Another acceptable option for ligation and division of the arteries is using the endovascular cutters. The specimen is then placed in a specimen bag. Prior to creating the abdominal wall incision graspers are placed on the specimen as well as the proximal and distal bowel. This avoids searching the abdomen once the pneumoperitoneum has been evacuated. The remainder of the procedure is similar to the dissection-facilitated procedure.

Near-Complete Laparoscopic Colectomy

In a near-complete procedure there is intracorporeal division of the mesocolon and bowel and an intracorporeal anastomosis as well. An abdominal incision is made only for delivering the specimen and/or inserting an anvil or anastomotic device. This is the most challenging technique of resection, and anastomosis and is recommended only after mastering the previously described techniques. When performing an intracorporeal anastomosis, there are numerous options. These include hand-sewn, biodegradable anastomotic device, stapled side-to-side functional end-to-end, and an anastomosis using the circular stapler.

The key step in a successful intracorporeal anastomosis is the alignment of the proximal and distal bowel limbs. If a hand-sewn anastomosis is being performed, the proximal and distal limbs are aligned end-to-end (Fig. 8). This is best achieved by the assistant holding the bowel with atraumatic graspers in the upper ports. The surgeon standing between the patient's legs (the laparoscope in the lower midline port) has his needle driver and grasper in the right and left lower quadrant ports. An additional upper midline port may be necessary to aid bowel alignment. A one- or two-layer running or simple interrupted anastomosis can be performed. This can also be performed using the Endo-Suture (Auto Suture, Norwalk, CN) suturing device (Fig. 9). The mesenteric defect is closed in a similar fashion by suture or hernia stapler.

A side-to-side, functional end-to-end stapled intracorporeal anastomosis is another option for a true transverse colectomy or extended right hemicolectomy. The two ends are aligned by the assistant with graspers in the upper ports such that the stapled ends are pointing caudad. Three stay sutures are placed, securing the proximal to the distal limb, and are cut long and clipped. The two limbs can now be manipulated by the assistant grasping these sutures. With the laparoscope in the lower midline port, the surgeon, standing between the patient's legs, introduces a grasper in the right lower quadrant port and a 60 mm endocutter in the right upper quadrant port. (The placement of the 60 mm endocutter requires lengthening the original 10 mm skin incision to 18 mm to accommodate this instrument.) The superior corner of the previously placed staple line of each bowel limb is excised, and the endocutter is initially introduced in a closed fashion (Fig. 10). After engaging the bowel it is fully opened, inserted, then closed and fired. After checking the lumen for hemostasis the remaining bowel defect is closed with suture or another application of an endovascular cutter.

At the conclusion of any of the above procedures the abdomen is copiously irrigated and suctioned. Hemostasis is assured. The pneumoperitoneum is evacuated and all trocars are removed under direct vision. All fascial incisions 10 mm or greater are carefully closed (Fig. 11).

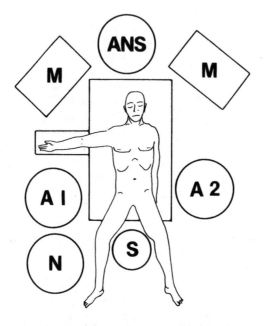

Fig. 1. Positioning of the patient and team. Patient in supine, modified lithotomy position position. *ANS*, Anesthetist; *S*, surgeon; *A1, A2*, assistants; *N*, nurse; *M*, monitor

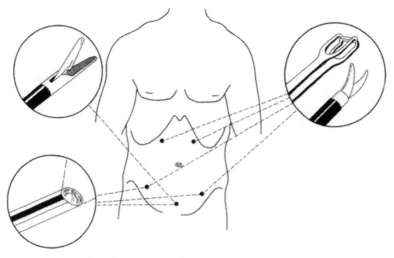

Fig. 2. Trocar sites and instrumentation

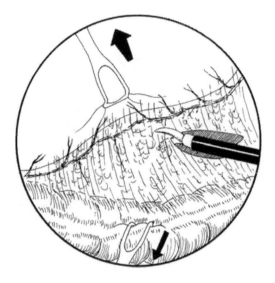

Fig. 3. A window is created in the gastrocolic omentum

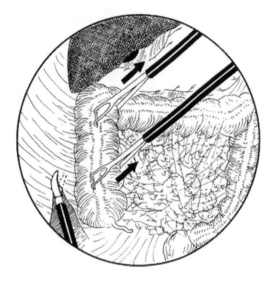

Fig. 4. Traction and countertraction are used for dissecting the hepatic and splenic flexure

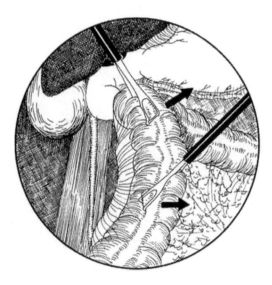

Fig. 5. The retroperitoneal portion of the duodenum is visualized by medial mobilization of the mesocolon

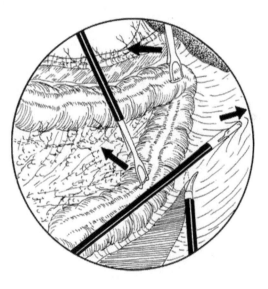

Fig. 6. Dissection of parietocolic attachments of the splenic flexure

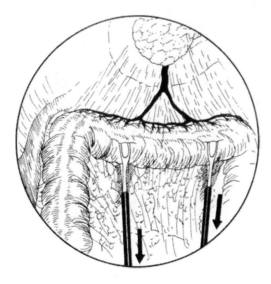

Fig. 7. The midcolic vessels are exposed by retracting the transverse colon

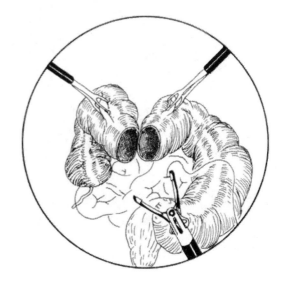

Fig. 8. Intracorporeal hand-sewn anastomosis

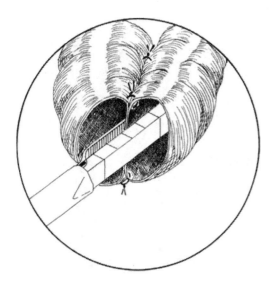

Fig. 9. A side-to-side mechanical anastomosis is performed

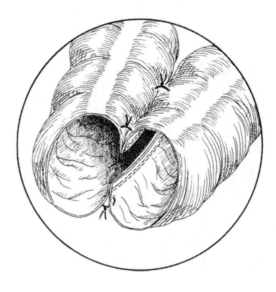

Fig. 10. View of the posterior wall of the anastomosis

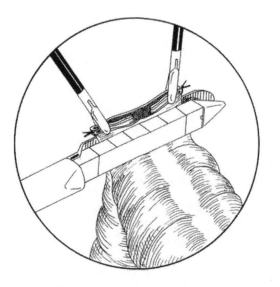

Fig. 11. Closure of the anterior wall of the anastomosis

Comments

1. The patient should be in a low lithotomy position. If the knees are raised too high, they interfere with the surgeon's instruments and arm movements.
2. Change the position of the operative table, i.e., reverse Trendelenburg, right side up, left side up, as often as necessary to assist operative exposure.
3. Always use a 30° angle laparoscope. Used properly, this provides much greater visualization than a 0° laparoscope.
4. During this procedure many instruments are moved in and out the trocar sleeves. If one hand is free, it should fix the trocar sleeve in position when changing instruments. The new instrument is directed to the exact position at which one was previously working. This avoids wasting time moving the laparoscope to find and redirect the new instrument as well as potential viscus injury from a blind insertion.
5. Make an effort to evacuate all blood at the conclusion of the procedure as this is not only a nidus for infection but also the source of significant postoperative pain. A good suction irrigation device is important. Such as the Probe Plus II (Ethicon, Cincinnati, OH) as it has interchangeable probes, electrocautery, and a 10-mm diameter suction.

References

Beart RW (1994) Laparoscopic colectomy: status of the art. Dis Colon Rectum 37:S47-S49

Cohen SM, Wexner SD (1994) Laparoscopic right hemicolectomy. Surg Rounds 627–635

Falk PM, Beart RW, Wexner SD et al (1993) Laparoscopic colectomy: a critical appraisal. Dis Colon Rectum 36:28–34

Pappas TN (1992) Laparoscopic colectomy – the innovation continues. Ann Surg 216:701–702

Phillips EH, Franklin M, Carroll BJ (1992) Laparoscopic colectomy. Ann Surg 216:703–707

Sackier JM (1993) Laparoscopic colon and rectal surgery. In: Hunter JG, Sackier JM (eds) Minimally invasive surgery. McGraw-Hill, New York pp 179–191

Schlinkert RT (1991) Laparoscopic-assisted right hemicolectomy. Dis Colon Rectum 34:1030–1031

Wexner SD, Cohen SM, Johansen OB et al (1993) Laparoscopic colorectal surgery: a prospective assessment and current perspective. Br J Surg 80:1602–1605

42 Laparoscopic Left Colectomy

M. Jacobs

Introduction

Laparoscopically guided colon surgery is extremely challenging but quite rewarding. Excellent visualization can be achieved once the techniques of retraction are learned. Extensive mobilization of the colon can be achieved without a xiphoid-to-pubis incision, and, once familiar with the retroperitoneum, an extensive mesenteric resection can be employed when necessary. Resection of the left colon is especially rewarding because the circular stapler can be placed per anus, facilitating the anastomosis and further decreasing the size of the abdominal incision to that necessary to remove the specimen.

Positioning of the Patient and Team

The patient is positioned in low lithotomy stirrups. The operating room table is placed in Trendelenburg and rotated toward the right side. Two monitors are used, one at the patient's left shoulder and the other at the left knee. The surgeon stands to the patient's right. The assistant stands at the left or between the legs, and the nurse stands next to the surgeon (Fig. 1).

Technique

Four 10- to 11-mm trocars are placed. (The pneumoperitoneum is initiated through an infraumbilical Veress puncture or via an open Hasson technique with abdominal insufflation to 15 mmHg.) The first trocar is placed infraumbilically, and a 10-mm 30° angle laparoscope is passed into the abdomen. An initial exploration is performed, inspecting the liver and the entire abdomen. The additional ports are placed under direct vision: one at the epigastrium, one suprapubic just to the left of the midline, and one at the left anterior axillary line at the level of the umbilicus (Fig. 2).

The camera is switched to the epigastric port and is held by the assistant, who also provides medial traction on the descending colon with a Babcock through the

left-sided cannula. The surgeon (standing on the right side) uses a Babcock through the umbilical trocar with the left hand and an endocautery scissors or hook dissector through the suprapubic cannula with the right hand (Fig. 3). The mobilization begins by incising the white line of Toldt at the level of the midsigmoid and proceeds proximally toward the splenic flexure (both surgeon and assistant look at the monitor at the patient's knee). The colon is bluntly dissected medially. The left ureter is identified at the pelvic brim and protected during the subsequent maneuvers.

When the splenic flexure is dissected, the operating room table is placed in reverse Trendelenburg position and rotated toward the right side. The laparoscope is now used through the left suprapubic port. The assistant moves between the patient's legs and holds the camera and provides lateral countertraction at the level of the phrenocolic and splenocolic ligaments. The surgeon uses a Babcock through the epigastric port and retracts the splenic flexure medially, placing the ligaments under tension so they can be transected with electrocautery scissors or electrocautery hook suction device or divided between clips placed through the umbilical cannula (Fig. 4). Both surgeon and assistant look at the monitor near the patient's head.

After transecting these ligaments the assistant provides traction with the Babcock at the inferior edge of the gastrocolic ligament. It is transected to the level of the midtransverse colon by the surgeon using the endoscissors or electrocautery hook suction device placed through the umbilical port (Fig. 5).

If the greater omentum is not to be removed (benign or palliative resection), it is easier for the assistant to hold the transverse colon inferiorly with the Babcock through the left-sided trocar and for the surgeon to hold the greater omentum superiorly providing countertraction with the Babcock through the epigastric port. The omentum is dissected from the transverse colon using the endoscissors through the umbilical cannula.

The mobilized colon is reflected laterally and the mesentery is placed under traction by the assistant using a Babcock grasper through the left-sided port. The camera remains in the left suprapubic trocar. The surgeon provides countertraction with a Babcock in the epigastric port and scores the mesentery from the level of the visualized left colic or inferior mesenteric artery if this is to be taken. These vessels are clearly seen bowing as violin strings after appropriate traction is applied on the mesentery (Fig. 6 a).

The mesentery is dissected proximally along its base to the level of the midtransverse colon with the scissors placed via the umbilical port. The left colic or inferior mesenteric artery is divided between clips that are applied through the umbilical port after the creation of a window at the base of the mesentery (Fig. 6 b). The mesentery is divided proximally until the left branch of the middle colic is once again identified by the bowing of these vessels when the mesentery is under traction and countertraction. When the extent of bowel resection is determined the smaller vessels and the marginal artery are transected between endoclips until the edge of the colon is reached at the site of proximal and distal transection sites, completing the intracorporeal devascularization (Fig. 6 c).

If the resection also includes the sigmoid colon, the suprapubic trocar is exchanged for a 33-mm trocar, and the 60-mm endolinear cutter is used to divide the colon at the rectosigmoid junction or appropriate location (Fig. 7). The bowel is then delivered through an enlarged left lateral trocar site (easily done since the splenic flexure and transverse colon are well mobilized). The bowel is then transected at the chosen proximal level (midtransverse colon; Fig. 8). The anvil of the circular stapler is placed into the proximal colon secured by a pursestring suture and replaced back into the abdominal cavity, and the abdominal wall incision is closed (Fig. 9). Reinsufflation is performed. The shaft of the stapler is placed into the rectum to the level of the staple line, opened, and the spike is extruded through the end of the bowel. The anvil and the stapler are attached, approximated, and fired, creating an end-to-end double-staple anastomosis (Fig. 10). The integrity of the anastomosis is checked by submerging the anastomosis in saline while insufflating air through a sigmoidoscope. The proximal colon must be occluded with an atraumatic clamp.

References

Cooperman AM, Katz V, Zimmon D, Botero G (1991) Laparoscopic colon resection: a case report. J Laparoendosc Surg 1 (4):221–224

Falk PM, Beart RW jr, Wexner BD, Thorson AG, Jagelman DG, Lavery IC, Johanson OB, Fitzgibbons RJ jr (1993) Laparoscopic colectomy: a critical appraisal. Dis Colon Rectum 36 (1):28–34

Franklin ME jr, Ramos R, Rosenthal D, Schuessler W (1993) Laparoscopic colon procedures. World J Surg 17 (1):51–56

Phillips EH, Franklin M, Carroll BJ, Fallas MJ, Ramos R, Rosenthal D (1992) Laparoscopic colectomy. Ann Surg 216 (6):703–707

Wilson T (1991) Laparoendoscopy for abdominal cancer. Med J Aust 155:275

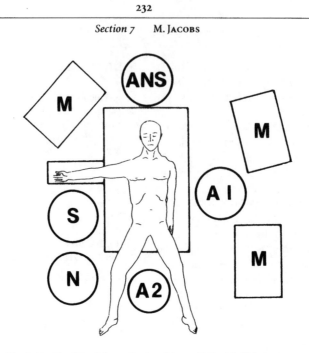

Fig. 1. Positioning of the patient and team. Patient in lithotomy position. *ANS*, Anesthetist; *S*, surgeon; *A1, A2*, assistants; *N*, nurse; *M*, monitor

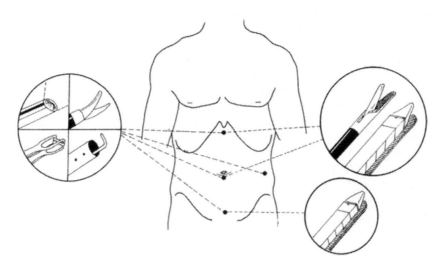

Fig. 2. Trocar sites and instrumentation

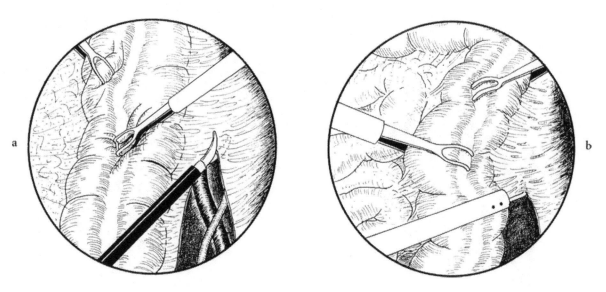

Fig. 3. Mobilization of distal (**a**) and proximal (**b**) lateral colon attachments

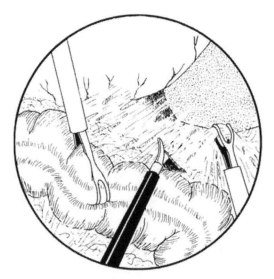

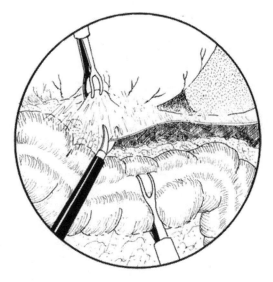

Fig. 4. Division of splenocolic ligament

Fig. 5. Division of gastrocolic ligament

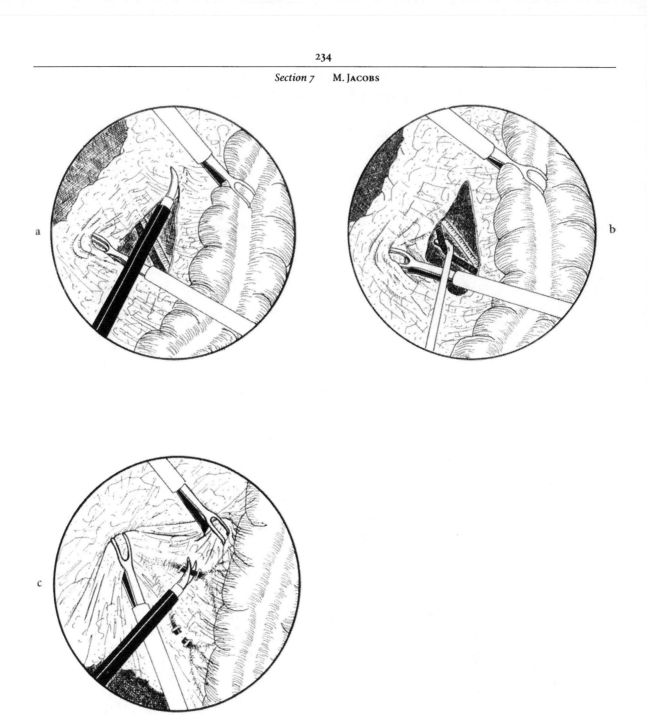

Fig. 6. a, b Dissection of inferior mesenteric artery and vein.
c Dissection of mesenteric vessels

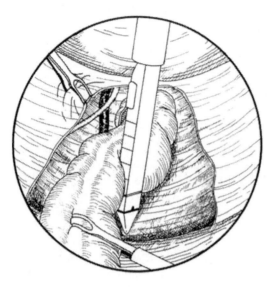

Fig. 7. Transection of the colon with the endocutter

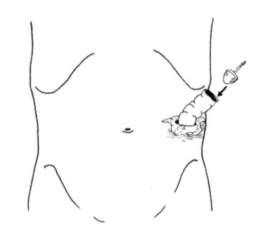

Fig. 8. Exteriorization of proximal colon limb

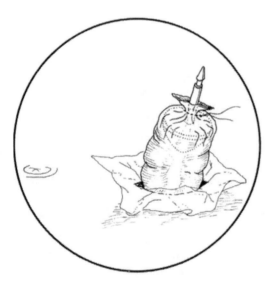

Fig. 9. Anvil of circular stapler secured externally and replaced into abdominal cavity

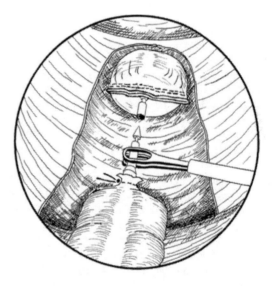

Fig. 10. Creation of end-to-end double-staple anastomosis

43 Laparoscopic Low Anterior Resection

A. Simons and R.W. Beart

Introduction

Preoperative evaluation of patients undergoing laparoscopic resection is identical to that for open colonic resection. Some feel more compelled to use computered tomography in evaluating the rest of the abdomen since manual exploration is not possible. Alternatively, intraoperative laparoscopic ultrasonography allows excellent examination of the parenchyma of the liver.

Positioning of the Patient and Team

The patient is placed in the combined position, much as for a low anterior resection (Fig. 1). In this position the perineum is accessible for use of the stapler or perhaps conversion to an abdominal perineal resection if necessary. The surgeon stands on the patient's right with the assistant standing on the side of the tumor.

Technique

The patient is given a bowel preparation and taken to the operating room. The patient must be prepared for the eventuality that the procedure cannot be completed laparoscopically. The procedure is initiated with a 10- to 11-mm port in the left upper quadrant (Fig. 2). This location is chosen because placing a camera through the umbilicus locates it directly over the origin of the inferior mesenteric artery. This is too close to see the artery well. Alternatively, the camera can be placed in the right upper quadrant, but the falciform ligament frequently makes entering the abdomen difficult. With the camera in position, a second 10- to 11-mm port site is placed in the suprapubic area, and two 5-mm ports are placed at the traditional colostomy sites (Fig. 2). It may be desirable to move these 5-mm ports somewhat closer to the pubic bone, but if they are too close to the 10- to 11-mm suprapubic port, the surgeon's hands may not work freely. The patient is placed in the steep Trendelenburg position and rotated to the right as far as possible. This allows the small bowel to be placed in the right upper quadrant with excellent exposure of the sigmoid.

Using a two-handed technique and using the 5-mm port on the right side of the abdomen and the suprapubic port, the surgeon initiates the procedure by grasping the peritoneal reflection of the sigmoid and incising the peritoneal reflection along the white line of Toldt (Fig. 3). This incision is carried to the splenic flexure and into the pelvis. It is important to mobilize the entire extent of the sigmoid. The sigmoid is then bluntly lifted from the retroperitoneum, identifying the gonadal vessels and the ureter (Fig. 4). Once these have been clearly identified, the bowel is laid back into its normal position and a peritoneal incision is made over the aorta and down over the right iliac vessel (Fig. 5). Using a combination of sharp and blunt dissection, the sigmoid mesentery is lifted off the retroperitoneum at the level of the bifurcation of the aorta.

The sacral promontory is identified and a "window" is created from the right side of the mesentery through to the dissection in the area on the left side of the mesentery (Fig. 6). Once this window is created, the mesentery can be elevated and the inferior mesenteric vessels are placed on traction. The inferior mesenteric vessels are bluntly dissected and isolated. The vein and artery are separated and clipped separately (Fig. 7). These vessels are divided carefully. They should be partially transected, and hemostasis should be confirmed before the vessels are completely divided. The ureter can once again be identified from both the right and left side of the mesentery.

A nerve-sparing procedure is possible. The sympathetic nerve can be identified at the level of the sacral promontory and dissected free from the mesentery. Once the sigmoid mesentery is mobilized and the inferior mesenteric vessels divided above the bifurcation of the aorta, traction is placed on the rectum, and perirectal tissues are dissected. This is carried out with the electrified scissors. The hypogastric vessels should be exposed, and this marks the lateral plane of dissection. Posteriorly, Waldeyer's fascia is easy to expose bluntly. Anteriorly, Denonvilliers' fascia should be incised and the vagina or prostate exposed (Fig. 8).

Once the dissection is carried 5 cm below the level of the tumor, the rectum mesentery can be divided with electrocautery. If any bleeders are identified, they can be clipped. Once the rectal wall is completely visualized, the rectum can be transected. The suprapubic port needs to be replaced with an 18-mm port, and a 60-mm endoscopic linear stapler can be placed through this port and the bowel transected (Fig. 9). This incision is enlarged, and the tumor and sigmoid colon are brought through a 5 cm incision in the suprapubic area. The mesenteric dissection is completed under direct visualization, and the anvil of the circular stapler is placed into the proximal bowel. Once this is secured, the bowel is returned to the abdominal cavity, and the incision is closed with a running absorbable monofilament suture.

The abdomen is reinsufflated and the circular staplers placed into the rectum via the anus. Under laparoscopic visualization the circular stapler is advanced until it is inserted to the level of the transected rectum (Fig. 10). The anvil shaft is advanced through the rectum and mated to the anvil from above. The stapler can then be closed. It is convenient at this point to look at the extent of tension on the descending colon, and if there is any tension, complete mobilization of the left colon and splenic flexure is appropriate. The stapler is then fired and removed. The abdomen can be carefully inspected and irrigated, and any blood clots should be removed. If desired, drains can be left in the presacral space. If there is any question about the completeness of the "donuts," air can be insufflated into the anus with the descending colon occluded by a clamp and the anastomosis under water. If there is no leak, all ports are then removed under direct vision, and ports larger than 5-mm are repaired with absorbable suture.

References

Beart RW jr (1994) Laparoscopic colectomy: status of the art. Dis Colon Rectum 37 [Suppl]:S47-S49

Braithwaite BD, Ritchie AWS, Earnshaw JJ (1994) Laparoscopic surgery for colorectal cancer. Br J Surg 81:313–316

Eltringham WK, Roe AM, Galloway SW, Mountford RA, Espiner HJ (1993) A laparoscopic technique for full thickness intestinal biopsy and feeding jejunostomy. Gut 34:122–124

Geis WP, Coletta AV, Verdeja J-C, Plasencia G, Ojogho O, Jacobs M (1994) Sequential psychomotor skills development in laparoscopic colon surgery. Arch Surg 129:206–212

Hoffman GC, Baker JW, Fitchett CW, Vansant JH (1994) Laparoscopic-assisted colectomy: initial experience. Ann Surg 219:732–743

Scoggin SD, Frazee RC, Snyder SK, Hendricks JC, Roberts JW, Symmonds RE, Smith RW (1993) Laparoscopic-assisted bowel surgery. Dis Colon Rectum 36:747–750

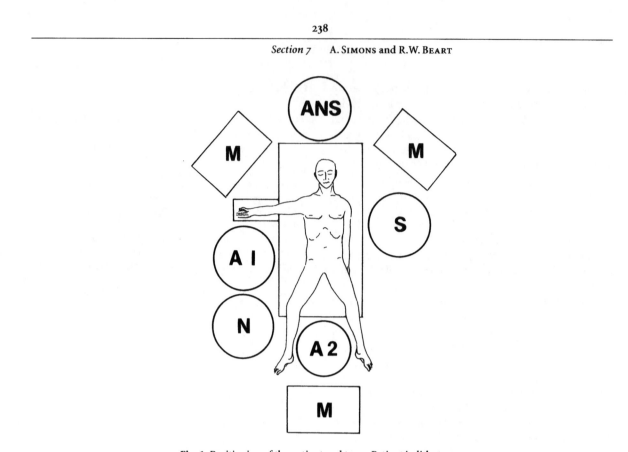

Fig. 1. Positioning of the patient and team. Patient in lithotomy position. *ANS,* Anesthetist; *S,* surgeon; *A1, A2,* assistants; *N,* nurse; *M,* monitor

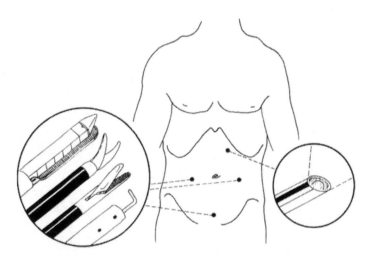

Fig. 2. Trocar sites and instrumentation

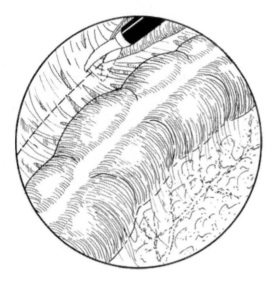

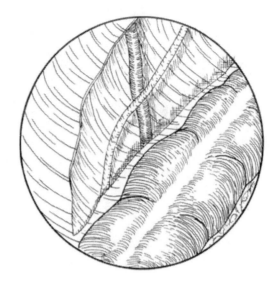

Fig. 3. Toldt's fascia is incised

Fig. 4. Identification of the ureter and iliac vessels

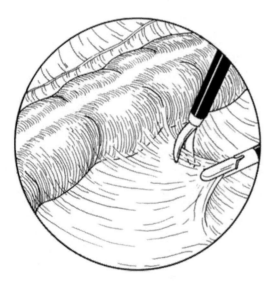

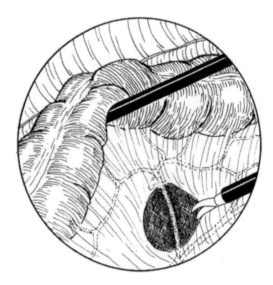

Fig. 5. Dissection of the mesenterium

Fig. 6. Dissecting a window at the mesenterium

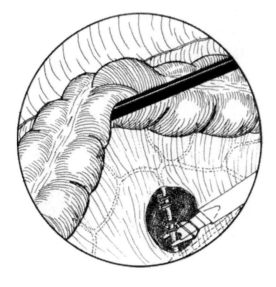

Fig. 7. Sigmoid vessels are divided

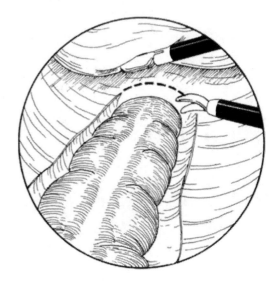

Fig. 8. Incising the peritoneum between the bladder and the rectum

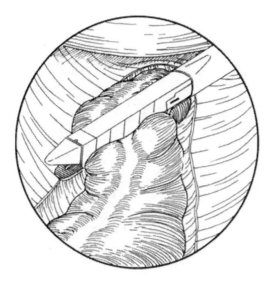

Fig. 9. The rectosigmoid colon is transected

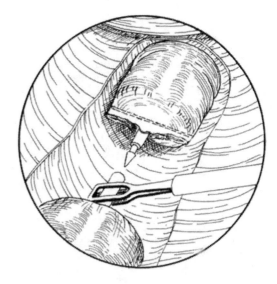

Fig. 10. The endoscopic mechanical anastomosis is being fashioned in the double stapled technique

44   Laparoscopic Abdominoperineal Rectum Extirpation

F. Köckerling, T. Reck, and I. Gastinger

Introduction

The most common indication for laparoscopic abdominoperineal rectum resection is a very low rectum carcinoma not higher than 4–5 cm above the dentate line. Advanced rectum carcinomas with wide infiltration of perirectal fatty tissue or adjacent structures (pT4) must be excluded. Enlargement of lymph nodes seen endosonographically does not necessarily represent a contraindication when a pelvic dissection – such as that in conventional surgery – is performed. An organ-preserving transanal full-thickness excision can be attempted in early tumor stages (T1) without infiltration of lymphatics, with a maximum tumor diameter of 2–3 cm, without ulceration, and with a G1-G2 tumor differentiation.

Positioning of the Patient and Team

For positioning of the patient and team, see Fig. 1

Technique

The bowel is prepared using a preoperative lavage with an isotonic solution (4–5 l per os). The addition of 50 g high molecular weight dextran per liter permits reduction of fluid resorption of up to 2 l. The patient is preoperatively referred to the stoma therapist, who selects and marks the appropriate site for the descendostomy. The patient is placed in a steep Trendelenburg position with slightly flexed hips; the 45°–50° angle ensures that the small bowel falls into the upper abdomen. A catheter is inserted into the bladder and taped to the thigh. Following digital examination the anus is closed with a pursestring suture to prevent spilling of tumor cells. The rima ani is maximally stretched and taped to facilitate the sacral portion of the operation. Sterile draping of the patient is the same as in conventional surgery, leaving free the abdomen from the xiphoid process to the symphysis and to the sides.

The laparoscopic abdominoperineal resection requires the well-coordinated efforts of a team consisting of two equally experienced surgeons, a very talented assistant to handle the video camera, a further assistant to aid the operators, and a scrub nurse with experience in laparoscopic surgery. The two operators stand to the left and right of the patient. Because of the deep Trendelenburg position of the patient, the video camera assistant cannot stand next to the operators but is placed instead next to the patient's head. The patient's left arm is covered; the right arm is used for venous and arterial access. A sterile drape is placed over a sturdy bracket to the left of the patient's head, thus permitting the video camera assistant to work undisturbed throughout the laparoscopic colorectal procedure.

The video unit, including the monitor, and the light source are placed between the patient's legs. The electrosurgical instruments are placed on the patient's right, and the instrument table and endoirrigators on the left (Fig. 1). Insertion of the five ports takes place in a semicircular pattern around the navel, the circle opening toward the lesser pelvis (Fig. 2). Puncture with the Veress needle and insertion of the optic trocar take place above the navel, somewhat to the left and lateral from the middle; this ensures an adequate distance to the lesser pelvis, on the one hand and, on the other, avoids insufflation of the ligamentum teres of the liver.

Four 12-mm working ports with screw fixation are inserted pairwise into the left and right lower abdomen. The use of 12-mm ports is necessary because the linear stapler can only be used through a 12-mm trocar and the most convenient angle of approach needed for the firing of the stapler changes throughout the operation. The preoperatively marked stoma site is used for the upper left working port. The operation commences when the operator reviews the abdomen and lesser pelvis through the 30° angle scope. The small bowel is pushed into the upper abdomen with the help of swabs on graspers. The Trendelenburg position can be made steeper in case the small bowel does not remain in place. Even the most extreme Trendelenburg positions have not caused us any problems. Finally, a view of the lesser pelvis is obtained.

In females the uterus and the adnexa must be lifted up in preparation for the later deep dissection of the lesser pelvis. To achieve this we use a ligature on a straight needle which has been inserted through the abdominal wall, which is then passed through the uterine latum ligament below the adnexa, turned 180°, and then inserted to the left of the uterus behind the left adnexa through the latum ligament. The needle is brought up to the abdominal wall and knotted; the uterus and the adnexa are thus lifted up to the abdominal wall. This technique permits a good view of the lesser pelvis even during mobilization.

Swabs on graspers are indispensable in further mobilization and dissection. Tissue can easily be stretched for mobilization with swabs on graspers without any risk of damage. In this manner injuries to the colon and rectum wall can especially be avoided. The mobilization begins by lysing of the fetal adhesions of the sigmoid to the lateral abdominal wall using diathermy instruments (Fig. 3). The sigmoid and descending colon are mobilized toward the left colonic flexure in such a way that a tension-free placement of the descendostomy can take place.

The peritoneum is cut along the fascia of Gerota; the mesosigmoid and descending mesocolon can thus be dissected from the fascia of Gerota and up to the aorta with swabs on graspers. Great care is taken to identify the left ureter at the site of its crossing with the left common iliac artery. If an adequate mobilization of the mesosigmoid up to the aorta can be performed, the sigmoid is folded toward the left and the peritoneum cut from the right above the level of the aorta and below the level of the inferior mesenteric artery and the superior rectal artery (Fig. 4). This creates an opening between the level of the aorta and the vessel axis of the superior rectal artery in the mesosigmoid (Fig. 5) through which a swab on a grasper can be inserted and the sigmoid and mesosigmoid lifted toward the abdominal wall.

The mobilization in a cranial direction and toward the trunk of the inferior mesenteric artery can now be continued. The mobilization in the layer between the aorta and the vessel stalk of the mesosigma is uncomplicated because it involves an avascular connective layer of the mesosigmoid. After identification of the trunk of the inferior mesenteric artery, it is encircled. The inferior mesenteric artery can be transected at the trunk either with the linear stapler or with clips (Fig. 6). Following transection of the inferior mesenteric artery at the trunk the upper (cranial) limit of the lymph node dissection is determined. A stepwise transection of the colon at the descending colon/sigmoid colon border (Fig. 7) and the mesocolon with the linear stapler takes place. After transection of the colon the end is pulled in a cranial direction with a grasper. The pelvic dissection commences. A U-shaped cut is made into the peritoneum around the rectum; the incision of the peritoneum should be made medially and somewhat caudally from the ureters. Through renewed lifting of the mesosigmoid with swabs on graspers, the dorsal fascial space between the fascia of

Waldeyer and the mesorectum is opened. The fine connective strands between the dorsal fascial space leaves can be cauterized, permitting opening of the dorsal fascial space and dissection up to the pelvic floor.

Anterior mobilization of the rectum takes place in males along the recess of Denonvilliers' fascia and in females along the same obliterated fascial space dorsal to the vagina. The bladder or the vagina is pushed ventrally with two swabs on graspers, the rectum is held under tension with the grasper and the fascial space dissected with the diathermy scissors or hook. Dissection should take place as deep as possible up to the pelvic floor. Division of the lateral ligaments with the medial rectal artery takes place following dorsal and ventral dissection in the fascial space of the rectum. To identify this artery swabs on graspers are inserted in the anterior and posterior fascial spaces, and the rectum is pulled to the opposite pelvic wall. The medial rectal artery thus comes into view and is stapled (Fig. 8). Following transection of the left and right medial rectal artery mobilization of the rectum in the lesser pelvis is completed by dividing the remaining lateral ligaments with the diathermy hook.

The abdominal portion of the operation is completed with the creation of the final stoma. For this the 12-mm port at the predetermined stoma site is replaced by a 20-mm retrieval port. The skin around the 12-mm port is cut in a circular fashion and the fascia incised with a cross. After placement of the 20-mm port the proximal colon end is pulled into the trocar sheath with the help of a sturdy grasper (Fig. 9). The pneumoperitoneum is deflated and the proximal colon end together with the trocar sheath can be pulled through the abdominal wall. The staple suture is opened at the abdomen with cautery and the final stoma is placed using single sutures.

Finally, the situation of the descending colon and its exit through the abdominal wall is reviewed through the intra-abdominal scope. Although the pneumoperitoneum has been released, the ports still remain in place to check for bleeding in the lesser pelvis during the sacral portion of the operation (Fig. 10). The sacral or perineal portion of the operation takes place as in conventional procedures. With increasing experience laparoscopic mobilization of the rectum can be carried out as far as the pelvic floor, so that only the levator ani on either side of the rectum need to be sacrally divided stepwise. The specimen is removed through the perineal wound. After completing the sacral portion a light pneumoperitoneum is created, and a search for bleeding in the sacral cavity is carried out from the abdomen. Bleeding can be controlled either with the diathermy clamp or with the endoclip instrument. At the end of the operation a drain is inserted over the left or right lower trocar sheath.

References

Köckerling F, Gostinger I, Schneider B, Krouse W, Gall FD (1993) Laparoscopic abdominoperineal excision of the rectum with high ligation of the inferior mesenteric artery in the management of rectal cancer. Surg Endosc 1:16–19

Phillips E, Franklin M, Carroll B, Fallas M, Ramos R, Rosenthal D (1992) Laparoscopic colectomy. Ann Surg 216 (6):703–707

Ottinger LW (1974) Fundamentals of colon surgery. Little Brown, Boston

Sackier JM, Berci G, Hiatt JR, Hortunian S (1992) Laparoscopic abdominoperineal resection of the rectum. Br J Surg 79 (11):1207–1208

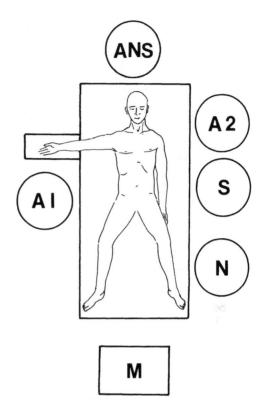

Fig. 1. Placement of the operating team and equipment. Patient in supine-reverse Trendelenburg position. *ANS*, Anesthetist; *S*, surgeon; *A*, assistant; *N*, nurse; *M*, monitor

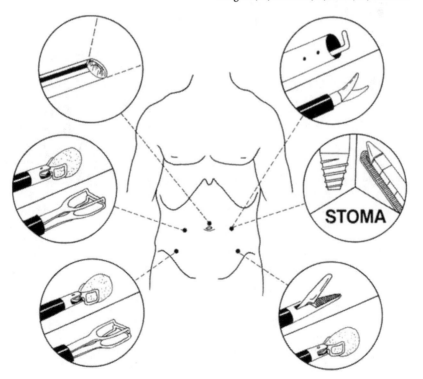

Fig. 2. Positioning of the ports

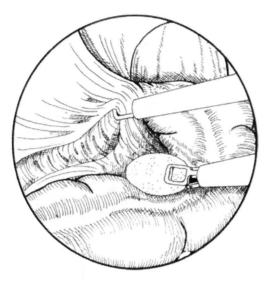

Fig. 3. Lysing of the fetal adhesions of the sigmoid to the lateral abdominal wall

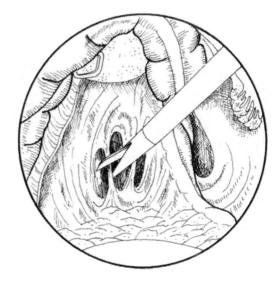

Fig. 4. Incision of the mesosigmoid below the vascular plane of the inferior mesenteric artery and the superior rectal artery

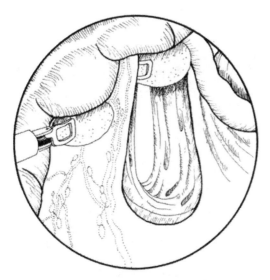

Fig. 5. An opening in the mesentery is created after incision of the mesosigmoid below the vascular plane of the inferior mesenteric artery and the superior rectal artery. Lifting of the mesosigmoid with a swab on a grasper in the mesenterial opening

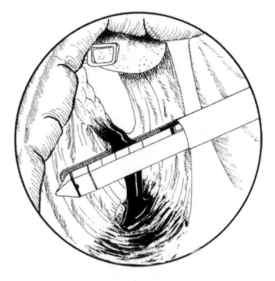

Fig. 6. Transection of the inferior mesenteric artery with the linear stapler

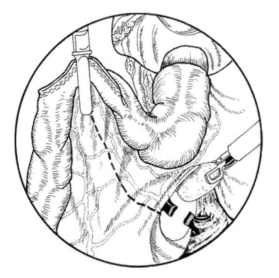

Fig. 7. Transection of the colon at the descending colon/sigmoid border with the linear stapler

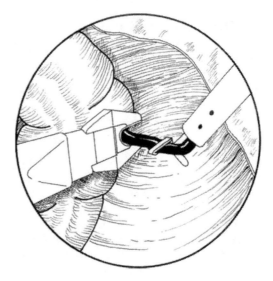

Fig. 8. Identification and clipping of the medial rectal artery in the stretched lateral ligament

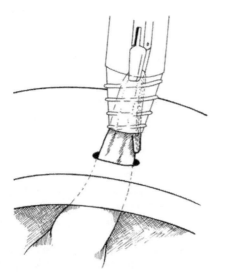

Fig. 9. Pulling the proximal colon end into the retrieval trocar

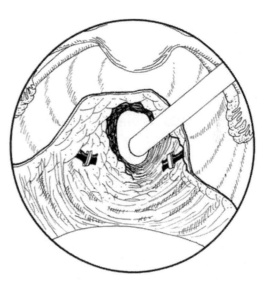

Fig. 10. Inspecting the lesser pelvis for any bleeding

45 Laparoscopic Rectopexy

F. Köckerling, T. Reck, and I. Gastinger

Introduction

The indications for laparoscopic rectopexy are identical to those of Well's rectopexy with laparotomy. The indication for a laparoscopic approach must consider any prior surgery, site of the incisions, and expected adhesions. Also, in cases of severe cardiac, pulmonary, or other risk factors for anesthesia with intubation we avoid an abdominal procedure and favor an extra-abdominal corrective operation. In addition to a general preoperative workup, sphincter pressure is measured. A defecogram and a rectoscopy are also part of the preoperative routine examinations. Any further pathological findings of the colon are excluded by means of colonoscopy or barium enema. If in addition to the prolapse of the rectum there is an elongated sigmoid, a sigmoid resection should be considered.

Positioning of the Patient and Team

For positioning of the patient and team, see Fig. 1

Technique

Preoperative colonic lavage is very important; a low-risk repair can thus be performed in the event of intraoperative trauma to the intestinal tract. The patient is placed on the operating table in a steep Trendelenburg position so that the small bowel falls into the upper abdomen, thus permitting a clear view up to the lesser pelvis. The patient is draped leaving the abdomen clear from the xiphoid to the symphysis and laterally. Placement of the operation team and equipment as well as of the ports is the same as that for abdominoperineal rectum resection (Figs. 1, 2).

Similar to the abdominoperineal resection, the uterus and adnexa are fixed to the anterior abdominal wall with a straight needle (chapter 44). In doing this a blocked view is avoided while the rectum is being mobilized. One thus obtains a good view of the lesser pelvis, with the internal hernia presenting as a protrusion of the Douglas peritoneum with peritonealization of the posterior wall of the vagina. As in laparoscopic abdominoperineal rectum resection, the sigmoid colon is mobilized by careful dissection of the embryonic adhesions on the lateral abdominal wall with cautery scissors. Stretching of the colon is also carried out gently, primarily with swabs on graspers. The mesosigmoid is separated from the fascia of Gerota as far as the aorta with the swabs on graspers. The left ureter is displayed at the site of crossing with the common iliac artery and vein medial to the spermatic or ovarian vein.

The dorsal mobilization of the rectum does not differ from that in conventional procedures. The mesorectum is lifted with a swab on a grasper from the left and ventrally, thus creating an entry to the dorsal fascial space (Fig. 3). The fine connective strands between the Waldeyer's fascia and mesorectum (dorsal fascial space) can now be seen and are transected, as far as possible, in the direction of the pelvic floor. If a further opening of the dorsal fascial space from the left is no longer possible, the sigmoid is folded over to the left and on the right; the lateral peritoneum of the colon is incised at the pelvic outlet. Swabs on graspers are placed beneath the mesentery which is then lifted to the anterior abdominal wall (Fig. 4).

To completely mobilize the rectum as far as the pelvic floor both lateral ligaments must be stepwise divided using accurate diathermy (Fig. 5). Larger vessels are closed with titanium clips and divided. Because the internal hernia has already caused a protrusion of the peritoneum of Douglas between the posterior vaginal wall and the anterior wall of the rectum, a dissection in the anterior fascial space can be usually avoided. In addition, extensive dissection can cause damage to the parasympathetic and sympathetic nerves. Adequate mobilization can be achieved with a generous dorsal mobilization of the rectum in the presacral space with bilateral transection of the lateral ligaments (Fig. 6).

Prolene mesh is cut extra-abdominally into the appropriate size (Fig. 7). Two or three holes are cut into the mesh to aid fixation with sutures or with the hernia stapler to the fascia of Waldeyer. The mesh is rolled up, placed into the abdomen through a working port, and unrolled at the sacrum (Fig. 8). There are several methods available for fixation of the mesh to the fascia of

Waldeyer, either with the hernia stapler (Fig. 8) or with intra- and extra-abdominal knotted single sutures (Fig. 9). In the latter the usual knotting technique is used, whereby the knots are made extra-abdominally and then pushed through the trocar with a knot-pusher. Three single knots are required to fix the mesh. The windows which have been cut into the mesh facilitate fixation under vision and help to avoid injury to the presacral venous plexus (Fig. 9).

After creation of a stable connection between the mesh and the fascia of Waldeyer the rectum is placed inside the mesh and stretched in a cranial direction with the help of swabs on graspers (Fig. 10). The lateral ends of the mesh can once again be cut to measure; here one must consider that only three-fourths of the rectum circumference should be enclosed by the mesh. Later development of stenoses can be thus avoided. The cranially stretched rectum can then be fixed to the lateral ends of the mesh with three or four knotted single sutures (Fig. 10). The needle should only enter the muscularis layer of the rectum and not the bowel lumen, which might lead to contamination of the mesh. If the stretched rectum has been properly fixed, the space of Douglas becomes significantly smaller (Fig. 11).

Following lavage of the lesser pelvis and a renewed search for bleeding, a drain is inserted into the lesser pelvis and its end pulled through a trocar incision. The remaining ports are removed under vision and the incisions closed in layers. Because foreign material has been inserted into the abdomen, the antibiotics which were administered prophylactically during the operation are given for an additional day. Light meals can be introduced after the first bowel movement, usually on the third postoperative day. It is important that straining at stool should be avoided; hence the use of a mild laxative as required.

References

Goligher, JC (1980) Surgery of the anus, rectum and colon, 4th edn. Balliere Tindall, London, pp 224–226

Lomas MI, Cooperman H (1972) Correction of rectal prolapse by use of polypropylene mesh. Dis Colon Rectum 15:416–420

Schlinkert RT, Beart RW jr, Wolf BG, Pemberton JH (1985) Anterior resection for complete rectal prolapse. Dis Colon Rectum 28:409–412

Wells C (1959) New operations for rectal prolapse. Proc R Soc Med 52:602–607

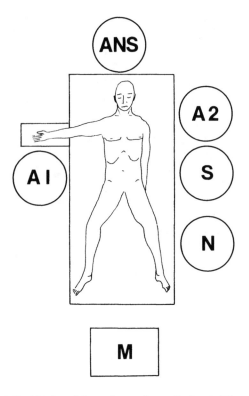

Fig. 1. Positioning of the patient and team. Patient in lithotomy position. *ANS*, Anesthetist; *S*, surgeon; *A*, assistant; *N*, nurse; *M*, monitor

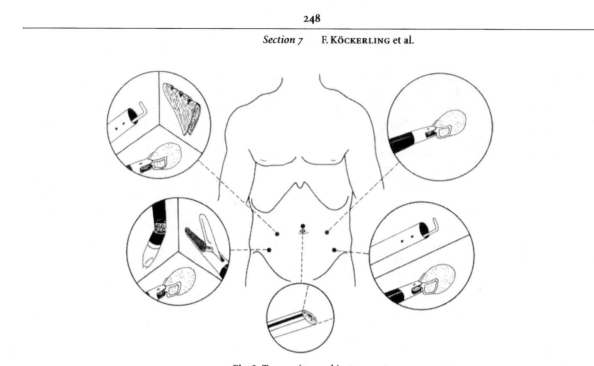

Fig. 2. Trocar sites and instruments

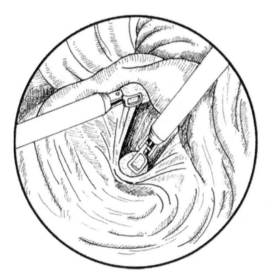

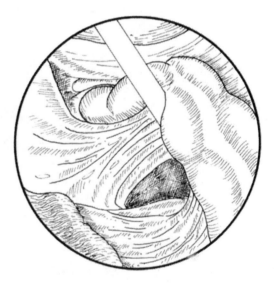

Fig. 3. Opening of the dorsal space with a swab on a grasper from the left following incision of the peritoneum and display of the ureter

Fig. 4. Swabs on graspers are placed beneath the mesosigmoid and used to lift it to the anterior abdominal wall

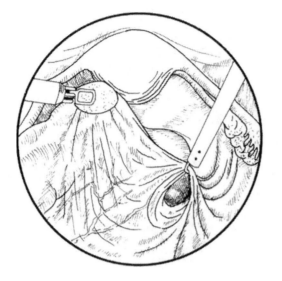

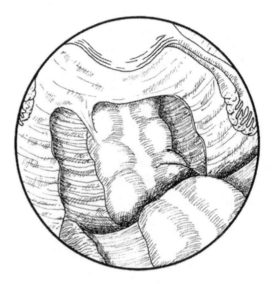

Fig. 5. Incision of the mesentery below the vascular axis from the right along the pelvic outlet

Fig. 6. Mobilization of the rectum as far as the pelvic floor by opening the dorsal space and by dividing the lateral ligaments on both sides

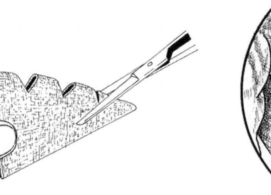

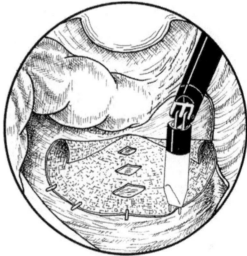

Fig. 7. The nonresorbable mesh material is cut into the required size and shape

Fig. 8. Unrolling of the mesh from the sacrum and the fascia of Waldeyer. Fixation of the upper edge of the mesh with the hernia stapler

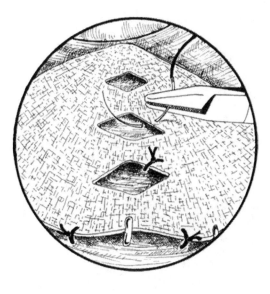

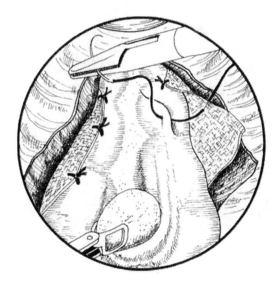

Fig. 9. Additional suturing of the mesh to the fascia of Waldeyer with extra-abdominally knotted single sutures

Fig. 10. Placement of the mobilized rectum inside the mesh and stretching of the rectum in a cranial direction with swabs on graspers. The lateral ends of the mesh are fixed to the rectum wall with three or four single sutures at the 10 and 2 o'clock axis

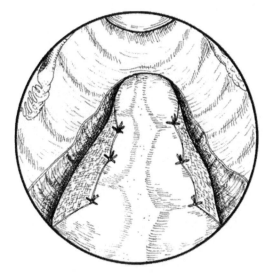

Fig. 11. The rectum wall appears to be stretched in the lesser pelvis following fixation of the lateral ends

46 Laparoscopic Hartmann's Procedure and Hartmann's Reversal Procedure

P. Reissman and S.D. Wexner

Introduction

The impact of laparoscopy on colorectal surgery has been steadily increasing. Procedures which were recently considered impossible are now performed universally as more experience has been gained, and advanced instrumentation has been made available. Hartmann's procedure originally consisted of segmental resection of the upper rectum or sigmoid, closure of the rectal stump, and creation of an end colostomy. Today, however, the procedure has diversified and is performed with a variable length of the closed stump (Hartmann's pouch) ranging from the rectum to the entire colon and is used to treat a variety of colorectal disorders. The procedure may be applicable instead of a primary anastomosis in patients with intra-abdominal sepsis, acute diverticulitis, complications of diverticular disease such as fistula or perforation, toxic colitis, obstructing or nonresectable tumor, ischemic colitis, perforation due to foreign body or trauma, volvulus, following resection in a poor general condition, and in any event of unprepared bowel. In other conditions such as inflammatory bowel disease, colitis or extensive ischemic colitis, a total abdominal colectomy with closure of the rectum and creation of an end ileostomy may be performed. The avoidance of primary anastomosis with its related risks in all of these conditions makes Hartmann's procedure a safe and attractive option.

The major disadvantage of Hartmann's procedure is the necessity of an additional operation for the restoration of bowel continuity. This second operation may also be associated with a high morbidity. With the recent advances in laparoscopic techniques and instrumentation, laparoscopic reversal of Hartmann's procedure has become an option. As mentioned above, a large variety of pathological conditions may lead the surgeon to close the distal stump of the rectum or colon and create an end colostomy or ileostomy. Therefore the laparoscopic reversal of Hartmann's procedure may have wider applications than Hartmann's procedure itself. Because all of these patients have an abdominal incision in addition to a stoma and may have significant adhesions, laparoscopy should be performed by an experienced and skillful team.

Positioning of the Patient and Team

The patient is placed in the modified lithotomy position. The legs are almost flat to avoid interference with the laparoscopic instruments during surgery. This position is important for several reasons: (a) this position enables the transanal introduction of a circular stapler in case the surgeon decides to perform a primary anastomosis; (b) it provides the option for intraoperative colonoscopy; (c) the colonoscope may also be used for retraction of the hepatic or splenic flexure, thereby facilitating the dissection of these segments; (d) rigid or flexible proctoscopy may be required to confirm that the margins of resection are adequate and free of inflammation, diverticular disease or tumor; and (e) if required, another assistant or the camera holder may be placed between the legs.

The operating room configuration is shown in Fig. 1. It is imperative to have two monitors placed on each side of the patient toward the legs for the convenience of the surgeon and assistants. As a general principle the surgeon, camera, operative field, and monitor should all be along one line for better orientation. Relocation of personnel and monitors is required if a more extensive resection such as extended or subtotal colectomy is performed.

Technique

A standard technique is used to create a pneumoperitoneum. If the patient has had a previous surgery, an open "Hasson" technique using a blunt-tipped trocar is used. Alternatively, the Veress needle may be inserted in any area remote to surgical scars. After pneumoperitoneum has been established with a pressure of 15 mmHg, eventually a 10- to 12-mm trocar is inserted at the umbilical site to be followed by a 0° laparoscope. Initial assessment and inspection of the abdominal cavity is performed. In case of adhesions which prevent adequate visualization the laparoscope may be driven to a "free" area where one or more additional trocars may be placed to facilitate adhesiolysis. If the procedure is considered possible, the patient is placed in a steep Trendelenburg and tilted to the right position. The placement of trocars and instruments is shown in Fig. 2. All ports are 10–12 mm in size as all instruments, including the suction and scissors used in laparoscopic colonic surgery, are 10 mm in diameter. It is important to place the lateral ports lateral to the rectus muscles to avoid epigastric artery injury. Furthermore, the ports should not be placed too close to one another to prevent "sword fighting." Body habitus may also dictate the port placement as the length of instruments is limited. The procedure is started with three trocars; however, to provide better traction or exposure, a fourth or rarely a fifth trocar may be required in the left lower quadrant or suprapubic location. Once the instruments and camera are in position, a thorough inspection of the abdominal cavity, pelvis and rectosigmoid colon is performed.

Mobilization of the sigmoid colon is the initial step. This step is performed only after adequate exposure with the small bowel retracted out of the pelvis and away from the surgical field. The principle of traction and countertraction is practiced for the incision of the lateral peritoneal attachments of the sigmoid (line of Toldt; Fig. 3). The surgeon retracts the sigmoid colon with an atraumatic clamp in his left hand and holds a 10-mm monopolar or bipolar laparoscopic electrocautery scissors in his right hand. Other 10-mm instruments such as a right-angle Kelly or Dennis clamp may also be used as needed. Additional traction is provided by the assistant who also uses an atraumatic clamp. Frequent repositioning is required since care is taken not to lock the clamp while grasping the bowel to avoid incidental enterotomy. The laparoscopic scissors may also be used to cauterize small vessels and to perform sharp or blunt dissection. When using the cautery it is crucial to completely visualize the tip of the scissors to prevent an inadvertent thermal injury. After additional mobilization is achieved, the left ureter must be identified by meticulous dissection according to the usual anatomic landmarks. Ureteric stents (regular or illuminated) can help identify the ureters in patients who have had previous pelvic or abdominal surgery with anticipated significant adhesions and fibrotic tissues.

The extent of colon mobilization is determined by the planned procedure. For sigmoidectomy the rectosigmoid, left colon, and splenic flexure are usually mobilized to provide sufficient length for a tension-free colostomy. It is helpful to mark the planned extent of resection distally and proximally by clips or hernia staples placed on the mesentery close to the colonic wall. This step allows reassessment during the dissection. Furthermore, the mobilization should be undertaken to an extent that the proximal marked site easily reaches the abdominal wall at the planned colostomy site without tension.

After sufficient mobilization has been achieved, the mesenteric vessels are dissected and divided by either clips (Fig. 4) or by laparoscopic linear vascular stapler devices. This maneuver is carried out while the colon is pulled toward the abdominal wall and medially so the mesenteric vessels are stretched and may be easily identified. "Windows" are created in avascular regions of the mesentery, followed by isolation of the vessels and division between clips or by linear stapler devices. The level of ligation of the mesenteric vessels is dictated by the underlying pathology. The commonly available 35-mm stapler may be introduced via a 12-mm port. Generally, if a port needs to be replaced by a larger sized one, a Seldinger technique is used with a 10-mm exchange rod after the skin incision is sufficiently enlarged. Although a linear stapler is more expeditious, it causes a significant increase in the cost of the procedure. Differently sized clips and staples are available, and these should be used as appropriate according to the vessel and tissue size. If hemostasis is inadequate after the use of either clips or stapler devices, an endoloop should be placed to control it. If the linear stapler is used, the tips should always be inspected before firing. This vision is achieved by a "flip over" maneuver of the colon toward the surgeon and while repositioning the scope lateral to the colon. The position of the ureter should also be verified again prior to stapler utilization.

Mesenteric dissection is carried out toward the distal margins until the colonic wall is completely isolated. Colonic division is performed intracorporeally by a 60-mm endoscopic linear cutter introduced through an 18-mm port (Fig. 5). This port should be in the right lower quadrant to provide easier access to the rectosigmoid. A rigid proctoscopy should be performed before the transection to ensure an adequate, disease-free rectal margin. After division of the rectosigmoid the staple line is inspected for hemostasis. Reinforcement with running or interrupted absorbable sutures may be performed. A long marking nonabsorbable stitch is placed at the tip of the closed rectal stump for easier identification in the future during the reversal procedure. If distal sigmoid is left attached to the rectum, it may be sutured to the abdominal wall to prevent its retraction into the pelvis. This may be pursued in patients with mucosal ulcerative colitis or Crohn's colitis who undergo subtotal colectomy and an end ileostomy as the initial stage of surgical therapy to be followed by either an ileorectal anastomosis or a completion proctectomy and creation of an ileoanal reservoir at a later stage.

The distal edge of the proximal colon is now grasped by a Babcock clamp for its later introduction through the incision of the stoma. At this stage the stoma site is addressed, and a 2 cm round skin incision is performed in one of the premarked positions. The anterior fascia is incised longitudinally. The rectus muscle is split, followed by a longitudinal incision of the posterior fascia to make an adequate opening for the stoma. The pneumoperitoneum is evacuated, and the proximal colon is now introduced through the incision by the laparoscopic Babcock clamp. Once it is identified at the stoma incision, the colon is grasped with a regular Babcock and gently pulled after the grasp of the laparoscopic Babcock is released. The stoma incision should be large enough to deliver the segment to be resected (Fig. 6). If this incision turns out to be too small, it may be extended. However, if the incision is too large, stomal prolapse or parastomal hernia may develop. Therefore, if the incision is extended, it may have to be partially sutured before the maturation of the colostomy. Small wound protectors may also be used to prevent direct contact between the specimen and the abdominal wall. After the proximal colon is delivered, an extracorporeal resection is performed and a colostomy is matured at the level previously marked by clips.

Alternatively, the proximal colon with the specimen may be delivered through a 33-mm port placed at the premarked stoma site using the Seldinger technique. If this option is pursued, the proximal colon is grasped by a Babcock and delivered through the transparent trocar. After the proximal colon is delivered, the trocar is removed and the specimen resected. Before maturing the colostomy it is important to incise the surrounding fascia to prevent strangulation of the colostomy since all trocars stretch the fascia.

The colostomy is matured in the standard fashion using chromic 3-0 sutures with slight eversion. After this step is concluded, the abdomen is reinsufflated for final inspection, irrigation of the pelvis, and to ensure that the descending colon has not been rotated. The procedure is complete after all the fascia in all port sites is sutured to prevent port site hernias (Fig. 7). This maneuver may be performed under laparoscopic guidance using one of the several instruments which are available or by direct suturing if the fascia can be adequately exposed. In elective cases the nasogastric or orogastric tube is removed immediately after the procedure while the Foley catheter is usually left for 24 h. In our experience, the majority of patients after elective laparotomy or laparoscopy may be started on a clear liquid diet the day following surgery and advanced to regular diet within the next 48 h.

Laparoscopic Reversal of Hartmann's Procedure

When Hartmann's procedure was originally introduced, reversal with closure of the stoma at a later time was not considered. Since then the majority of patients who undergo Hartmann's procedure are reoperated upon for reversal and establishment of intestinal continuity. The only patients who retain a permanent stoma are those with unresectable extensive malignancy, those with fecal incontinence who are not candidates for sphincter reconstruction, those with intractable irradiation or Crohn's proctitis, and debilitated patients in a general poor condition. The optimal timing for stoma closure is controversial and varies from patient to patient; a period of 3–6 months is usually recommended but should be extended according to the patient's condition. Thorough investigations of both the rectal stump and the proximal colon are mandatory before reversal is considered. This is to exclude previously undiagnosed pathology such as concomitant malignancy, new pathology such as stricture formation or residual pathology such as diverticulosis or inflammation. Care should be taken not to be misled by diversion colitis, which resolves after intestinal continuity has been established. These investigations should be performed by either endoscopic or contrast studies.

Standard mechanical bowel preparation is undertaken prior to the reversal, including phosphate enemas of the rectal stump. The preparation for surgery, positioning of the patient, and the room setup are identical to those of Hartmann's procedure. Intraoperative ureteric stent insertion is extremely helpful. The initial step is to dissect the stoma free of the abdominal wall using an ordinary surgical technique. Subsequently, any adhesions in the proximity of the fascia are lysed under direct vision to ensure a free space before the introduction of the laparoscope. After sufficient mobilization of the stoma is achieved, the edges are trimmed and the anvil and the 29- or 33-mm circular stapler device are introduced and a pursestring suture placed (Figs. 8, 9). Any excess mucosa is trimmed to avoid interference during the anastomosis. If the vascular supply to the stoma is compromised during the dissection, a limited resection may be required.

Subsequently, the proximal colon containing the anvil is placed into the abdominal cavity. Several # 0 polydioxane fascial sutures are placed, but not tied. A 33-mm trocar is introduced through the incision and one or two of the fascial sutures are tied to prevent CO_2 leak; the peritoneal cavity is now insufflated. As in any other laparoscopic procedure, the abdominal cavity and pelvis are inspected. Adhesions from the previous procedure are very frequently present and should be carefully lysed using blunt and sharp dissection. At least three additional 10- to 12-mm ports are placed under laparoscopic visualization, preferably in similar locations as in Hartmann's procedure.

After adequate exposure is achieved by lysis of adhesions and retracting the small bowel out of the pelvis, attention is paid to both the proximal colon and the rectal stump. The proximal colon is inspected for sufficient mobilization to provide a tension-free anastomosis. Additional mobilization is frequently required by incising the lateral peritoneal attachments, including mobilization of the splenic flexure or transverse colon. Another resection may be shown to be required by the preoperative or intraoperative findings of additional or residual disease. The rectal stump must be clearly identified and free from adhesions to other organs. Rigid proctoscopy may be performed to facilitate the rectal stump dissection. This step may be easier if the rectal stump was tagged by a long, nonabsorbable stitch during the initial Hartmann's procedure.

After both the rectal stump and the proximal colon are cleared and confirmed for a safe, well-vascularized and tension-free anastomosis, the anvil is grasped with a specially designed modified Allis clamp (Ethicon Endosurgery, Cincinnati, OH) which is introduced through the right upper port. The circular stapler is introduced transanally and laparoscopically guided to reach the end of the rectal stump at the previous staple line. The shaft is now advanced carefully and should pierce the rectal stump close to this previous stapler line. After the shaft is completely exposed, the anvil is guided toward the pelvis and attached (Fig. 10). Once the anvil is securely attached to the circular stapler device, the laparoscope is placed in the right lower port for better visu-

alization while the circular stapler device is approximating the two ends of the colon and the anastomosis is fired. Care should be taken to ensure proper alignment of the descending colon with the rectal stump, and that no adjacent organs or tissues are trapped while closing the stapler device.

In cases of a short rectal stump in women, special attention must be paid to prevent injury to the posterior vaginal wall. After the anastomosis is created, the circular stapler is gently removed, and the proximal and distal donuts are carefully inspected for completeness. The pelvis is now irrigated with saline to cover the anastomosis and a straight atraumatic Dennis clamp is used to occlude the proximal colon while the anastomosis is tested for air leak by transanal air insufflation. If no leak is noted, the fluid is aspirated, final inspection of the pelvis and abdominal cavity is performed, and the ports are removed; the fascia at all port sites is closed. The skin at the colostomy site is left open.

In the unique cases of a long distal colonic stump (left or transverse) with a proximal end ileostomy or colostomy, a laparoscopic-assisted reversal procedure may be performed. The anastomosis is be performed extracorporeally after the two ends (stoma and distal colon) are mobilized and brought out of the abdominal wall through an incision. This incision may be carried out in continuity with the stoma incision or in a remote area, according to the anatomical findings.

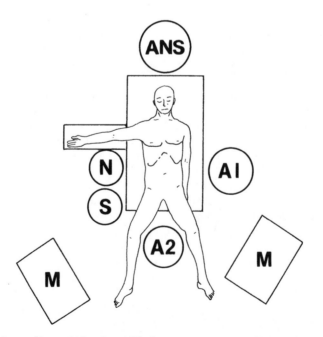

Fig. 1. Positioning of the patient and team. Patient in modified lithotomy position. *ANS*, Anesthetist; *S*, surgeon; *A1*, assistant; *N*, nurse; *M*, monitor. If a more extended colectomy is performed, relocation of personnel and monitors is required

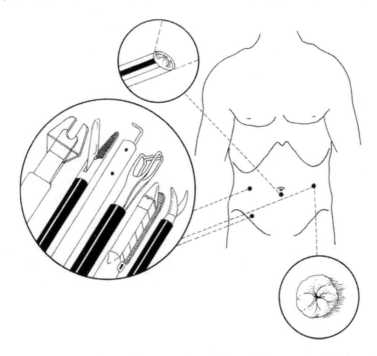

Fig. 2. Port site and instrument placement in laparoscopic Hartmann's procedure. All ports are 10–12 mm to provide flex-ibility with instrumentation. If required, an additional left lower quadrant or suprapubic port may be used

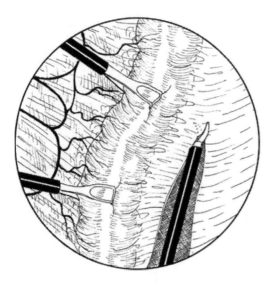

Fig. 3. Incision of the lateral peritoneal attachment of the sigmoid using scissors combined with cautery while the colon is retracted medially

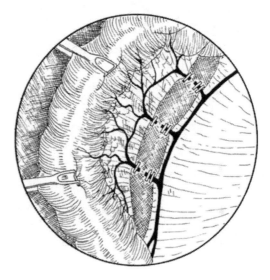

Fig. 4. The mesenteric vessels are isolated and divided by 10-mm clips

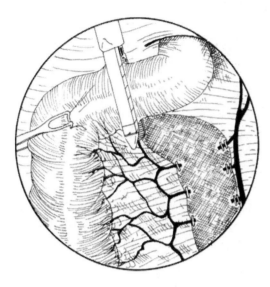

Fig. 5. Transection of the rectosigmoid junction using a 60-mm linear stapler

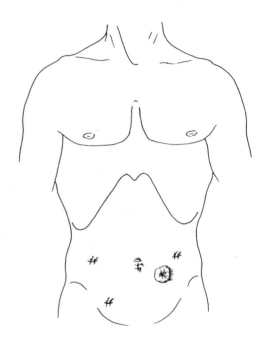

Fig. 7. The colostomy has been matured. The procedure is complete

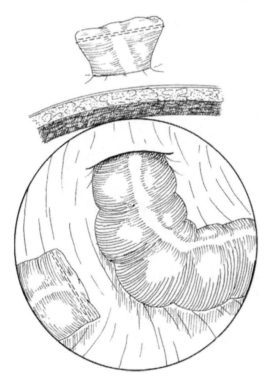

Fig. 6. The proximal colon including the specimen is gently pulled out through the colostomy incision

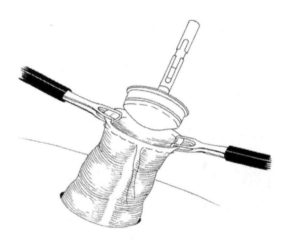

Fig. 8. Laparoscopic reversal of Hartmann's procedure. The colostomy is separated from the abdominal wall and completely mobilized

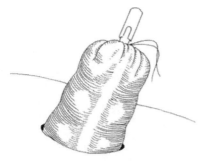

Fig. 9. After the edge is trimmed, an anvil of 29- or a 33-mm circular stapler is introduced and a pursestring suture is placed

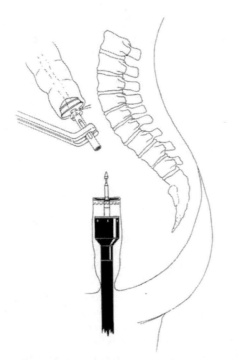

Fig. 10. The circular stapler has been passed transanally and the anvil is guided to be attached for creation of an end to end double stapled anastomosis

Comments

Since it was originally described in 1921, Hartmann's procedure has diversified to include various procedures which all result in either an end colostomy or ileostomy and a distal rectal or colonic stump. However, the majority of these procedures are performed as emergency or urgent ones, and therefore the role of laparoscopy may be limited. Conversely, the laparoscopic reversal of Hartmann's procedure may have much wider applications. The reversal procedure is always elective after the patient is thoroughly investigated and well prepared. Although technically challenging, laparoscopic reversal of Hartmann's procedure has proven to be feasible and safe. Early results of this procedure showed comparable morbidity and mortality to open procedures with the potential benefits of decreased postoperative pain, shorter duration of ileus and hospitalization, earlier return to normal activity, and enhanced cosmesis. However, prospective randomized trials with longer follow-up are required before final conclusions may be reached regarding the benefits of laparoscopic versus open Hartmann's or Hartmann's reversal procedures.

References

Haas PA, Haas GP (1988) A critical evaluation of the Hartmann's procedure. Am Surg 56:380–384

Larach SW, Hellinger MD (1994) The evolving role of laparoscopic technique in the performance of Hartmann's procedure. Surg Oncol Clin North Am 3:717–730

Reissman P, Teoh TA, Piccirillo M, Nogueras JJ, Wexner SD (1994) Colonoscopic-assisted laparoscopic colectomy. Surg Endosc 8:1352–1353

Roe AM, Prabhue S, Ali A et al (1991) Reversal of Hartmann's procedure: timing and operative technique. Br J Surg 78:1167–1170

Sosa JL, Sleeman D, Puente I, McKenney MG, Hartmann R (1994) Laparoscopic assisted colostomy closure after Hartmann's procedure. Dis Colon Rectum 37:149–152

Wexner SD, Cohen SM, Johansen OB, Nogueras JJ, Jagelman DG (1993) Laparoscopic colorectal surgery: a prospective assessment and current perspective. Br J Surg 80:1602–1605

47 Transanal Endoscopic Microsurgery

G. Buess and B. Mentges

Introduction

Endoscopic microsurgery is at the moment the most advanced procedure in the field of intraluminal surgery. At the same time, endoscopic microsurgery, which has been in clinical routine use since 1983, was the first complex endoscopic operation to be routinely applied in gastrointestinal surgery. The procedure is performed using the operative rectoscope from Wolf. A number of endoscopic instruments have been designed for transanal endoscopic microsurgery. CO_2 insufflation must be performed either by the use of the Wolf endosurgical combination, or by the Orest System from Dornier. Other systems cannot be used because of the small gas volume in the rectum. Dissection is best performed using the Erbe combination instrument. This instrument allows optimal handling and electronically controlled switching between the bipolar cutting mode and the monopolar coagulation mode (needle is pulled backward to allow monopolar coagulation). Suction is always provided due to the roller pump.

Positioning of the Patient and Team

The patient is in the lithotomy prone, side position (Fig. 1). Rectoscopy using a rigid instrument must be performed to determine the position of the patient on the operating table – this depends on the site of the tumor, which must be at the bottom of the optic field during surgery. An intraluminal ultrasound examination should be performed preoperatively in patients whose tumors are located in the higher rectum out of reach of the palpating finger. General anesthesia is the basic rule. The operative rectoscope is introduced by manual air insufflation and the tumor is localized (Fig. 1). The position of the rectoscope is fixed by a Martin retractor. The operative instruments and optics are introduced and connected to the different lines (Figs. 2, 3).

Technique

The type of excision depends on the type and position of the tumor. The standard is full-thickness excision because tearing of the tumor is prevented, and precise histological evaluation is possible. In the case of carcinoma inside an adenoma full-thickness excision is mandatory to guarantee complete excision. Full-thickness excision at the anterior wall above 10 cm is not possible because of the contact to the intraperitoneal cavity. The resection line for the dissection is defined by placing marking dots using a high-frequency cautery device (Fig. 4). The line should be 5 mm long for adenomas and at least 10 mm long for early cancers. After placement of the marking dots the bowel wall is transected to the appropriate layer by use of the standard technique. A monopolar cutting device is used. When a bleeder occurs, the suction device, which is positioned at the entrance of the rectoscope, is advanced, and the bleeder is localized and stopped by monopolar coagulation (Fig. 4).

Much more convenient is the use of the Erbe combination instrument. Pressing the yellow foot pedal advances the bipolar needle of the instrument, which allows precise dissection. In the case of a bleeder, pressing the blue foot pedal automatically pulls the needle backward, which allows the combination of suction and monopolar coagulation. Dissection from the perirectal tissue is usually performed in a layer close to the longitudinal muscles of the bowel wall, the tumor lifted upward (Fig. 5). All resulting bleeders must be stopped immediately by monopolar coagulation to guarantee optimal overview during the whole procedure. The defect is closed by transverse continuous suture, using monofilament thread. The suture starts at the right corner (Fig. 6). At the end of the suture a silver clip is placed onto the thread (Fig. 6). The clip is a fast, safe, and secure substitute for knotting.

47 Transanal Endoscopic Microsurgery

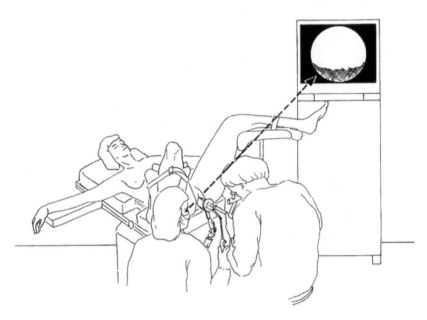

Fig. 1. Positioning of the patient and team

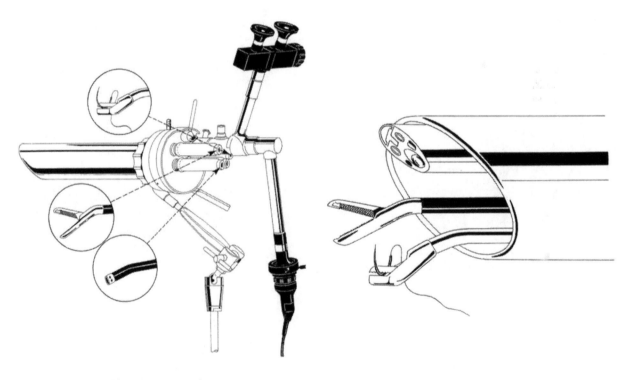

Fig. 2. Instrument sites

Fig. 3. Instrumentation

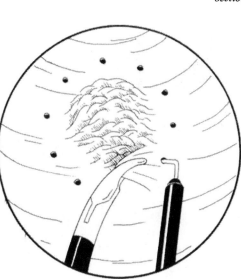

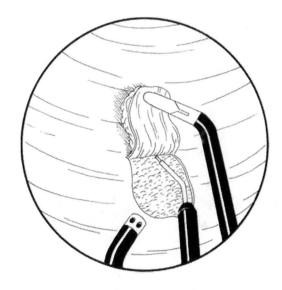

Fig. 4. Area to be resected is marked with electrocautery

Fig. 5. Full thickness dissection of the lesion

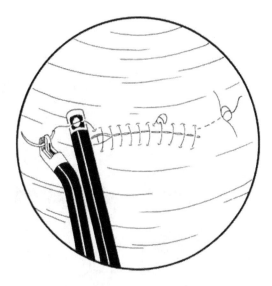

Fig. 6. Closure of the full thickness defect

Comment

Sessile adenomas and early rectal cancers are the main indications for transanal endoscopic microsurgery. In Germany there is broad agreement that sessile adenomas with a diameter of more than 2 cm located within the reach of a rigid rectoscope should be resected not by the snare (because of the risk of incomplete removal) but by rectoscopic full-thickness excision. Full-thickness excision is not possible in locations close to the dentate line and on the intraperitoneal part of the anterior rectal wall above 10 cm from the anal verge. In these areas mucosectomy or partial wall excisions should be performed.

Early rectal cancers are an indication when a pT1 cancer according to Hermanek is suspected. This should be the case in clinical stage 1 tumors. Additionally, on endoluminal ultrasound examination the muscular layer of the bowel should not have been reached. Histological examination should demonstrate good or moderate differentiation. Full-thickness excision is the standard rule in all cases of local excision of rectal cancer. In early cancers we perform a partial wall excision close to the dentate line. At the anterior wall above 10 cm laparotomy and anterior rectal resection is indicated. A cancer should not be excised locally at this area.

Clinical application started in 1983. In Tübingen between August 1989 and May 1993, adenomas were resected in 190 patients and carcinomas in 75. The complication rate in adenomas which required surgical reintervention was 3%, and postoperative mortality was 0.4%. Recurrent adenomas were found in 2% of patients. Salm surveyed 44 German clinics in 1994 and collected data on 1900 patients treated by transanal endoscopic microsurgery. In 433 of these a carcinoma was resected with curative or palliative intent. The overall complication rate was 6.3%, and 2.3% had to undergo a surgical reintervention.

References

Bueß G (1992) Endoluminal rectal surgery. In: Operative manual of endoscopic surgery. Cuschieri A, Bueß G, Périssat J (eds) Springer, Berlin Heidelberg New York, pp 303–325

Bueß G, Hutterer F, Theiss J, Boebel M, Isselhardt W, Pichlmaier H (1984) Das System für die transanale endoskopische Rektumoperation. Chirug 55:677–680

Cuschieri A, Bueß G (1992) Introduction and historical aspects. In: Operative manual of endoscopic surgery. Cuschieri A, Bueß G, Périssat J (eds) Springer, Berlin Heidelberg New York, pp 3–5

Mason AY (1976) Rectal cancer: the spectrum of selective surgery. Proc R Soc Med 69:237–244

Mentges B, Bueß G, Raestrup H, Manncke K, Becker HD (1994) Indications and technique for TEM (transanal endoscopic microsurgery). Endosc Surg 5:247–250

Salm R, Lampe H, Bustos A, Matern U (1995) Experience with TEM in Germany. Endosc Surg Allied Technol 5(2):251–255